Polyester Drug Delivery Systems

Polyester Drug Delivery Systems

Editor: Trystan Worrell

FOSTER ACADEMICS
www.fosteracademics.com

www.fosteracademics.com

FOSTER ACADEMICS

Cataloging-in-Publication Data

Polyester drug delivery systems / edited by Trystan Worrell.
p. cm.
Includes bibliographical references and index.
ISBN 978-1-64646-558-3
1. Polymeric drug delivery systems. 2. Drug delivery systems. 3. Polymers in medicine.
4. Polyesters. I. Worrell, Trystan.
RS201.P65 P65 2023
615.1--dc23

Foster Academics,
118-35 Queens Blvd., Suite 400,
Forest Hills, NY 11375, USA

ISBN 978-1-64646-558-3 (Hardback)

Contents

Preface

Polyester refers to a category of synthetic polymers built up from several chemical repeating units connected together by ester (CO-O) groups. They include both naturally occurring chemicals like those found in insects and plants, and synthetic chemicals like polybutyrate. Polyesters exhibit a diverse range of properties and useful applications. They are used as building blocks in drug delivery vehicles due to their properties of biodegradability and biocompatibility. Poly(caprolactones) (PCL), poly(dioxanone)s (PDO), poly(valerolactone)s (PVL), poly(lactide)s (PLA), poly(lactide-co-glycolide) (PLGA), poly(butyrolactone)s (PBL) and poly(glycolide)s (PGA) are some common polyesters utilized in drug delivery applications. The usage of polyester drug delivery systems may enhance bioavailability and pharmacokinetic properties, enable local administration, and prevent medication deactivation. This book elucidates prospective developments with respect to polyester drug delivery systems. Scientists and students actively engaged in the study of these drug delivery systems will find it full of crucial and unexplored concepts.

The information shared in this book is based on empirical researches made by veterans in this field of study. The elaborative information provided in this book will help the readers further their scope of knowledge leading to advancements in this field.

Finally, I would like to thank my fellow researchers who gave constructive feedback and my family members who supported me at every step of my research.

Editor

1

PLA/PLGA-Based Drug Delivery Systems Produced with Supercritical CO_2—A Green Future for Particle Formulation?

Gauri Gangapurwala [1,2], Antje Vollrath [1,2], Alicia De San Luis [1,2,3] and Ulrich S. Schubert [1,2,*]

1 Laboratory of Organic and Macromolecular Chemistry (IOMC), Friedrich Schiller University Jena, Fürstengraben 1, 07743 Jena, Germany; gauri.gangapurwala@uni-jena.de (G.G.); antje.vollrath@uni-jena.de (A.V.); alicia.de.san.luis.gonzalez@uni-jena.de (A.D.S.L.)
2 Jena Center for Soft Matter (JCSM), Friedrich Schiller University Jena, Philosophenweg 7, 07743 Jena, Germany
3 POLYMAT and Kimika Aplikatua Saila, Kimika Fakultatea, University of the Basque Country UPV/EHU, Joxe Mari Korta Zentroa, Tolosa Hiribidea 72, 20018 Donostia-San Sebastián, Spain
* Correspondence: ulrich.schubert@uni-jena.de.

Abstract: Supercritical carbon dioxide (SC-CO_2) can serve as solvent, anti-solvent and solute, among others, in the field of drug delivery applications, e.g., for the formulation of polymeric nanocarriers in combination with different drug molecules. With its tunable properties above critical pressure and temperature, SC-CO_2 offers control of the particle size, the particle morphology, and their drug loading. Moreover, the SC-CO_2-based techniques overcome the limitations of conventional formulation techniques e.g., post purification steps. One of the widely used polymers for drug delivery systems with excellent mechanical (T_g, crystallinity) and chemical properties (controlled drug release, biodegradability) is poly (lactic acid) (PLA), which is used either as a homopolymer or as a copolymer, such as poly(lactic-*co*-glycolic) acid (PLGA). Over the last 30 years, extensive research has been conducted to exploit SC-CO_2-based processes for the formulation of PLA carriers. This review provides an overview of these research studies, including a brief description of the SC-CO_2 processes that are widely exploited for the production of PLA and PLGA-based drug-loaded particles. Finally, recent work shows progress in the development of SC-CO_2 techniques for particulate drug delivery systems is discussed in detail. Additionally, future perspectives and limitations of SC-CO_2-based techniques in industrial applications are examined.

Keywords: drug delivery systems; polymeric microparticles; polymeric nanoparticles; polylactic acid (PLA); poly(lactic-*co*-glycolic) acid (PLGA); supercritical carbon dioxide (SC-CO_2)

---

1. Introduction

The targeted treatment of diseases with drug-loaded carriers is becoming a substantial reality in clinical practice [1]. Diverse nano- and micrometer-sized systems based on liposomes, polymeric nanoparticles (NPs), dendrimers, and micelles are on their way to change modern medicine. The sustainability of the production of these systems, however, is still a challenge.

Conventional production strategies for the preparation of drug-loaded liposomes [2,3] or particles [4,5] usually involve organic solvents, such as tetrahydrofuran or ethyl acetate, which are often considered a health risk and contribute to environmental risks [6]. Thus, they have to be removed from the final product, together with the excess of stabilizers, by additional purification or cleaning procedures [7] which is usually followed by freeze-drying or lyophilization that leads to dry powdered product [8]. Consequently, there is an increasing demand for efficient alternative strategies that rely on sustainable chemistry and can replace (potentially) toxic organic solvents, and which additionally, offer advantages in biodegradation, waste reduction, time and energy efficiency, and in the use of renewable raw materials [9,10]. One method that is attracting significant attention in recent years is the supercritical fluid (SCF) technology, in particular the liposome and particle formulation with supercritical carbon dioxide (SC-CO_2) [11]. SC-CO_2 is the most economical, chemically stable, and benign compound in its supercritical state, and of high interest to replace common organic solvents.

This review describes the properties and applications of SC-CO_2 as solvent, anti-solvent, and extraction compound for the production of drug-loaded particles, focusing on poly (lactic acid) (PLA) and its copolymer system, poly (lactide-*co*-glycolide) (PLGA). These are among the most established polymers in the pharmaceutical field [12,13]. PLA is a biocompatible aliphatic homopolymer that is approved by the food and drug association agency (FDA) for a wide range of biomedical and pharmaceutical applications, such as bone replacements scaffolds, sutures and stable particle systems [14,15]. It has two enantiomeric forms, L- and D-, along with an optically inactive meso-form. PLA can directly be synthesized via different methods such as polycondensation, ring-opening polymerization or enzymatic polymerization of the lactic acid monomer, whereby the ring-opening polymerization provides the best control over the polymerization, yielding higher molar mass PLA [16]. The latter allows tuning the stereo-chemistry of the L- and D- forms in the final polymer, which influences the molar mass and dispersity, the mechanical and thermal properties of PLA, particularly crystallinity, and the degradation behavior [16]. Additionally, it also can facilitate the tuning of the melting temperature (T_m) and the glass transition temperature (T_g) by varying the content of L-form of PLA [16]. The pure L-PLA (so-called PLLA) has attracted much attention from the pharmaceutical industry because of its high crystallinity. The naturally occurring degradation of PLA occurs via hydrolysis and by breaking of the ester bonds due to enzymatic degradation. This property renders it as a suitable polymeric carrier for drug molecules in nanomedicine. Furthermore, its high elasticity and tensile strength make it suitable for biomedical replacement devices and tissue engineering [16].

The use of lactic acid in combination with glycolic acid (GA) yields PLGA, which also has a contribution in this review as copolymer derivative of PLA. PLGA systems are extensively studied as sustainable drug delivery systems, thanks to their biocompatibility, biodegradability, particle size, morphology, and drug release properties in various in vivo and in vitro systems [17]. Its polymeric properties, such as the degradation rate and T_g, can be fine-tuned by adjusting the LA:GA content ratio [7,18,19].

This review provides an overview of PLA/PLGA-based drug delivery particle systems produced with SC-CO_2 techniques till the present date (November 2020), including a detailed description of the latest studies published since 2014 with details of polymer characteristics, encapsulated drugs, and rationales of the studies.

2. Carbon Dioxide as Supercritical Fluid

SC-CO_2 is presently very popular as a green alternative for several applications including extraction, production of polymers, removal of residual solvents or monomers and formulation of polymeric particles, foams or scaffolds [20]. The word "supercritical" defines the state of the solvent, which is a prerequisite for using it in the areas mentioned above. This physical state was already described in 1822 by Cagnaird de la Tour, who observed the disappearance of the boundaries between the liquid and gaseous phases when increasing the temperature far above the boiling point of water [21]. The author described the critical pressure and critical temperature concepts, including the critical point (Figure 1). SCFs impart valuable physicochemical properties such as low viscosity, high diffusivity, and high compressibility that are a combination of the liquid and gaseous states of the compound and are largely influenced by a slight change in pressure and temperature. The generation of SCFs is a reversible process; i.e., SCF goes back to liquid or gaseous phase depending on the pressure and temperature of the system. Examples of commonly known SCFs are CO_2, acetone, chlorodifluoromethane, ethanol, hexane, propane, pentane, toluene as well as water. The supercritical conditions for acetone, ethanol, propane, toluene, and water are hard to achieve due to the high pressure and temperature required. Moreover, water in its supercritical state is highly corrosive and harsh [22]. On the contrary, CO_2 can achieve its supercritical state at "mild" conditions, T = 31 °C and P = 73 bar. Additionally, it is non-toxic, chemically stable, non-flammable, presents low surface tension and is cost-effective.

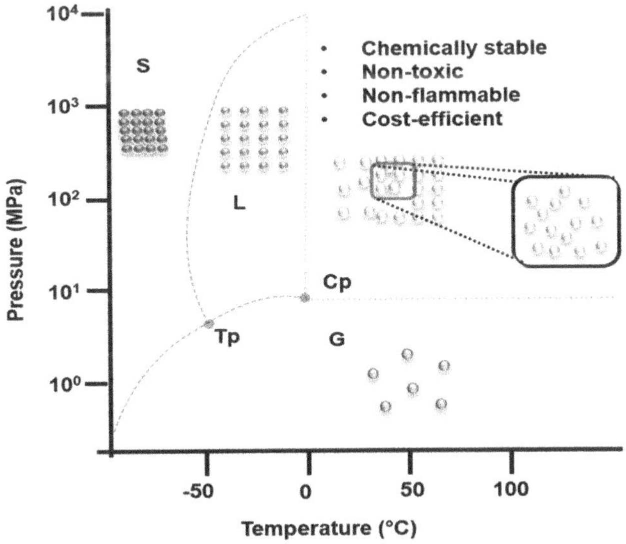

Figure 1. Phase diagram of carbon dioxide (CO_2) (not to scale). S, L, and G denote the solid, liquid and gaseous phases respectively. Cp denotes the critical pressure point (31 °C, 7.3 Mpa) and Tp denotes the triple point (−56 °C, 0.5 MPa) for CO_2.

3. Solubility of Polyesters in SC-CO_2

In the light of prior research and studies, SC-CO_2 is an established solvent for small molecules but not for organic polymers. Also, SC-CO_2 is nonpolar and aprotic and hence exhibits certain selective solubility for ionic and polar compounds as well as for higher molar mass polymers [23]. The solubility of a polymer in SC-CO_2 depends on its chemical structure as well as on its physicochemical and mechanical properties, e.g., molar mass, end groups (e.g., fluorine, amine), the architecture (branched or linear), T_g and crystallinity. However, it also depends on the experimental conditions, such as pressure, temperature, and the use or not of a co-solvent in the system. The most important parameters influencing the solubility of a polymer in SC-CO_2 are presented in Figure 2. Moreover, the main parameters for the solubility of polyesters are briefly discussed in the following.

Compared to other polymer classes such as fluoropolymers, polyesters such as PLA generally reveal a limited solubility in SC-CO_2, which was explained among other factors by their lower chain flexibility [23]. Nevertheless, the solubility of the polyesters can be positively influenced, e.g., by decreasing the molar mass and dispersity of the polymer. It was demonstrated that a high molar mass PLA with M_w = 128 kDa was not soluble in SC-CO_2 even at high-pressure conditions, above P = 1398 bar [24]. However, it was possible to process a low molar mass PLA with M_w = 5.5 kDa in SC-CO_2 at P = 250 bar and T = 65 °C without the addition of any co-solvent, e.g., for the formulation of particles [25]. Additionally, the introduction of terminal groups, such as carboxyl, hydroxyl, acetate, or fluorine groups that modify the interactions between the polymer and the CO_2 molecule, plays an important role in the solubility properties of the polymer. For instance, J. Gregorowicz et al. confirmed that there is an influence of molar masses and terminal groups on the solubility by illustrating the difference of solubility between two different molar mass PLLA polymers with two different terminal groups. The study suggests that for low molar mass systems, the solubility is predominantly controlled by the end groups rather than by the molar mass [25].

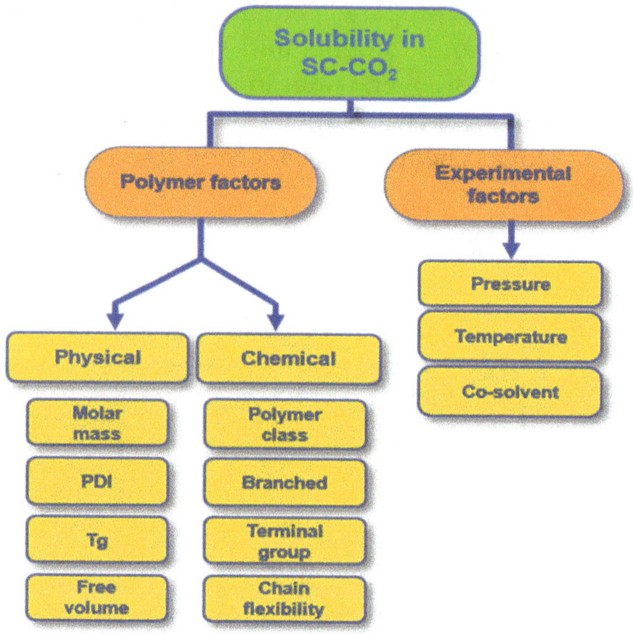

Figure 2. Parameters that influence the solubility of a polymer in SC-CO_2 divided into the two main categories "polymer factors" and "experimental factors" with their illustrated subgroups.

Furthermore, the architecture of the polymer and subsequently its free volume plays a vital role in the solubility in SC-CO_2. The free volume refers hereby to the free spaces left in the solid state of the polymeric chain at the molecular level [26]. The free volume of the polymer chain is directly proportional to the polymer chain flexibility, and leads to higher solvent diffusion and enhanced solubility in the SC-solvent. Influenced by the architecture, the free volume of a highly branched polymer is higher and, thus, it is more likely to be soluble compared to a linear polymer [27,28]. However, even if the polymer is branched, it was found that with increasing dispersity the solubility decreases, independent of the molar mass [23]. The solubility difference between linear and hyperbranched polymers, including polyesters, is not yet studied with similar molar masses. However, it is reported that the solubility of hyperbranched polymers can be positively influenced by a shorter chain length including the addition of several acetate or fluorine moieties as terminal groups [29,30].

Prior literature also emphasized that the T_g and the crystallinity are both related to the free volume of the polymer (T-T_g). Therefore, lower T_g corresponds to higher chain flexibility of the polymer and a higher free volume which in turn, corresponds to an increased solubility [27]. Additionally, the stereochemistry represents an important factor for the solubility: semi-crystalline PLLA presenting a T_g of 55 to 60 °C and amorphous PDLA with a T_g of 50 to 60 °C have different mechanical properties and different solubility behavior. Some authors have also recognized that the T_g tends to decrease with increasing the pressure and the temperature, which makes the polymer more susceptible to solvation by SC-CO_2 [16]. Moreover, the self-interactions within the polymer structure also contribute whereby, the solubility in SC-CO_2 is higher if the self-interactions are weaker compared to the interactions between the SC-CO_2 and the polymer [23,27]. In principle, the intermolecular and intramolecular interactions are controlling the process of mixing and solubility. Finally, the solubility of a polymer is determined by the density of SC-CO_2, which is dependent on the process parameters and tends to elevate with pressure. With increasing pressure, the polymer solubility is likely to be enhanced.

However, if the polymer remains insoluble in SC-CO_2, even under high-pressure conditions, polar co-solvents such as ethanol or acetone are used. The addition of these solvents contributes to decrease the difference in the free volume between the polymer and the SCF solvent and, hence, to increase the solubility of the polymer in the system [27].

Moreover, the thermodynamic equations of state (EOS) (e.g., Sanchez-Lacombe EOS) are extensively applied, in combination with the experimental protocols, to predict the solubility of polymers in SC-CO_2 [31,32]. Predicting the conditions under which the polymer will dissolve might help to obtain a basic understanding of the solubility and SC-CO_2/polymer interactions. Likewise, efforts to study the phase behavior of various polymers-SCF have been attempted [28,33].

At this point, there are still open questions about the solubility of polymers in SC-CO_2. However, the SC-CO_2 is exploited for PLA and its copolymer PLGA to obtain drug-loaded carriers. In the next sections, various processes using SC-CO_2 to produce polymeric particles will be described in detail.

4. SC-CO_2 Techniques and Important Formulation Parameters

4.1. Rapid Expansion of Supercritical Solution (RESS)

Early studies on the RESS process were reported already in the late 1980s. This technique is based on the rapid depressurization of supercritical solutions containing the solute, SC-CO_2 acts as a solvent. The solute in the process can be either inorganic or organic materials, from which morphologies such as particles, thin films and powders can be attained [34,35]. The development of the process was supported by mathematical modelling and experimentally proven by J. W. Tom and P. Debendetti, who confirmed its potential to formulate polymeric monodisperse particles [31,36]. Kim et al. further illustrated the possibilities to use the RESS technique for the formulation of drug-loaded particles by the co-precipitation of biodegradable PLLA with drugs, such as naproxen. A wide range of sizes from 10 to 75 μm and especially, naproxen microparticles of 2 to 5 μm attached to >20 μm sized PLLA particles were obtained [37]. Additionally, seminal contributions made in the past twenty years suggest that the RESS technique can be exploited for the micronization of various hydrophobic pharmaceuticals to improve their dissolution behavior with the advantage of no residual solvent in the final product [38,39].

The RESS technique is, theoretically, a single-step solvent free (or minimal amount of organic co-solvent) particle production process, based on the high-speed expansion of the solubilized mixture of solute (polymer or polymer + drug) and the supercritical solvent (Figure 3). The process thermodynamically favors adiabatic conditions within the system [31]. However, the theoretical principle can be divided into two significant steps. At first the solute (e.g., drug or polymer) is supersaturated under supercritical conditions with SC-CO_2. In the second step, the supersaturated solute solution is expanded rapidly through a small orifice into a vessel under depressurized conditions. The density of the solute and the solvent power of the CO_2 rapidly decreases, resulting in particles/precipitate formation (polymer or drug). The solubility of the solute is of vital importance since supersaturation is the main factor for the initiation of particle nucleation and growth, and influences the final size and morphology of the particles. Therefore, and as mentioned previously in this manuscript, for some poorly soluble solutes a co-solvent can be used to improve the interaction between the solute and the solvent [40,41].

The final particle properties in the system can be controlled by varying the process parameters. Among many process parameters, one of the most widely used approaches in the existing literature is the study of the effect of pre-expansion variables, which include pressure and temperature [42,43]. Another important process variable that can influence the properties of the particles is the size of the nozzle, which is located in the expansion vessel. In particular, the nozzle length to nozzle diameter ratio (L/D ratio) is important [44]. Previous theoretical modelling investigations have shown that increasing the nozzle diameter (D) the particle size decreases at constant pressure [45].

A recent modification of RESS is the expansion of the supercritical solution directly in liquid solvents, so-called RESOLV [46–48]. In this process, the SC-CO_2 solution containing the solute is directly expanded in a liquid to prevent aggregation of the precipitated product. The liquid in which it is expanded may or may not contain a stabilizer.

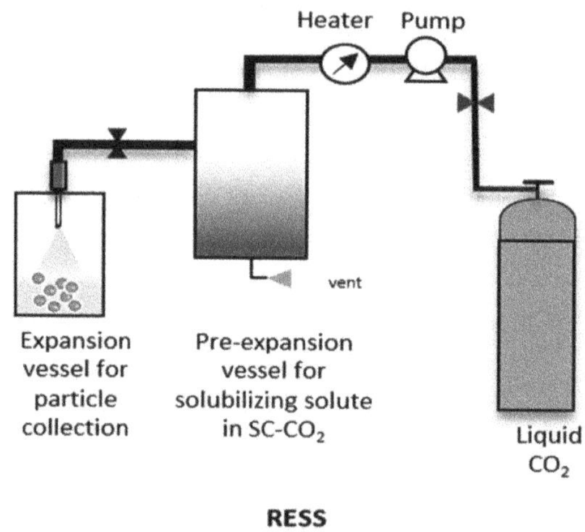

Figure 3. Schematic representation of the RESS process.

4.2. Supercritical Anti-Solvent (SAS), Gas Anti-Solvent (GAS) and Modifications

The application of SC-CO_2 as an anti-solvent was introduced in the early 1990s, to obtain particles from drugs and to encapsulate active agents like such as into polymeric carriers, which limits the RESS process [49]. Examples of anti-solvent processes are SAS, GAS, and solution-enhanced dispersion by supercritical fluid (SEDS). The principle of all anti-solvent-based processes is similar, they depend on the diffusivity of SC-CO_2 into the organic solvent in which the solute is solubilized. Therefore, these methods exploit the low solubility of the solute in SC-CO_2, in which the solute precipitates, and the high affinity between the organic solvent and SC-CO_2, obtaining high mass transfer rates [50]. This causes a decrease in the density of the organic solvent containing the solute which in turn, leads to a decrease in the solvation power of the solvent and causes nucleation and precipitation of the solute in the form of particles. The organic solvent is eliminated from the system along with the SC-CO_2 [50].

On one hand, in GAS (batch mode) the solute-solvent mixture is poured in a high-pressure vessel and subsequently, the SC-CO_2 is injected until the desired pressure is achieved. On the other hand, in SAS (semi-continuous mode) the organic solvent-solute mixture and the SC-CO_2 are injected simultaneously [46,51] (Figure 4). Unlike RESS, in these cases, the mixture of phases and the precipitation of the final particles occurs in the same vessel. M. Kalani et al. and Reverchon et al. explained in depth the influence of the pressure, temperature, initial concentration of the solution, the type of organic solvent and the polymer:drug ratio on the process and final product [50–52]. In particular, small drug molecules can be easily processed using SAS. For example, various antibiotics (griseofulvin, ampicillin, amoxicillin, and tetracycline) and organic solvent combinations (*N*-methyl pyrrolidone, dimethyl sulfoxide, ethyl alcohol and methylene chloride) were tested [39,53]. The authors demonstrated that the choice of the organic solvent is one of the crucial factors for the success of particle formation via anti-solvent techniques. However, these techniques are not limited to the pure drug application and can be also applied for the formulation of drug-loaded polymer particles, as shown by Salmaso et al. and M. Kalani et al. [54,55]. Similar to the RESOLV modification for RESS, is the supercritical assisted injection in liquid anti-solvent (SAILA) process for SAS since the final product is obtained in suspension [56].

Finally, in the solution-enhanced dispersion by supercritical fluids (SEDS) method two co-axial nozzles are used and SC-CO_2 is employed as both anti-solvent and dispersing agent [57]. This allows the possibility of using two types of solutions (aqueous and organic) simultaneously, facilitating the encapsulation of water-soluble drugs, such as 5-fluorouracil (5-Fu) or morphine, in a polymeric system [58,59]. The miscibility between the aqueous phase and SC-CO_2 during the process can be increased by adding an aqueous phase-miscible modifier (e.g., ethanol) soluble in SC-CO_2. However, one of the most important factors in the process is the ratio between the flow rates of the organic solution, the aqueous solution and the modifier which has to be fine-tuned [59].

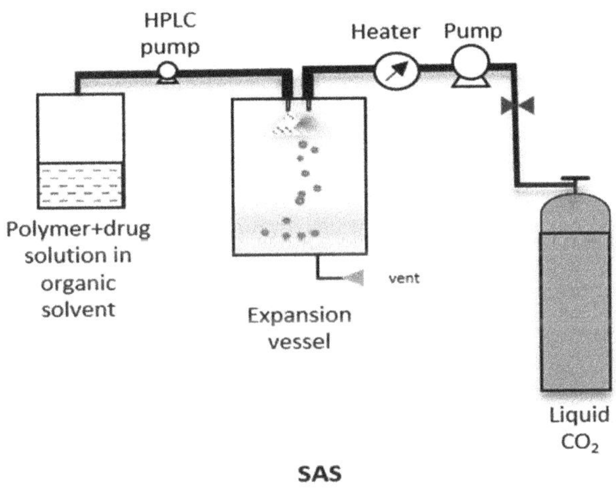

Figure 4. Schematic representation of SAS process.

4.3. *Particles from Gas Saturated Solutions (PGSS)*

PGSS is a well-established technique for the production of particles or drug carriers from polymers that are capable of absorbing SC-CO_2 but are not easily soluble as solutes. Few commonly known solutes include polyesters (e.g., PLLA and PLGA), poly(vinylpyrrolidone) and poly(ethylene glycol) (PEG) [57]. In this case, the SC-CO_2 acts as solute and is supersaturated by the melted mixture of the polymer and the drug [29,60] (Figure 5). The supersaturated gas is expanded and the molten polymer-drug material is precipitated based on the Joule–Thompson effect [61].

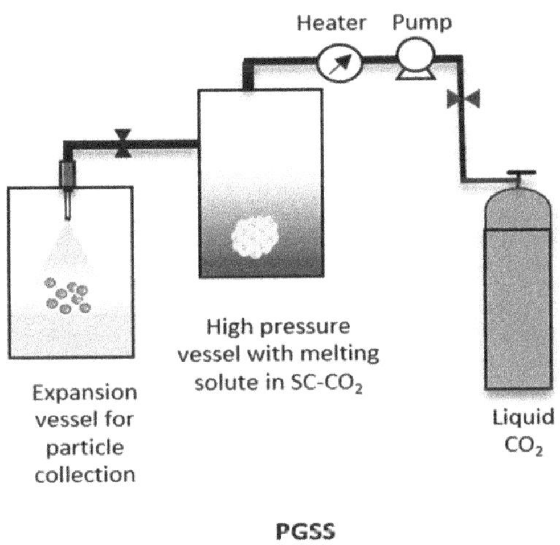

Figure 5. Schematic representation of PGSS process.

4.4. *Supercritical Fluid Extraction Emulsions with SC-CO_2 (SFEE)*

Finally, the SFEE method exploits the solubility of organic solvents in SC-CO_2, whereby the diffusion and solubility depend on several parameters, including the temperature and pressure of the system [62]. In this process, a polymer-drug emulsion is formed, and the organic solvent is extracted with SC-CO_2 (Figure 6). The advantage of this process relies on the combination of the conventional emulsion process followed by subsequent solvent extraction using SC-CO_2. The final particle size depends on the emulsion droplet size which at the same time, depends on the technique used for generating the droplets, sonicator, or homogenizer [63,64].

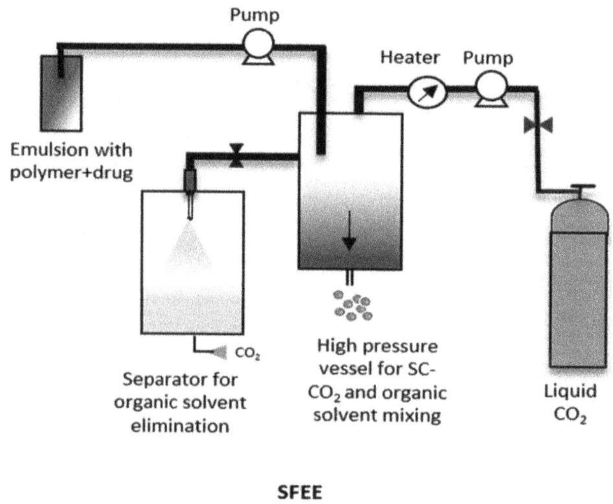

Figure 6. Schematic representation of SFEE process.

4.5. Advantages and Limitations of the SCF Techniques

In the previous sections, the techniques in which SC-CO_2 can be used as solvent, anti-solvent or solute were described in detail together with some representative examples. To complete this analysis, Table 1 shows a comparison of all these techniques focusing on the advantages and limitations of each of them.

Table 1. Overview of advantages and limitations of the SC-CO2-based techniques.

SCF Technique	Advantages	Limitations
RESS, RESOLV	Single-step particle production. No/low amount of organic solvent required. Final product properties can be controlled by controlling the process parameters. The final product is free of residual solvent.	Solute should be solid or amorphous. The solubility of solute is selective for low molecular weight polymer and small molecules.
SAS, GAS, SEDS	Milder process parameters (temperature and pressure required) compared to RESS. Overcomes the limitation of solute solubility in SC-CO_2. Encapsulation of labile active substances is possible.	Use of organic solvent. Some biopolymers tend to plasticize in presence of SC-CO_2.
PGSS	Organic solvent free process. Homogeneous product obtained. Encapsulation of labile active substances is possible.	Particle aggregation can occur during the product formation. Nozzle blockage can occur.
SFEE	Wider range of biopolymers can be processed including PCL and PMMA. Encapsulation of hydrophobic drugs, proteins and essential oils is possible. Monodisperse particle production.	Multiple steps required. Organic solvent is used.

5. Drug-Loaded PLA/PLGA Particles Using SC-CO_2

The previous section was intended to provide a basic understanding of the principles of SC-CO_2-based techniques. This section, on the other hand, serves as an overview of completed studies related to the production of drug delivery systems consisting of PLA/PLGA-based polymers until recently. The use of SC-CO_2 for the formulation of polyester particles was first attempted by J. W. Tom and P. G. Debenedetti in 1991. Since then, many advances have been made in the formulation of drug-loaded polymeric systems. A summary of drug-loaded PLA and PLGA-based particles prepared via SC-CO_2 is shown in Table 2. Furthermore, those studies that were published from 2014 are described in detail in the following pages.

Table 2. Overview of (drug-loaded) PLA/PLGA particles obtained using SC-CO_2.

SCF Technique	Polymer; Molar Mass (kDa)	Cargo/ Drug	Overview	Ref/Year
RESS, SAS	PLLA; 5.5 PDLLA; 5.3	-	Production of MPs of PLLA, PDLLA and PGA via successful processing of polyhydroxy polymers.	[36]/ 1991
RESS	PLLA; 10	Pyrene	Production of composite particles using RESS: variation of production parameters and use of pyrene as a model compound for coprecipitation with PLLA.	[65]/ 1994
RESS	PLLA; 2	Naproxen	Microencapsulation of Naproxen in PLLA. Application of specific equation of the state theory for a prediction of the parameters: EOS modeling of the process parameters was successfully correlated with the experimental results.	[37]/ 1996
ASES	PLLA; 102	Hyoscine butyl bromide, indomethacin, piroxicam and thymopentin	The Aerosol solvent extraction system (ASES) technique was used to produce drug/polymer particles using various model drugs. Drug-loaded PLLA MPs with sizes below 50 μm were obtained.	[66]/ 1996
PCA	PLLA; 100	Gentamycin, rifamycin and naltrexone	The PCA method with ion pairing as a preliminary stage was used to encapsulate drugs into PLLA. Their release profile was revealed indicating matrix-controlled diffusion for particles produced by PCA.	[49]/ 1997
SEDS	PDLLA; n/d PLLA; n/d PLGA; n/d	-	Successful preparation of PDLLA, PLLA, PLGA and PCL MPs using SEDS technique.	[67]/ 1999
GAS	PLLA; 102	Insulin	Preparation of insulin-loaded PEG-PLLA NPs with varying content and molar mass of PEG. The low molar mass PEG improved the morphology of the co-precipitation product and drug release kinetics.	[68]/ 2001
SAS	PLLA; 29	Diuron	Production of diuron loaded PLLA MPs ranging from 1–5 μm by single-step SAS process. A different concentration of diuron and PLLA in the system affected the final morphology of the product.	[69]/ 2001
ASES	PLLA; 50	4-Hydroxy-benzoic acid	Drug-loaded PLLA MPs with sizes between 2 to 3 μm and loading capacities of 9.2% and 15.6% were achieved (for *p*-hydroxybenzoic acid and lysozyme).	[70]/ 2002

Table 2. *Cont.*

SCF Technique	Polymer; Molar Mass (kDa)	Cargo/ Drug	Overview	Ref/Year
PCA	PLLA; 100	Budesonide	Preparation of budesonide loaded PLLA MPs was successful. The obtained product particles showed ~80% encapsulation efficiency (EE) and were studied in vitro prior to in vitro drug release analysis.	[71]/ 2002
GAS	PLLA; 102	Insulin	Production and in vitro investigation of insulin-loaded PEG-PLLA particles with sizes <1 µm. The PEG content was varied observing that the loading capacity of insulin was inversely proportional to the molar mass of PEG.	[72]/ 2004
GAS	PLLA; 102	Nissin	Formulation of nissin loaded PLLA particles with antibacterial activity via GAS technique proving its potential for protein encapsulation.	[54]/ 2004
Pressure quenching	PLGA (50/50); 96 (65/35); 10 (75/25); 97 PLLA; 160	Deslorelin	Drug encapsulation into PLGA polymer particles of different compositions. PLGA (50/50) was found to work the best; The sizes of the drug-loaded particles ranged from 2.2 to 13.8 µm. PLLA was not used further. The technique proved to maintain the integrity of the active substance, low residual solvent and sustained release of the final product.	[73]/ 2004
SC-CO_2 assisted plasticization and spraying	PDLLA; 8	Ribonuclease-A, lysozyme, insulin, and calcitonin	Successful encapsulation of proteins in PDLLA MPs. PDLLA was first plasticized using SC-CO_2, then the drug was mixed with it and the molten mixture was sprayed to obtain dry particles. The particles retained the enzymatic activity of insulin and calcitonin which was confirmed by biological assays.	[74]/ 2005
SSI	PDLLA; 9	Indomethacin	Indomethacin was impregnated on PDLLA NP carriers maintaining the size between 190 to 290 nm and spherical morphology of the particles with up to 6.6 wt% of the drug	[75]/ 2005
SAS	PLLA; 2 PLLA; 50 PLGA (50:50); 48	Bupivacaine hydrochloride	Encapsulation of bupivacaine hydrochloride in PLLA (M_W = 2 kDa) MPs. Varying the ratios of the PLGA/PLLA polymer content, two different levels of bupivacaine HCl (5 and 10%) were used and particles of 4 to 10 µm in geometric mean diameter were obtained. A controlled drug release was observed for up to 7 days.	[76]/ 2006

Table 2. *Cont.*

SCF Technique	Polymer; Molar Mass (kDa)	Cargo/ Drug	Overview	Ref/Year
SEDS	PLLA; 100 PLGA; 100	Paclitaxel	PLLA, $PLGA_{(50/50)}$ and mixtures of both (PLLA/$PLGA_{(50/50)}$) were co-precipitated with paclitaxel to obtain MPs. The size of the MPs was influenced by the feed ratio. Final drug loading was between 14.1 and 16.3%. The release rate depended on the ratio of PLLA/PLGA in the final product.	[77]/ 2008
SAS	PLLA; 85–160	Rifampicin	Formulation of rifampicin loaded PLLA NPs with varying PLLA:drug ratios. The average particle size was <5 µm. A lower polymer content resulted in more irregular shaped particles, but a higher polymer content decreased the drug loading. 7 to 80% of polymer content particles were found to show a more controlled release of the drug without an initial burst.	[78]/ 2008
SEDS	PLLA; 100 PLGA; 100	Indomethacin	Indomethacin loaded PLLA/$PLGA_{(50/50)}$ MPs with 2.35 µm size were produced. Release studies revealed diffusion-controlled release in early stage and bioerosion in later. In vitro cell studies revealed the activity of IDMC-PLLA/PLGA particles on the non-small cell lung cancer cell line.	[79]/ 2008
SEDS	PLLA;100	SiO_2 NP 5-Fluorouracil	5-Fluorouracil was adsorbed on SiO_2 NPs which were then co-precipitated with PLLA. Spherical smooth particles with a size of ~530 nm were obtained. The EE was claimed to be 80.53%. The technique proved to be efficient for the preparation of drug-loaded MPs with controlled release of the drug.	[80]/ 2009
SAS	PLLA; 100	5-Azacytidine	The drug was encapsulated in PLLA MPs final sizes were ~2 µm. Optimal conditions of 40 °C and 11 MPa, and a CO_2 flow rate of 30 mL/min were used to obtain 5-Azacytidine loaded MPs with 95% drug entrapment. The drug release profiles in acid and basic medium were reported as well as the stability of the entrapped drug.	[81]/ 2009
RESOLV	PLLA; 11	Retinyl palmitate	Retinyl palmitate was encapsulated in PLLA yielding particle sizes in the range of 40 to 110 nm and an average loading of 0.9 to 6.2%. The entrapment efficiency increased with increasing the pre-expansion temperature and the concentration of drug, but the size of the NPs was affected by the degree of saturation.	[47]/ 2009

Table 2. *Cont.*

SCF Technique	Polymer; Molar Mass (kDa)	Cargo/ Drug	Overview	Ref/Year
SEDS	PLLA; 50 PLLA-PEG; 70-5	siRNA	siRNA loaded L-PLA and PEG-PLA particles with a size range between 100 to 300 nm and 600 to 700 nm respectively were obtained. Furthermore, the drug release was found to be dependent on the polymer used. The in vivo sustained release was successfully studied without affecting the biological activity of the siRNA.	[82]/ 2010
SAA	PLLA; 85–140	-	Spherical MPs of PLLA were produced in the size range of 1 to 1.5 μm. BSA was also processed and spherical particles with retained biological activity were obtained. The process was hence claimed to be suitable for thermolabile compounds.	[83]/ 2011
RESS + SEDS	PLA-PEG-PLA; 29	-	The study revealed the advantages of combined SEDS and RESS technique for processing partially soluble polymers obtaining particles with sizes of ~2 μm. The process parameters controlled the morphology and size of the final product during the process.	[84]/ 2011
Reverse emulsion SEDS	PLLA-PEG; 25:5; 50:5; 100:5	5-Fluorouracil	Drug/copolymer emulsion with varying ratios of PLLA:PEG (organic phase) were formed with the subsequent SC-CO_2 spraying. The drug-loaded particles revealed a size ≤ 1 μm and were efficient to inhibit the growth of tumor in animal studies by 51.92%, which is higher than the free 5-Fluorouracil. This technique proved to be efficacious for the encapsulation of hydrophilic compounds.	[58]/ 2012
SAA	PEG-PLA; 7.7–9.7; 8.1–23.1	-	Spherical MPs of PLLA were produced in the size range of 1 to 1.5 μm. BSA was also processed and spherical particles with retained biological activity were obtained. The process was therefore claimed suitable for thermolabile compounds.	[85]/ 2012
SpEDS	PLLA; 77	Fe_3O_4 NPs Methotrexate	Production of methotrexate loaded PLLA MPs via drug and polymer co-precipitation on Fe_3O_4 NPs was presented. Particle size decreased with increase in Fe_3O_4 content. The EE was 60.8% and a sustained released was observed. The SpEDS process was successful in the production of magnetic particles.	[86]/ 2012

Table 2. *Cont.*

SCF Technique	Polymer; Molar Mass (kDa)	Cargo/ Drug	Overview	Ref/Year
SEDS	PLLA; 10 PLLA-PEG; 50, 100, 200	Lysozyme	Lysozyme loaded PLLA/PLLA-PEG MPs with varying sizes were produced. The particles size and drug loading were affected by the PEG content and by the M_W of the PLLA. However, the structure of the initial polymer did not change during the SEDS processing confirming that protein or labile compounds can be processed using this technique.	[87]/ 2012
SAS	PLLA; n/d	Paracetamol	The process parameters for the encapsulation of paracetamol into PLLA MPs were investigated. Final particle sizes varied with increasing pressure or temperature. A sustained drug release was observed over 4 weeks proving that SAS can be promising for the production of drug-loaded vehicles.	[88]/ 2012
SEDS	PLLA; 100	Morphine	Morphine loaded PLLA (MF-PLLA) spherical MPs with a mean diameter of 2.45 µm were prepared using the optimum conditions of 17.5/2.5 aqueous solution, ethanol and DCM ratio. The calculated drug loading was 4.73 ± 0.34%. The release profile revealed a burst release in first 4 h and slow-release until 168 h.	[89]/ 2012
ASES	PLLA; 50 and 100; mPEG-PLLA various ratios	Leuprolide acetate	Leuprolide acetate loaded MPs using PLLA and mPEG-PLLA were studied regarding the polymer molar mass, the block length and the drug:polymer ratio. The increase of the PEG length in the copolymer increased the particles size from 2.86 to 5.63 µm. The study showed the influence of the varying factors on the final product morphology and size.	[90]/ 2012
SEDS	PLLA; 100 PLLA-PEG-PLLA; n/d	Morphine	Morphine was encapsulated in PLLA-PEG-PLLA particles with particle size range of 2.04–5.73 µm. The influence of the process parameters and the content of PEG on the final product was studied. The highest EE of ~87% was obtained at drug:polymer ratio of 1:10 with 3% PEG and at 120 bar and morphine concentration of 8 mg/mL. The release rate was faster by increasing PEG content in the final product.	[59]/ 2013

Table 2. *Cont.*

SCF Technique	Polymer; Molar Mass (kDa)	Cargo/ Drug	Overview	Ref/Year
RESOLV	PLGA (85/25); n/d	Fenofibrate	PLGA was co-precipitated with fenofibrate obtaining particles with sizes of ~3 μm. The most suitable stabilizer was SDS driving to a particles size of ~0.89 μm. Furthermore, coprecipitation of PLGA and fenofibrate was attempted with SDS as a stabilizer, where the structures obtained were comparatively non agglomerated and in the size range below 1 μm. Increasing the number of depressurization cycles resulted in the agglomeration of the final product.	[91]/ 2013
SAS	PLLA; 100	10-Hydroxycamptothecin	Encapsulation of 10-hydroxycamptothecin into PLLA NPs with subsequent in vitro release studies is shown. The loading capacity of the particles was influenced by the solvent combination used. The loaded particles produced with suitable conditions were spherical in shape with 794 nm (mass median diameter) size with a loading capacity of 13.3%. The in vitro release investigation proved that the increase in the concentration of PLLA influences the controlled release and loading capacity of the drug.	[92]/ 2013
PCA	PLLA; 50	Lysozyme	Lysozyme loaded PLLA MPs were produced with irregular shape, in a size range of 16.9 ro 18.8 μm and with a porosity of 78.2–86.3%. Further characterization also revealed no changes in the structure or activity of the active compound during the process, proving the suitable for processing and encapsulation of labile materials.	[93]/ 2013
RESS + SAS	PLLA; n/d	-	RESS and SAS techniques were applied to PLLA for the production of MPs and revealed that the technique had a major influence on the morphology and size of the particles. Spherical particles were obtained with SAS process, which was then chosen for further investigation. The size of the particles was largely dependent on the initial concentration, flow rate, process temperature and pressure in the SAS process.	[94]/ 2013

Table 2. *Cont.*

SCF Technique	Polymer; Molar Mass (kDa)	Cargo/ Drug	Overview	Ref/Year
SC-CO_2 infusion pressure quench technique	PLLA; n/d PLGA; n/d	Bevacizumab	Bevacizumab was coated on PLLA NPs that were further encapsulated into porous PLGA microparticles by exposing the mixture to SC-CO_2. The Bevacizumab loaded PLLA particles (265 nm) were infused in porous PLGA of 1.67 µm. The sustained release proved to be effective for 4 months with retained signaling protein activity (Vascular endothelial growth factor).	[95]/ 2013
SSI	PLLA; 100	5-Fluorouracil	PLLA MPs were prepared and impregnated with 5-fluorouracil. The resulting size was 0.68 µm. The impregnation efficiency was influenced by the pressure, temperature, and co-solvent concentration. The highest impregnation efficiency observed was 12 µg/mg at 60 °C and 100 bar without cosolvent and 60 µg/mg with 4 mol % of cosolvent.	[96]/ 2013
SAS	PLLA; n/d	Ibuprofen	Co-precipitation of ibuprofen and PLLA resulting in MPs with sizes between 0.9 to 1.8 µm and up to 10.1% drug loading. It was observed that increasing the pressure and decreasing the temperature decreased the particles size. The maximum amount of drug remained on the surface of the particles, which was confirmed by release rates and FTIR, XRD and DSC analysis.	[97]/ 2014
SAS	PLLA; n/v	Naproxen	Co-precipitation of naproxen and PLLA yielded MPs with a size of 1.2 µm and 13.2% drug loading. A slow controlled release was observed compared to free drug. The pressure had an inverse effect on the final particle size. The drug:polymer ratios did not influence the release rate of the profiles and the pH value of the external medium.	[98]/ 2014
SAS-EM	PLGA; 50	Curcumin	Production of curcumin loaded PLGA particles with modified SAS whereby the polymer-drug solution was ultrasonicated before spraying to enhance the mixing which resulted in a higher drug loading and improved yield.	[99]/ 2014

Table 2. *Cont.*

SCF Technique	Polymer; Molar Mass (kDa)	Cargo/ Drug	Overview	Ref/Year
SAS-EM	PLGA; 50	Curcumin	Optimization of the process parameters to obtain curcumin coated PLGA (75:25) NPs. The influence of the solvent type, the initial concentration of solute, the CO_2 flow rates, the curcumin:PLGA ratio and the ultra-sonication power was investigated. Loading, size distribution and yield of the final curcumin coated PLGA NPs improved with increasing the ultrasonic power and high solvent flow rates.	[100]/ 2014
SEDS	PEG-PLLA; 27	Paclitaxel	Encapsulation of paclitaxel into a folic acid (FA)-PEG-PLLA copolymer for tumor targeting yielded MPs with sizes between 2.4 and 2.9 μm and a drug loading of 7 to 9%. The FA content influenced the EE obtaining the highest (23%) for a FA:polymer ratio of 0.6:1. The PTX-FA-PEG-PLLA particles showed higher uptake in tumor cell lines while the distribution of the drug was found to be specifically higher in tumor tissues. In vivo studies revealed that FA conjugated particles were more effective compared to the unconjugated particles.	[101]/ 2015
SAS	PLLA; n/d	Zidovudine	Zidovudine-loaded PLLA particles (dry dispersions) were formulated. The nine possible combinations from three variables of the process parameters (drug ratio, pressure, temperature) were tested. The batch with 1:2 (Zidovudine–PLLA) ratio, at 45 °C and 85 bar gave 91.5% yield, with 40% drug content. Intestinal permeability studies revealed drug permeability of approximately 9.9%, which was higher than that of pure Zidovudine (3.8%).	[102]/ 2015
PCA	PLLA; 50	Insulin	Insulin-loaded PLLA porous MPs with sizes of ~4 μm were produced. The insulin encapsulation was found to be the highest with the lowest concentration of drug (5 wt. %). The physicochemical characterization revealed no major chemical changes in insulin but only minor changes in the secondary structure. The hypoglycemic activity was retained and sustained released was observed.	[103]/ 2015

Table 2. *Cont.*

SCF Technique	Polymer; Molar Mass (kDa)	Cargo/ Drug	Overview	Ref/Year
SAS	PLLA; n/d.	17α-Methyltestosterone	Drug-loaded particles were produced and the in vitro drug release behavior was investigated. The study shows the use of SAS for the encapsulation of a hormone in biodegradable systems. The investigation leads to the conclusion that increasing the drug ratio concerning the polymer the drug entrapment increased but also led to aggregation in the final product.	[104]/ 2016
SAILA	PLLA; 28 PLGA; 20	Piroxicam	The drug encapsulation capacity of PLLA and PLGA was compared using piroxicam as the model drug. Particles of 1.53 µm ± 0.53 size were obtained from PLGA and broader distribution was obtained from PLA with 1.76 µm ± 1.05 size particles. Preliminary encapsulation studies revealed an EE of 60% and controlled release of up to 5 days.	[105]/ 2016
Rapid expansion of subcritical solution	PLLA; 4.7	Tetrahydro curcumin	Various drug:PLLA ratios on the particle morphology and stability of drug after processing were investigated. The average particle size was ~80 to 110 nm and the loading capacity varied between ~13 and 25%. It was shown that the loading capacity was directly proportional to the expansion temperature and the drug:polymer weight ratio, but inversely proportional to the expansion temperature. While the size of the particles had no major effect of process conditions.	[106]/ 2016
SAS	PLLA; n/d	Tamoxifen citrate	Encapsulation of tamoxifen citrate into PLLA particles was studied resulting in 280 nm size particles and in a high EE of 94%. Compared to the conventional encapsulation process, the SAS process provided the advantage of single-step processing.	[107]/ 2017
SAILA	PLGA (75:25); 20	Piroxicam; indomethacin; diclofenac	Various drug-loaded PLGA particles were produced with narrow distributions and sizes ranging from 0.3 to 2.5 µm. A higher drug ratio, temperature and pressure resulted in co-precipitation of the drug and polymer. A low EE was observed for the drugs that had more solubility in anti-solvent medium and also for higher process temperature.	[108]/ 2017

Table 2. *Cont.*

SCF Technique	Polymer; Molar Mass (kDa)	Cargo/ Drug	Overview	Ref/Year
SAS	PLLA; 100	Gefitinib	The production of gefitinib (GFB) loaded PLLA particles resulted in being influenced by the solution flow rate affecting the loading of the GFB. The highest drug loading obtained with optimized conditions was 15.8% with an EE of 94% in spherical particles with D_{50} of 2.48 µm. GFB loaded MPs revealed a lower crystallinity compared to raw GFB. A sustained release over the time was measured which then was complemented with the in vitro anti-tumor experiments, where the encapsulated particles were more effective than raw GFB.	[109]/ 2017
PCA	PLLA; 50	Insulin	Preparation of insulin-loaded and -unloaded porous PLLA NPs at 80 bar and 35 °C (INS) with a solution flow rate of 4 mL min^{-1}. The INS loading was determined to be 4.85% and the EE 97%. The particles revealed a porous, rough surface and sizes of 16 ± 3.14 µm for PLLA PM and 19.03 ± 3.05 µm for INS-PLLA PM as mean geometric diameter. The authors showed in vivo hypoglycemic effects for pulmonary delivery of INS-PLLA PMs compared to an untreated group supported with sustained release.	[110]/ 2019
SAS	PLLA; n/d	5-Fluorouracil	The production of pure drug particles and drug-loaded PLLA particles yielded particles with sizes from 220 to 670 nm depending on the process conditions. The highest drug loading capacity obtained was of 42% at 50 °C and 120 bar pressure. The organic solution mixture also influenced the particles sizes.	[111]/ 2019

Abbreviations: Aerosol solvent extraction system (ASES); compressed anti-solvent (PCA); gas anti-solvent (GAS); microparticle (MP); nanoparticle (NP); n/d—not determined; n/a—not applicable; poly(L-lactic acid) (PLLA); poly(D-lactic acid) (PDLA); poly(D,L-lactic acid) (PDLLA); poly(glycolic acid) (PGA); poly(lactic-*co*-glycolic)acid (PLGA); poly(ethylene glycol) (PEG); poly(caprolactone) (PCL); rapid expansion of supercritical solution (RESS); rapid expansion of supercritical solution in liquid solvent (RESOLV); supercritical assisted atomization (SAA); supercritical assisted injection in liquid antisolvent (SAILA); supercritical anti-solvent (SAS); supercritical anti-solvent precipitation with enhanced mass transfer (SAS-EM); supercritical fluid emulsion extraction-continuous (SFEE-C); solution-enhanced dispersion by supercritical fluids (SEDS); encapsulation efficiency (EE).

5.1. Drug-Loaded Particles Using SAS

In 2014, A. Montes et al. exploited SAS for the encapsulation of the anti-inflammatory drugs ibuprofen and naproxen into PLLA and Eudragit (a methacrylate-based copolymer) particles using dichloromethane (CH_2Cl_2) and acetone as solvents, respectively [97]. For ibuprofen-loaded particles, mild operating conditions with P = 120 to 200 bar and T = 40 to 50 °C were applied. Although the conditions were similar, the Eudragit particles revealed a much smaller size, in the range of 160 ± 0.03 nm, compared to the loaded PLLA particles, with a size of 1.3 ± 0.7 µm. The maximum achieved ibuprofen loading was similar in both cases with 10% for PLLA and 8% for Eudragit. It was further observed that as the polymer to drug ratio increased (from 1:1 to 1:5), the final drug load decreased and the particle size increased. Similar results were shown for naproxen-loaded PLLA and Eudragit particles [98]. For PLLA particles, sizes between 600 nm to 1.43 µm and 13% as the highest drug loading were reported.

In a further development of the SAS process, F. Zahibi and co-workers aimed for uniform particles with smaller size distribution and an increased drug loading along with a high particle yield. The authors proposed a sonication step before the expansion of the mixture, during the mixing of SC-CO_2 and the solvent [100]. The intermediate mixing supported the mutual diffusion and combination of the solvent and the solute achieving a higher supersaturation, which resulted in smaller and more uniform particles. The authors investigated the influence of several variables, such as the flow rate of the organic mixture, the polymer:drug ratio and the ultrasonication power (W), on the yield, the drug loading, and the size of the final product. They observed that an increase in the solution flow rate resulted in a decrease in the mean size of the particles but in an increase of the drug loading. A similar effect was observed when the ultrasonic power increased from 120 to 240 W. This increase in the ultrasonic power enabled an efficient mixing that led to a higher mass transfer. However, if the ultrasonic power was further increased to 300 W, the opposite effect occurred and the average size of the particles increased and the drug loading decreased. This was explained as a result of the heat generation due to the high ultrasonic power. Further influencing parameters such as the static agitation time or the influence of the molar ratio of CO_2 to organic solvent were explored. The increase of the static agitation time to six seconds considerably affected the loading compared to non-static agitation. In addition, a higher molar ratio of CO_2 to solvent led to smaller and more uniform particles due to higher supersaturation.

In 2015 and 2018, anti-solvent techniques similar to SAS were applied to produce insulin-loaded PLLA porous microspheres, as reported by A.-Z. Chen et al. and Lin et al. [103,110]. The former group used a modification of a process described in 2007. This procedure was based on the spraying through a coaxial nozzle of the polymer-drug solution, previously pressurized with SC-CO_2 in a second high-pressure vessel, causing the formation of droplets due to supersaturation [112]. In the work reported here, the authors first formed an emulsion with PLLA dissolved in CH_2Cl_2 and insulin dissolved in the water phase. The authors obtained particles with an aerodynamic diameter of 4.31 µm. In the latter study, an insulin loading of around 5% and encapsulation efficiency (EE) of 97% was reported by subjecting the INS-PLLA emulsion to the process described above. The conditions applied for the process were P = 80 bar and T = 35 °C using a flow rate of 4 mL/min. The resulting particles revealed a rough surface and a mean diameter of 16 ± 3 µm if no drug was present, whereas they were found to be slightly larger, with a size of 19 ± 3 µm, when insulin was encapsulated. Subsequent in vitro and in vivo studies proved the biocompatibility and the desired hypoglycemic effects for pulmonary delivery of the prepared insulin-PLLA particles with a sustained drug release.

In another study, anti-retroviral drugs presenting low permeability, high dissolution rate and low bioavailability such as zidovudine (3′-azido-2′3′-dideoxythymidine) were considered for their encapsulation into PLLA using SAS, to obtain solid dispersions that improve intestinal absorption [102]. Briefly described, three different zidovudine:PLLA ratios (2:1, 1:1 and 1:2) were formulated in ethanol using three different pressures (P = 135, 100 and 85 bar) while keeping the temperature constant at 45 °C for all runs. At 85 bar the loading capacity (LC) of the particles was calculated to 13%, 23% and

7%, respectively. Although the EE was higher for the drug:polymer ratio of 1:2, ex vivo experiments that evaluated the intestinal permeability proved higher zidovudine permeation for the 1:1 ratio. This result indicates that the use of SAS method allows the modification of suitable polymeric carrier systems in terms of absorption and dissolution properties of the drug [102].

More recently, P. S. C. Sacchetin et al. attempted the production of PCL/PLA particles for the controlled release of the hydrophobic steroidal drug 17α-methyltestosterone with SAS [104]. The influence of the PCL content in the PCL/PLA particles and of different ratios of steroidal drug to PCL/PLA ratio were studied at P = 800 bar and T = 40 °C. With increasing the amount of PCL from 1:9 to 1:1 (ratio related to PLA) the size of particles increased up to 53 μm. Likewise, the EE increased from 20 to 51%. On the other hand, a higher amount of 17α-methyltestosterone in the system led to amorphous powder formation with an increase in the mean diameter from 23 to 54 μm. The release of the steroid from the particles was proven at different pH values simulating gastrointestinal conditions.

The successful production of a controlled delivery system with tamoxifen (TAM) as payload using SAS at P = 130 bar and T = 38 °C was further reported by D. Alias and co-workers [107]. To confirm the chemical and physical stability of the drug before and after the process, the authors compared the characteristics of unprocessed TAM, encapsulated TAM, and micronized TAM. The Fourier transform-infrared (FTIR) data revealed that the SAS process did not affect the chemical composition of TAM and that no free TAM was observed in the encapsulated sample. Regarding the morphology, TAM loaded particles were spherical with a smooth surface and amorphous compared to the unprocessed TAM, indicating an improvement of the NP dissolution in water. Finally, the product was free of residual solvent confirming the potential of SC-CO_2 in the production of drug delivery systems with no post formulation purification steps needed. Similar studies with gefitinib as anti-cancer drug have been attempted using SAS to obtain gefitinib loaded dry powdered inhalers [109]. Lin et al. optimized thereby various system parameters, such as the solvent:co-solvent ratio of CH_2Cl_2 and EtOH (ranging from 0 to 0.5), the concentration of PLLA, the flow rate of the polymer-drug solution (F = 0.5 to 1.6 mL/min), as well as the pressure (P = 90 to 120 bar) and the temperature (T = 33 to 48 °C). The flow rate revealed the highest impact on the final gefitinib loading, and at optimized conditions (CH_2Cl_2/EtOH ratio = 0.2, c= 5 mg/mL, F = 1.2 min/mL, T = 48 °C and P = 90 bar) spherical particles with an average diameter of 2.5 μm, a LC of 16% and an EE of 94% were obtained. It was further shown that the crystallinity decreased compared to unprocessed gefitinib and that no solvent traces were left in the final product. Gefitinib loaded PLLA MPs revealed that a sustained release over the time was more effective at lower concentrations compared to raw gefitinib.

A recent study used a mixture of dimethyl sulfoxide (DMSO) and CH_2Cl_2 (ratio 1:1 *v/v* %) within the SAS process for the production of PLLA-coated 5-Fu [111]. The temperature-pressure conditions for various runs were 35 and 50 °C and 120, 150 and 180 bar, keeping the other process parameters such as the solution concentration and flow rates, unchanged. The obtained size for the coated particles varied from 0.6 to 1.2 μm (at 35 and 50 °C respectively) and the drug load ranged from 32 to 42%, whereby the best results were observed at 50 °C and 180 bar. The dissolution profile clearly showed a slower release rate from the PLLA-coated 5-Fu particles compared to the micronized particles.

5.2. Drug-Loaded Particles Using Modified SAS

Although the conventional SAS technique proved to be promising over the years for drug-loaded PLA-based delivery systems, many authors also used SEDS and the modified SAS technique SAILA for this goal. The SEDS technique that uses two co-axial nozzles and enables the simultaneous introduction of two different solutions was used to formulate PLLA-based particles with and without the presence of drugs, e.g., morphine, 5-Fu and paclitaxel [59,91,101]. Paclitaxel was encapsulated into PEG-PLLA and folate (FA) conjugated FA-PEG-PLLA polymer with varying the content of FA (0.3, 0.60 or 0.9 to 1.0) using CH_2Cl_2 as organic solvent [101]. Scanning electron microscopy (SEM) images of paclitaxel-loaded and -unloaded particles are displayed in Figure 7. The final particle sizes ranged between 2.3 and 3.5 μm. The highest EE was 23% and was obtained with the lowest drug:FA-PEG-PLLA ratio of 0.3:1.

However, it was reported that the ratio of 0.6:1 with encapsulated paclitaxel proved to be more effective in vivo due to the targeting effect.

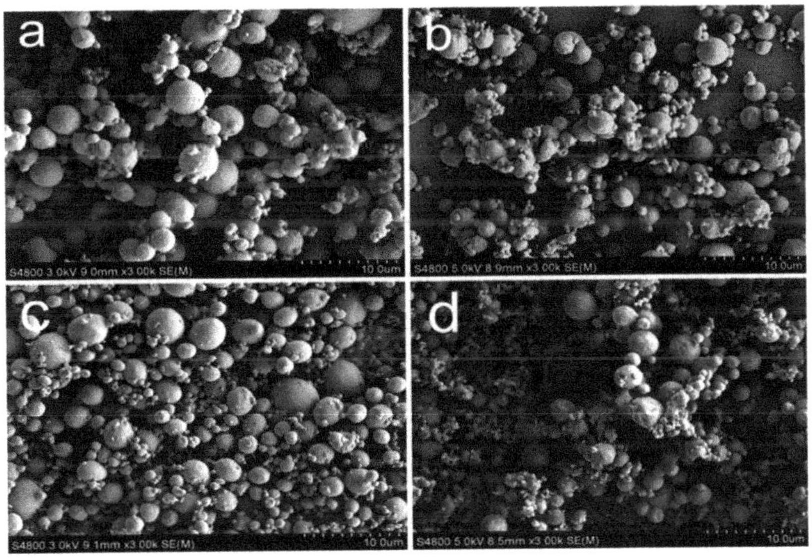

Figure 7. SEM images of microparticles prepared using the SEDS process. (**a**) FA-PEG-PLLA, (**b**) paclitaxel-loaded FA-PEG-PLLA (90% FA), (**c**) PEG-PLLA and (**d**) paclitaxel-loaded PEG-PLLA (scale 10 μm).

On the other hand, SAILA was applied by Campardelli et al. to demonstrate the successful production of an aqueous suspension of PLGA MPs loaded with the anti-inflammatory lipophilic drug piroxicam [105]. In preliminary experiments, the authors used PLGA and PLA as carriers and studied different process parameters, such as temperature (T = 60 to 80 °C), gas to liquid ratio (G/L ratio = 1 to 2.6) as well as various polymer concentrations at constant pressure (P = 80 bar). Spherical, smooth particles of both polymers in the sub-micron region (d = 0.4 ± 0.1 μm) and micron region (2.1 ± 0.8 μm) were produced, whereby the final particle size decreased from the micro-region just by increasing the G/L ratio to 2.6. Piroxicam-loaded PLGA particles with a size of 1.3 μm ± 0.3 and an EE of 60% could be produced by using a PLGA concentration of 2.5 mg/mL and a polymer: drug ratio of 1:20 (settings: P = 80 bar, T= 80 °C, G/L ratio = 1.6). R. Campardelli et al. also proposed the same technique to co-precipitate the anti-inflammatory drugs indomethacin and diclofenac, additionally to piroxicam with PLGA at 80 bar, 60 °C and using a gas to liquid ratio of 1.4 [108]. Particles in the range of 2 to 3 μm with an EE between 64% and 86% were obtained for all active payloads. The piroxicam-loaded PLGA system was further studied with varying the polymer:drug ratio and the concentration of the polymer solution. With increasing the polymer:drug ratio (5:1, 10:1 and 20:1) the size and dispersity of the particles decreased, as represented in Figure 8. The particle size could be further decreased by reducing the initial polymer concentration from 10 mg/mL to 2.5 mg/mL. However, it was noticed that the larger particles revealed slower release rates.

5.3. Drug-Loaded Particles Using Supercritical Fluid Emulsion Extraction (SFEE)

Another SC-CO_2 assisted approach adopted at present and often used to obtain drug-loaded particles, with no or low residual solvent content, is the supercritical fluid emulsion extraction (SFEE) technique that was already mentioned earlier in Section 4.4. The SFEE process is based on the formation of an emulsion and posterior subjection to SC-CO_2 in atomized form. The event increases the contact opportunities between SC-CO_2 and the oil phase, causing the precipitation of the polymer-drug mixture in particle form due to a mass transfer mechanism [63]. Thus, critical aspects concerning the solvent removal after formulation in conventional emulsion method can be avoided [61].

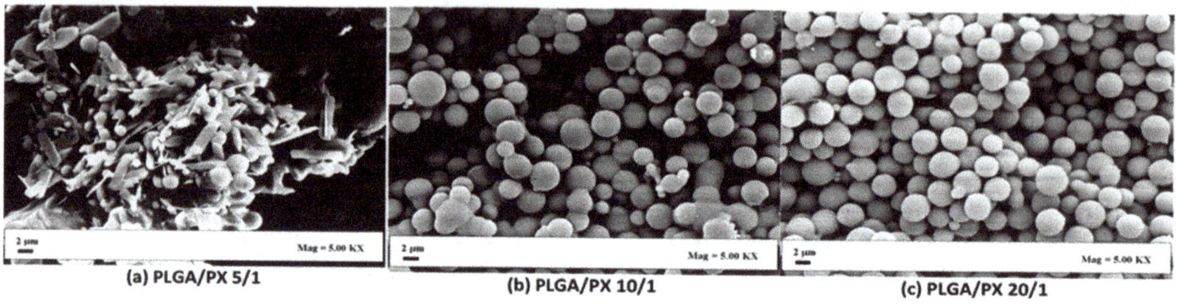

Figure 8. Piroxicam-loaded PLGA particles produced by SAILA with varying polymer/drug ratio of (**a**) 5:1 (**b**) 10:1 and (**c**) 20:1 (scale 2 µm). Reprinted with permission from [108], Elsevier, 2017.

The most recent study using SFEE was published in 2019 by C. Gimenez-Rota et al. [113]. In this report, β-carotene is encapsulated together with the anti-oxidants α-tocopherol and rosmarinic acid into PLLA and PLGA particles [113]. Experiments with several different double emulsions and various external phases were shown in this study. The SFEE process was carried out at 80 bar and 37 °C throughout all the experiments with a constant liquid-gas ratio of 0.1. The final sizes for the loaded PLLA particles ranged from 0.5 to 1.4 µm, whereby the influence of the droplet size of the emulsion on the final particle size was successfully demonstrated (see Figure 9). If the droplet size in the PLLA emulsion was about 2.1 µm, a final particle size of 1.4 µm was obtained. For a droplet size of 1.2 µm in the emulsion, the final PLLA particles revealed a size of 0.3 µm. The EE was calculated to be 72% and 62%, respectively. For PLGA, the same droplet sizes (2.1 and 1.2 µm) were tested and particles of 2 and 0.3 µm with an EE of 52% and 62%, respectively, were reported. The authors also mention that the use of a water-miscible solvent such as acetone failed to provide a stable emulsion and concluded that the SFEE process depends on the solvent and the carrier selected in the system. An overview of further research studies which used the SFEE technique for the removal of the organic solvents is presented in Table 3.

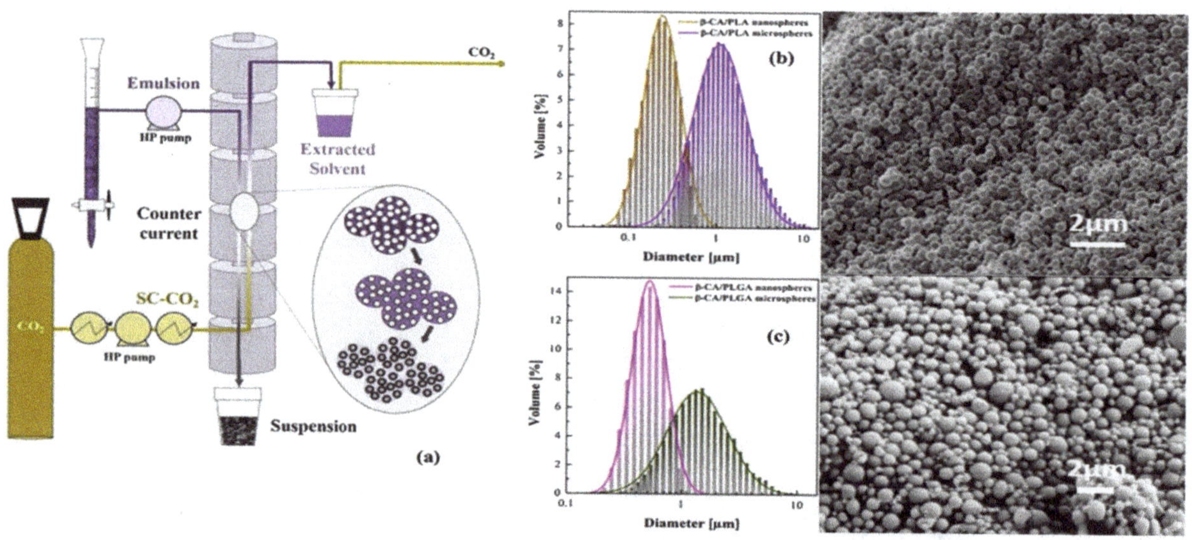

Figure 9. Left side. Schematic representation of the SFEE process (**a**). Size distributions of PLA (**b**) and PLGA (**c**) particles showing the possibility of varying particle sizes by modification of the initial droplet size in the emulsion. **Right side**: SEM images of PLLA loaded particles obtained from the emulsion after application of the SFEE method. Reprinted with permission from [113], Elsevier, 2019.

Table 3. Overview of loaded PLA/PLGA particles obtained using the supercritical fluid emulsion extraction (SFEE) method during the purification process.

Technique	Polymer; Molar Mass (kDa)	Cargo	Overview	Ref/Year
SFEE	PLGA (50:50); 42–65	Lysozyme	The influence of various emulsion technique parameters on the morphology of lysozyme loaded $PLGA_{(50/50)}$ particles was studied. The particle sizes ranged from 0.1 to 1.7 µm. Among three different encapsulation methods, the in situ suspension emulsion was found to be most efficient with an EE of 48.5%.	[114]/ 2009
SFEE	PLGA (50/50); 42–65	Ketoprofen	Encapsulation of ketoprofen into PLGA particles applying first a conventional emulsion technique and subsequently SFEE was examined. Particles revealed a final particle size of 100–200 nm. The higher ketoprofen content reduced the stability and EE over time. Suspended co-formulation was speculated to be metastable and provided important information for the limit of the overloaded formulations.	[115]/ 2009
SFEE	PLGA (75/25); 60–120	Piroxicam; diclophenac sodium	Single and double emulsion techniques were compared with varying the emulsion process parameters in the encapsulation of piroxicam and diclophenac sodium into PLGA particles. Drug-loaded particles with sizes between 1 to 3 µm were obtained with EEs of 88% and 97% for diclofenac sodium and piroxicam, respectively. The SFEE proved to be an efficient technique for the production of drug-loaded particles.	[116]/ 2010
SFEE	PLGA (75/25); 20	Retinyl acetate	The production of retinyl encapsulated PLGA (75:25) NPs via batch and continuous mode of operation was tested. The continuous mode was more efficient and yielded 3.3 to 4.5 µm sized particles with high EEs of 80 to 90%. In this study, the mass transfer phenomenon of the process was exploited.	[117]/ 2011
SFEE-C	PLLA; 28 PLGA (75/25); 20	-	PLLA, PLGA (75/25) and PCL particles were prepared by the application of various process parameters. Operating conditions of 38 °C, 80 bar and L/G ratio of 0.1 resulted in particles of PLA, PCL and PLGA with a mean size of 233 nm, 342 nm and 212 nm, respectively. The influence of various polymer concentrations on the final particle sizes and distributions were studied.	[118] 2013
SFEE-C	PLGA (50/50); 44	Insulin	Insulin-loaded PLGA MPs were produced using double emulsion and tested on rat embryonic cell for viability and drug release studies. Particles sizes resulted between 2 to 3 µm and revealed no degradation of the insulin which maintained further the activity in the cells.	[64]/ 2013
SFEE	PLGA (75/25); n/d	Celecoxib	Celecoxib loaded PLGA (75/25) MPs of 10.5 µm size were produced with a drug loading of 10.9%. These particles were found to be more stable and had higher accumulation levels of celecoxib to the targeted area compared to the conventional particles.	[119]/ 2013

Table 3. *Cont.*

Technique	Polymer; Molar Mass (kDa)	Cargo	Overview	Ref/Year
SAA and SFEE-C	PLGA (50/50); 38–54	Hydrocortisone acetate	The rapid recrystallization of hydrocortisone acetate while encapsulation into PLGA and continuous emulsion processing were resolved and particles of ~3 μm with an EE of 75% were obtained.	[120]/ 2013
SFEE	PLLA; 60 PLGA (75/25); 20	β-Carotene, α-tocoferol, rosmarinic acid	Drugs were encapsulated in the polymeric carriers to improve their shelf life and stability. The solvent was removed at 80 bar and 37 °C. The encapsulation of β-carotene in PLGA, as well as co-encapsulation of α-tocoferol and β-carotene, was possible resulting in range of sizes 0.3 to 4.3 μm (for PLLA and PLGA) with improved shelf life of the drugs. Rosmarinic acid encapsulation was limited to low efficiencies.	[113]/ 2019
SFEE	PLLA; n/d	Rhodamine B	Rhodamine B loaded emulsion microbeads were prepared and exposed to SFEE. The size of the microbeads was 1 ± 0.2 μm. Human monocytes showed uptake of loaded microbeads. The technique provided an excellent alternative to the conventional technique with improved product quality and reduced residual solvent.	[11]/ 2019

Abbreviations: Microparticle (MP); nanoparticle (NP); n/d—not determined; n/a—not applicable; poly(L-lactic acid) (PLLA); poly(D-lactic acid) (PDLA); poly(D,L-lactic acid) (PDLLA); poly(lactic-*co*-glycolic)acid (PLGA); poly(caprolactone) (PCL); supercritical fluid emulsion extraction-continuous (SFEE-C); solution-enhanced dispersion by supercritical fluids (SEDS); supercritical assisted atomization (SAA).

6. Industrial Application of Using SC-CO_2 Processes for the Production of Drug-Loaded Particles

The supercritical fluid-based technologies are categorized as the bottoms-up approaches for the formulation of drug delivery systems in environmentally friendly conditions. Although the process seems simple, previous work has shown that there cannot be universally applicable conditions and that they must be specifically optimized for each polymer/drugs system. To date, SC-CO_2 is the best choice as SCF for the pharmaceutical industry, but the SC-CO_2-based techniques raise questions that are not yet answered for scale-up processes, e.g., the GMP cost estimation, calculation for estimation of parts of GMP equipment, together with the above-mentioned lack of standard processing conditions [121].

Theoretical modelling predictions try to find the answer to understand the phase equilibria of a system with multiple components. These studies could also answer the questions of the compatibility/solubility of the solutes in the SCF, make hydrodynamic modelling of the fluid flow through the capillary and microparticle nucleation and help in the development to have better control over the final product properties. However, this is still in progress and additionally, these theoretical answers also need experimental data to correlate the predictions with the experimental results and in the end, offer a suitable process for practical use [122].

So far, only a few processes such as SFEE were implemented and patented for the production of fine particles, and certainly more intensive and rigorous research is required [123,124]. A review from P. Sheth et al. has focused on the application of the SCF technologies for NP systems in the pharmaceutical industry. The authors nicely presented various industrial-scale leaders for the production of NPs which also includes SFC-based industries [57]. Nevertheless, it is obvious that although the advantages of the SC-CO_2-based processes are numerous, many gaps in knowledge still need to be bridged. Thus, further investigations and evaluations of the process parameters are urgently needed to realize a broad and successful application of this technology in the near future.

7. Conclusions

The techniques described above demonstrate the enormous potential of SC-CO_2 for the production of PLA and PLGA-based drug delivery systems, including solid dispersions, formulations for oral delivery as well as inhalations. SC-CO_2 offers the advantages of being non-toxic and inexpensive and is the right step in the direction of green chemistry for the production of drug carrier systems. PLA and PLGA particles in the micro-and nanometer range can be produced by techniques that involve SC-CO_2 as solvent (RESS, RESOLV), anti-solvent (SAS, SEDS, SAILA) or extractant (SFEE), depending on the SC-CO_2 compatibility with the system materials and the desired product [61,79]. However, after the study of the various scientific articles, it is evident that the anti-solvent techniques are a popular choice for particle formulations. The low solubility (and low polarity) of PLA and its copolymer in SC-CO_2 can be blamed for this challenge in techniques based on SC-CO_2 acting as a solvent, such as RESS. Hence, the inclination toward anti-solvent techniques such as SAS, SAILA, and along with PGSS are explored and investigated owing to the advantages of SC-CO_2.

The design and formulation of drug-loaded biodegradable particles with improved control over the system are still in progress. Exploiting the solvent/anti-solvent properties of SC-CO_2 for the particle formation is thereby challenging. The major obstacles for wide-scale applications of SC-CO_2-based techniques are the limited choice of soluble biopolymers, the tendency of some polymers to plasticize during processing, the compatibility of organic solvents and the technical apparatus. At the same time, the principles of the particle formation and size distributions are dependent on the solute-solvent properties and the thermodynamics of the system. There are numerous unknown variables involved in the system, which indicates the necessity for solutions for the transfer of technology or upscaling. The application of theoretical modelling tools to understand phase equilibria, which are not covered in this overview, is expected to fill the gaps in the present research [125,126].

With thorough experimental investigations and correlating the findings with appropriate theoretical modelling predictions, the SC-CO_2-based processes can be a reality in the coming years for the production of polymer-based drug delivery systems if enough energy and focus is set on this technology.

Acknowledgments: This work was supported by the Deutsche Forschungsgemeinschaft (DFG) via the Collaborative Research Center SFB 1278 "PolyTarget" project number 316213987, A04. Furthermore, Alicia De San Luis acknowledges the financial support from the Basque Government (Programa postdoctoral de perfeccionamiento de personal investigator doctor 2018–2019).

Abbreviations

CO_2	Carbon dioxide
CH_2Cl_2	Dichloromethane
DMSO	Dimethyl sulfoxide
DSC	Differential scanning calorimetry
EE	Encapsulation efficiency
FA	Folate
FDA	Food and drugs association
FTIR	Fourier transform infrared spectroscopy
5-FU	5-Florouracil
GA	Glycolic acid
GAS	Gas antisolvent solution
G/L	Gas/liquid
GMS	Glyceryl monostearate
L/D	Length/diameter
LA	Lactic acid
LC	Loading capacity
MP	Microparticle
µm	Micrometer
Mn	Molar mass
NP	Nanoparticle
Nm	Nanometer
kDa	Kilodalton
P	Pressure
PCL	Poly(caprolactone)
PCA	Pressure compressed antisolvent
PEG	Poly (ethylene glycol)
PDLA	Poly (D-lactic acid)
PLLA	Poly (L-lactic acid)
PLGA	Poly (lactic-*co*-glycolic acid)
P_C	Critical pressure
RESS	Rapid expansion of supercritical solution
RESOLV	Rapid expansion of supercritical solution in liquid
SAA	Supercritical assisted atomization
SAS	Supercritical antisolvent
SAILA	Supercritical antisolvent in liquid
SAS-EM	Supercritical antisolvent- enhanced mass transfer
SC-CO_2	Supercritical carbon dioxide
SCF	Supercritical fluid
SDS	Sodium dodecyl sulfate
SEDS	Solution-enhanced dispersion solvent
SEM	Scanning electron microscopy

SFEE	Supercritical fluid emulsion extraction
T	Temperature
T_g	Glass transition temperature
T_m	Melting temperature
TAM	Tamoxifen
TEM	Transmission electron microscopy

References

1. Farjadian, F.; Ghasemi, A.; Gohar, O.; Roointan, A.; Karimi, M.; Hamblin, M.R. Nanopharmaceuticals and nanomedicines currently on the market: Challenges and opportunities. *Nanomedicine (London)* **2019**, *14*, 93–126. [CrossRef] [PubMed]
2. Panahi, Y.; Farshbaf, M.; Mohammadhosseini, M.; Mirahadi, M.; Khalilov, R.; Saghfi, S.; Akbarzadeh, A. Recent advances on liposomal nanoparticles: Synthesis, characterization and biomedical applications. *Artif. Cells Nanomed. Biotechnol.* **2017**, *45*, 788–799. [CrossRef] [PubMed]
3. Chang, H.-I.; Yeh, M.-K. Clinical development of liposome-based drugs: Formulation, characterization, and therapeutic efficacy. *Int. J. Nanomed.* **2012**, *7*, 49–60. [CrossRef]
4. Schubert, S.; Delaney, J.T.; Schubert, U.S. Nanoprecipitation and nanoformulation of polymers: From history to powerful possibilities beyond poly(lactic acid). *Soft Matter* **2011**, *7*, 1581–1588. [CrossRef]
5. Rosca, I.D.; Watari, F.; Uo, M. Microparticle formation and its mechanism in single and double emulsion solvent evaporation. *J. Control. Release* **2004**, *99*, 271–280. [CrossRef] [PubMed]
6. Byrne, F.P.; Jin, S.; Paggiola, G.; Petchey, T.H.M.; Clark, J.H.; Farmer, T.J.; Hunt, A.J.; Robert McElroy, C.; Sherwood, J. Tools and techniques for solvent selection: Green solvent selection guides. *Sustain. Chem. Process.* **2016**, *4*, 7. [CrossRef]
7. Shkodra-Pula, B.; Grune, C.; Traeger, A.; Vollrath, A.; Schubert, S.; Fischer, D.; Schubert, U.S. Effect of surfactant on the size and stability of PLGA nanoparticles encapsulating a protein kinase C inhibitor. *Int. J. Pharm.* **2019**, *566*, 756–764. [CrossRef]
8. Konan, Y.N.; Gurny, R.; Allemann, E. Preparation and characterization of sterile and freeze-dried sub-200 nm nanoparticles. *Int. J. Pharm.* **2002**, *233*, 239–252. [CrossRef]
9. Raston, C. Renewables and Green Chemistry. *Green Chem.* **2005**, *7*, 57. [CrossRef]
10. Butler, M.; Olga, K. Introduction. In *Green Chemistry Guide*; Butler, M., Rivin, J.M., Eds.; National Pollution Prevention Roundtable: Los Angeles, CA, USA, 2015; pp. 1–5. Available online: https://www.lacitysan.org/san/sandocview?docname=cnt022546 (accessed on 19 November 2020).
11. Ciaglia, E.; Montella, F.; Trucillo, P.; Ciardulli, M.C.; Di Pietro, P.; Amodio, G.; Remondelli, P.; Vecchione, C.; Reverchon, E.; Maffulli, N.; et al. A bioavailability study on microbeads and nanoliposomes fabricated by dense carbon dioxide technologies using human-primary monocytes and flow cytometry assay. *Int. J. Pharm.* **2019**, *570*, 118686. [CrossRef]
12. Englert, C.; Pröhl, M.; Czaplewska, J.A.; Fritzsche, C.; Brendel, J.C.; Majdanski, T.C.; Yildirim, T.; Schubert, S.; Gottschaldt, M.; Windhab, N.; et al. Pharmapolymers in the 21st century: Synthetic polymers in drug delivery applications. *Prog. Polym. Sci.* **2018**, *87*, 107–164. [CrossRef]
13. Shive, M.S.; Anderson, J.M. Biodegradation and biocompatibility of PLA and PLGA microspheres. *Adv. Drug Deliv. Rev.* **1997**, *28*, 5–24. [CrossRef] [PubMed]
14. Kumari, A.; Yadav, S.K.; Yadav, S.C. Biodegradable polymeric nanoparticles based drug delivery systems. *Colloids Surf. B Biointerfaces* **2010**, *75*, 1–18. [CrossRef] [PubMed]
15. Mondal, D.; Griffith, M.; Venkatraman, S.S. Polycaprolactone-based biomaterials for tissue engineering and drug delivery: Current scenario and challenges. *Int. J. Polym. Mater.* **2016**, *65*, 255–265. [CrossRef]
16. Farah, S.; Anderson, D.G.; Langer, R. Physical and mechanical properties of PLA, and their functions in widespread applications—A comprehensive review. *Adv. Drug Deliv. Rev.* **2016**, *107*, 367–392. [CrossRef]
17. Reul, R.; Tsapis, N.; Hillaireau, H.; Sancey, L.; Mura, S.; Recher, M.; Nicolas, J.; Coll, J.-L.; Fattal, E. Near infrared labeling of PLGA for in vivo imaging of nanoparticles. *Polym. Chem.* **2012**, *3*, 694–702. [CrossRef]
18. Makadia, H.K.; Siegel, S.J.; Hirenkumar, M.; Steven, S. Poly Lactic-co-Glycolic Acid (PLGA) as Biodegradable Controlled Drug Delivery Carrier. *Polymers* **2012**, *3*, 1377–1397. [CrossRef]

19. Danhier, F.; Ansorena, E.; Silva, J.M.; Coco, R.; Breton, A.L.; Préat, V. PLGA-based nanoparticles: An overview of biomedical applications. *J. Control. Release* **2012**, *161*, 505–522. [CrossRef]
20. DeSimone, J.M.; Tumas, W. *Green Chemistry Using Liquid and Supercritical Carbon Dioxide*; Oxford University Press: New York, NY, USA, 2003.
21. Berche, B.; Henkel, M.; Kenna, R. Fenômenos críticos: 150 anos desde Cagniard de la Tour. *Rev. Bras. de Ensino de Fis.* **2009**, *31*, 2602-1–2602-4. [CrossRef]
22. Williams, J.R.; Clifford, A.A. *Introduction to Supercritical Fluids and Their Applications*; Humana Press: Totowa, NJ, USA, 2003; pp. 1–16. [CrossRef]
23. Girard, E.; Tassaing, T.; Marty, J.-D.; Destarac, M. Structure-Property Relationships in CO2-philic (Co)polymers: Phase Behavior, Self-Assembly, and Stabilization of Water/CO2 Emulsions. *Chem. Rev.* **2016**, *116*, 4125–4169. [CrossRef]
24. Conway, S.E.; Byun, H.S.; McHugh, M.A.; Wang, J.D.; Mandel, F.S. Poly(lactide-co-glycolide) solution behavior in supercritical CO2, CHF3, and CHClF2. *J. Appl. Polym. Sci.* **2001**, *80*, 1155–1161. [CrossRef]
25. Gregorowicz, J.; Bernatowicz, P. Phase behaviour of L-lactic acid based polymers of low molecular weight in supercritical carbon dioxide at high pressures. *J. Supercrit. Fluids* **2009**, *51*, 270–277. [CrossRef]
26. Wilson, R.; George, S.C.; Kumar, S.A.; Thomas, S. Liquid Transport Characteristics in Polymeric Systems. In *Transport Properties of Polymeric Membranes*; Elsevier B.V.: Amsterdam, The Netherlands, 2018; pp. 3–13. [CrossRef]
27. Kirby, C.F.; McHugh, M.A. Phase Behavior of Polymers in Supercritical Fluid Solvents. *Chem. Rev.* **1999**, *99*, 565–602. [CrossRef] [PubMed]
28. Rindfleisch, F.; DiNoia, T.P.; McHugh, M.A. Solubility of Polymers and Copolymers in Supercritical CO_2. *J. Phys. Chem.* **1996**, *100*, 15581–15587. [CrossRef]
29. Suttiruengwong, S.; Rolker, J.; Smirnova, I.; Arlt, W.; Seiler, M.; Luderitz, L.; Perez de Diego, Y.; Jansens, P.J. Hyperbranched polymers as drug carriers: Microencapsulation and release kinetics. *Pharm. Dev. Technol.* **2006**, *11*, 55–70. [CrossRef]
30. Gregorowicz, J.; Fras, Z.; Parzuchowski, P.; Rokicki, G.; Kusznerczuk, M.; Dziewulski, S. Phase behaviour of hyperbranched polyesters and polyethers with modified terminal OH groups in supercritical solvents. *J. Supercrit. Fluids* **2010**, *55*, 786–796. [CrossRef]
31. Debenedetti, P.G.; Tom, J.W.; Kwauk, X.; Yeo, S.-D. Rapid Expansion of Supercritical Solutions (Ress)—Fundamentals and Applications. *Fluid Phase Equilib.* **1993**, *82*, 311–321. [CrossRef]
32. Türk, M. Formation of small organic particles by RESS: Experimental and theoretical investigations. *J. Supercrit. Fluids* **1999**, *15*, 79–89. [CrossRef]
33. Fahmy, S.M. *Solubility of Fluorinated Polymers in Supercritical Carbon Dioxide*; Westphalian University of Applied Sciences Aachen: Aachen, Germany, 2005.
34. Petersen, R.C.; Matson, D.W.; Smith, R.D. Rapid Precipitation of Low Vapor-Pressure Solids from Supercritical Fluid Solutions—The Formation of Thin-Films and Powders. *J. Am. Chem. Soc.* **1986**, *108*, 2100–2102. [CrossRef]
35. Matson, D.W.; Fulton, J.L.; Petersen, R.C.; Smith, R.D. Rapid Expansion of Supercritical Fluid Solutions—Solute Formation of Powders, Thin-Films, and Fibers. *Ind. Eng. Chem. Res.* **1987**, *26*, 2298–2306. [CrossRef]
36. Tom, J.W.; Debenedetti, P.G. Formation of biodegradable PLA microparticles using rapid expansion of SC-CO2. *Biotechnol. Progr.* **1991**, *7*, 403–411. [CrossRef] [PubMed]
37. Kim, J.-H.; Paxton, T.E.; Tomasko, D.L. Microencapsulation of naproxen using rapid expansion of supercritical solutions. *Biotechnol. Prog.* **1996**, *12*, 650–661. [CrossRef]
38. Charoenchaitrakool, M.; Dehghani, F.; Foster, N.R.; Chan, H.K. Micronization by rapid expansion of supercritical solutions to enhance the dissolution rates of poorly water-soluble pharmaceuticals. *Ind. Eng. Chem. Res.* **2000**, *39*, 4794–4802. [CrossRef]
39. Hermsdorf, D.; Jauer, S.; Signorell, R. Formation and stabilization of ibuprofen nanoparticles by pulsed rapid expansion of supercritical solutions. *Mol. Phys.* **2007**, *105*, 951–959. [CrossRef]
40. Matsuyama, K.; Donghui, Z.; Urabe, T.; Mishima, K. Formation of L-poly(lactic acid) microspheres by rapid expansion Of CO2 saturated polymer suspensions. *J. Supercrit. Fluids* **2005**, *33*, 275–281. [CrossRef]

41. Yildiz, N.; Tuna, S.; Döker, O.; Calimli, A. Micronization of salicylic acid and taxol (paclitaxel) by rapid expansion of supercritical fluids (RESS). *J. Supercrit. Fluids* **2007**, *41*, 440–451. [CrossRef]
42. Satvati, H.R.; Lotfollahi, M.N. Effects of extraction temperature, extraction pressure and nozzle diameter on micronization of cholesterol by RESS process. *Powder Technol.* **2011**, *210*, 109–114. [CrossRef]
43. Reverchon, E.; Donsi, G. Salicylic-Acid Solubilization in Supercritical Co2 and Its Micronization by Ress. *J. Supercrit. Fluids* **1993**, *6*, 241–248. [CrossRef]
44. Wolff, S.; Beuermann, S.; Türk, M. Impact of rapid expansion of supercritical solution process conditions on the crystallinity of poly(vinylidene fluoride) nanoparticles. *J. Supercrit. Fluids* **2016**, *117*, 18–25. [CrossRef]
45. Helfgen, B.; Turk, M.; Schaber, K. Hydrodynamic and aerosol modelling of the rapid expansion of supercritical solutions (RESS-process). *J. Supercrit. Fluids* **2003**, *26*, 225–242. [CrossRef]
46. Reverchon, E.; Adami, R. Nanomaterials and supercritical fluids. *J. Supercrit. Fluids* **2006**, *37*, 1–22. [CrossRef]
47. Sane, A.; Limtrakul, J. Formation of retinyl palmitate-loaded poly(L-lactide) nanoparticles using rapid expansion of supercritical solutions into liquid solvents (RESOLV). *J. Supercrit. Fluids* **2009**, *51*, 230–237. [CrossRef]
48. Pathak, P.; Meziani, M.J.; Desai, T.; Sun, Y.-P. Nanosizing drug particles in supercritical fluid processing. *J. Am. Chem. Soc.* **2004**, *126*, 10842–10843. [CrossRef] [PubMed]
49. Falk, R.; Randolph, T.W.; Meyer, J.D.; Kelly, R.M.; Manning, M.C. Controlled release of ionic compounds from poly (L-lactide) microspheres produced by precipitation with a compressed antisolvent. *J. Control. Release* **1997**, *44*, 77–85. [CrossRef]
50. Kalani, M.; Yunus, R. Application of supercritical antisolvent method in drug encapsulation: A review. *Int. J. Nanomed.* **2011**, *6*, 1429–1442. [CrossRef] [PubMed]
51. Reverchon, E. Supercritical antisolvent precipitation of micro-and nano-particles. *J. Supercrit. Fluids* **1999**, *15*, 1–21. [CrossRef]
52. Byrappa, K.; Ohara, S.; Adschiri, T. Nanoparticles synthesis using supercritical fluid technology—Towards biomedical applications. *Adv. Drug Deliv. Rev.* **2008**, *60*, 299–327. [CrossRef]
53. Reverchon, E.; Della Porta, G. Production of antibiotic micro- and nano-particles by supercritical antisolvent precipitation. *Powder Technol.* **1999**, *106*, 23–29. [CrossRef]
54. Salmaso, S.; Elvassore, N.; Bertucco, A.; Lante, A.; Caliceti, P. Nisin-loaded poly-L-lactide nano-particles produced by CO2 anti-solvent precipitation for sustained antimicrobial activity. *Int. J. Pharm.* **2004**, *287*, 163–173. [CrossRef]
55. Kalani, M.; Yunus, R.; Abdullah, N. Optimizing supercritical antisolvent process parameters to minimize the particle size of paracetamol nanoencapsulated in L-polylactide. *Int. J. Nanomed.* **2011**, *6*, 1101–1105. [CrossRef]
56. Campardelli, R.; Oleandro, E.; Adami, R.; Reverchon, E. Polymethylmethacrylate (PMMA) sub-microparticles produced by Supercritical Assisted Injection in a Liquid Antisolvent. *J. Supercrit. Fluids* **2014**, *92*, 93–99. [CrossRef]
57. Sheth, P.; Sandhu, H.; Singhal, D.; Malick, W.; Shah, N.; Kislalioglu, M.S. Nanoparticles in the pharmaceutical industry and the use of supercritical fluid technologies for nanoparticle production. *Curr Drug. Deliv.* **2012**, *9*, 269–284. [CrossRef] [PubMed]
58. Zhang, C.; Li, G.; Wang, Y.; Cui, F.; Zhang, J.; Huang, Q. Preparation and characterization of 5-fluorouracil-loaded PLLA-PEG/PEG nanoparticles by a novel supercritical CO2 technique. *Int. J. Pharm.* **2012**, *436*, 272–281. [CrossRef] [PubMed]
59. Chen, F.; Yang, Y.; Yin, G.; Huang, Z.; Yao, Y.; Chen, X.; Liao, X.; Gu, J.; Gao, H. Preparation, characterization and in vitro release properties of morphine-loaded PLLA-PEG-PLLA microparticles via solution enhanced dispersion by supercritical fluids. *J. Mater. Sci. Mater. Med* **2013**, *24*, 1693–1705. [CrossRef]
60. Fraile, M.; Martin, A.; Deodato, D.; Rodriguez-Rojo, S.; Nogueira, I.D.; Simplicio, A.L.; Cocero, M.J.; Duarte, C.M.M. Production of new hybrid systems for drug delivery by PGSS (Particles from Gas Saturated Solutions) process. *J. Supercrit. Fluids* **2013**, *81*, 226–235. [CrossRef]
61. Soh, S.H.; Lee, L.Y. Microencapsulation and Nanoencapsulation Using Supercritical Fluid (SCF) Techniques. *Pharmaceutics* **2019**, *11*, 21. [CrossRef]
62. Sekhon, B.S. Supercritical fluid technology: An overview of pharmaceutical applications. *Int. J. PharmTech. Res* **2010**, *2*, 810–826.

63. Chattopadhyay, P.; Huff, R.; Shekunov, B.Y. Drug encapsulation using supercritical fluid extraction of emulsions. *J. Pharm. Sci.* **2006**, *95*, 667–679. [CrossRef]
64. Porta, G.D.; Falco, N.; Giordano, E.; Reverchon, E. PLGA microspheres by Supercritical Emulsion Extraction: A study on insulin release in myoblast culture. *J. Biomater. Sci. Polym. Ed.* **2013**, *24*, 1831–1847. [CrossRef]
65. Tom, J.W.; Debenedetti, P.G.; Jerome, R. Precipitation of Poly(L-Lactic Acid) and Composite Poly(L-Lactic Acid)—Pyrene Particles by Rapid Expansion of Supercritical Solutions. *J. Supercrit. Fluids* **1994**, *7*, 9–29. [CrossRef]
66. Bleich, J.; Muller, B.W. Production of drug loaded microparticles by the use of supercritical gases with the aerosol solvent extraction system (ASES) process. *J. Microencapsul.* **1996**, *13*, 131–139. [CrossRef] [PubMed]
67. Ghaderi, R.; Artursson, P.; Carlfors, J. Preparation of biodegradable microparticles using solution-enhanced dispersion by supercritical fluids (SEDS). *Pharm. Res.* **1999**, *16*, 676–681. [CrossRef] [PubMed]
68. Elvassore, N.; Bertucco, A.; Caliceti, P. Production of insulin-loaded poly(ethylene glycol)/poly(l-lactide) (PEG/PLA) nanoparticles by gas antisolvent techniques. *J. Pharm. Sci.* **2001**, *90*, 1628–1636. [CrossRef] [PubMed]
69. Taki, S.; Badens, E.; Charbit, G. Controlled release system formed by supercritical anti-solvent coprecipitation of a herbicide and a biodegradable polymer. *J. Supercrit. Fluids* **2001**, *21*, 61–70. [CrossRef]
70. Tu, L.S.; Dehghani, F.; Foster, N.R. Micronisation and microencapsulation of pharmaceuticals using a carbon dioxide antisolvent. *Powder Technol.* **2002**, *126*, 134–149. [CrossRef]
71. Martin, T.M.; Bandi, N.; Shulz, R.; Roberts, C.B.; Kompella, U.B. Preparation of budesonide and budesonide-PLA microparticles using supercritical fluid precipitation technology. *AAPS PharmSciTech* **2002**, *3*, 1–11. [CrossRef]
72. Caliceti, P.; Salmaso, S.; Elvassore, N.; Bertucco, A. Effective protein release from PEG/PLA nano-particles produced by compressed gas anti-solvent precipitation techniques. *J. Control. Release* **2004**, *94*, 195–205. [CrossRef]
73. Koushik, K.; Kompella, U.B. Preparation of large porous deslorelin-PLGA microparticles with reduced residual solvent and cellular uptake using a supercritical carbon dioxide process. *Pharm. Res.* **2004**, *21*, 524–535. [CrossRef]
74. Whitaker, M.J.; Hao, J.; Davies, O.R.; Serhatkulu, G.; Stolnik-Trenkic, S.; Howdle, S.M.; Shakesheff, K.M. The production of protein-loaded microparticles by supercritical fluid enhanced mixing and spraying. *J. Control. Release* **2005**, *101*, 85–92. [CrossRef]
75. Liu, H.; Finn, N.; Yates, M.Z. Encapsulation and sustained release of a model drug, indomethacin, using CO(2)-based microencapsulation. *Langmuir* **2005**, *21*, 379–385. [CrossRef]
76. Lee, S.; Kim, M.S.; Kim, J.S.; Park, H.J.; Woo, J.S.; Lee, B.C.; Hwang, S.J. Controlled delivery of a hydrophilic drug from a biodegradable microsphere system by supercritical anti-solvent precipitation technique. *J. Microencapsul.* **2006**, *23*, 741–749. [CrossRef] [PubMed]
77. Kang, Y.; Yin, G.; Ouyang, P.; Huang, Z.; Yao, Y.; Liao, X.; Chen, A.; Pu, X. Preparation of PLLA/PLGA microparticles using solution enhanced dispersion by supercritical fluids (SEDS). *J. Colloid Interface Sci.* **2008**, *322*, 87–94. [CrossRef] [PubMed]
78. Patomchaiviwat, V.; Paeratakul, O.; Kulvanich, P. Formation of inhalable rifampicin-poly(L-lactide) microparticles by supercritical anti-solvent process. *AAPS PharmSciTech* **2008**, *9*, 1119–1129. [CrossRef] [PubMed]
79. Kang, Y.; Yin, G.; Ouyang, P.; Huang, Z.; Yao, Y.; Liao, X.; Chen, A.; Pu, X. Preparation, characterization and in vitro cytotoxicity of indomethacin-loaded PLLA/PLGA microparticles using supercritical CO_2 technique. *Eur. J. Pharm. Biopharm.* **2008**, *70*, 85–97. [CrossRef] [PubMed]
80. Chen, A.-Z.; Li, Y.; Chen, D.; Hu, J.-Y. Development of core-shell microcapsules by a novel supercritical CO_2 process. *J. Mater. Sci. Mater. Med.* **2009**, *20*, 751–758. [CrossRef] [PubMed]
81. Argemí, A.; Vega, A.; Subra-Paternault, P.; Saurina, J. Characterization of azacytidine/poly(L-lactic) acid particles prepared by supercritical antisolvent precipitation. *J. Pharm. Biomed. Anal.* **2009**, *50*, 847–852. [CrossRef]
82. Jacobson, G.B.; Gonzalez-Gonzalez, E.; Spitler, R.; Shinde, R.; Leake, D.; Kaspar, R.L.; Contag, C.H.; Zare, R.N. Biodegradable nanoparticles with sustained release of functional siRNA in skin. *J. Pharm. Sci.* **2010**, *99*, 4261–4266. [CrossRef]

83. Adami, R.; Liparoti, S.; Reverchon, E. A new supercritical assisted atomization configuration, for the micronization of thermolabile compounds. *Chem. Eng. J.* **2011**, *173*, 55–61. [CrossRef]
84. Chen, A.-Z.; Zhao, Z.; Wang, S.-B.; Li, Y.; Zhao, C.; Liu, Y.-G. A continuous RESS process to prepare PLA-PEG-PLA microparticles. *J. Supercrit. Fluids* **2011**, *59*, 92–97. [CrossRef]
85. Adami, R.; Liparoti, S.; Izzo, L.; Pappalardo, D.; Reverchon, E. PLA-PEG copolymers micronization by supercritical assisted atomization. *J. Supercrit. Fluids* **2012**, *72*, 15–21. [CrossRef]
86. Chen, A.-Z.; Li, L.; Wang, S.-B.; Lin, X.-F.; Liu, Y.-G.; Zhao, C.; Wang, G.-Y.; Zhao, Z. Study of Fe3O4-PLLA-PEG-PLLA magnetic microspheres based on supercritical CO_2: Preparation, physicochemical characterization, and drug loading investigation. *J. Supercrit. Fluids* **2012**, *67*, 139–148. [CrossRef]
87. Chen, A.-Z.; Pu, X.-M.; Yin, G.-F.; Zhao, C.; Wang, S.-B.; Liu, Y.-G.; Wang, G.-Y.; Kang, Y.-Q. Study of lysozyme-polymer composite microparticles in supercritical CO_2. *J. Appl. Polym. Sci.* **2012**, *125*, 3175–3183. [CrossRef]
88. Kalani, M.; Yunus, R. Effect of Supercritical Fluid Density on Nano-encapsulated Drug Particle Size using the Supercritical Anti-solvent Method. *Int. J. Nanomed.* **2012**, *7*, 2165–2172. [CrossRef] [PubMed]
89. Zhang, Y.-Z.; Liao, X.-M.; Yin, G.-F.; Yao, Y.-D.; Chen, X.-C.; Yuan, P.; Huang, Z.-B.; Gu, J.-W. Preparation of water soluble drugs-loaded microparticles using modified solution enhanced dispersion by supercritical CO_2. *Powder Technol.* **2012**, *221*, 343–350. [CrossRef]
90. Jung, I.-I.; Haam, S.; Lim, G.; Ryu, J.-H. Preparation of peptide-loaded polymer microparticles using supercritical carbon dioxide. *Biotechnol. Bioprocess Eng.* **2012**, *17*, 185–194. [CrossRef]
91. Dalvi, S.V.; Azad, M.A.; Dave, R. Precipitation and stabilization of ultrafine particles of Fenofibrate in aqueous suspensions by RESOLV. *Powder Technol.* **2013**, *236*, 75–84. [CrossRef]
92. Wang, W.; Liu, G.; Wu, J.; Jiang, Y. Co-precipitation of 10-hydroxycamptothecin and poly (L-lactic acid) by supercritical CO_2 anti-solvent process using dichloromethane/ethanol co-solvent. *J. Supercrit. Fluids* **2013**, *74*, 137–144. [CrossRef]
93. Kang, Y.-Q.; Zhao, C.; Chen, A.-Z.; Wang, S.-B.; Liu, Y.-G.; Wu, W.-G.; Su, X.-Q. Study of Lysozyme-Loaded Poly-L-Lactide (PLLA) Porous Microparticles in a Compressed CO(2) Antisolvent Process. *Materials* **2013**, *6*, 3571–3583. [CrossRef]
94. Montes, A.; Gordillo, M.D.; Pereyra, C.; de la Ossa, E.J.M. Supercritical CO_2 precipitation of poly(L-lactic acid) in a wide range miscibility. *J. Supercrit. Fluids* **2013**, *81*, 236–244. [CrossRef]
95. Yandrapu, S.K.; Upadhyay, A.K.; Petrash, J.M.; Kompella, U.B. Nanoparticles in porous microparticles prepared by supercritical infusion and pressure quench technology for sustained delivery of bevacizumab. *Mol. Pharm.* **2013**, *10*, 4676–4686. [CrossRef]
96. Zhan, S.; Chen, C.; Zhao, Q.; Wang, W.; Liu, Z. Preparation of 5-Fu-Loaded PLLA Microparticles by Supercritical Fluid Technology. *Ind. Eng. Chem. Res.* **2013**, *52*, 2852–2857. [CrossRef]
97. Montes, A.; Gordillo, M.D.; Pereyra, C.; De los Santos, D.M.; de la Ossa, E.J.M. Ibuprofen-polymer precipitation using supercritical CO_2 at low temperature. *J. Supercrit. Fluids* **2014**, *94*, 91–101. [CrossRef]
98. Montes, A.; Kin, N.; Gordillo, M.D.; Pereyra, C.; Ossa, E.J.M.d.l. Polymer-naproxen precipitation by supercritical antisolvent (SAS) process. *J. Supercrit. Fluids* **2014**, *89*, 58–67. [CrossRef]
99. Zabihi, F.; Xin, N.; Jia, J.; Chen, T.; Zhao, Y. High Yield and High Loading Preparation of Curcumin-PLGA Nanoparticles Using a Modified Supercritical Antisolvent Technique. *Ind. Eng. Chem. Res.* **2014**, *53*, 6569–6574. [CrossRef]
100. Zabihi, F.; Xin, N.; Li, S.; Jia, J.; Cheng, T.; Zhao, Y. Polymeric coating of fluidizing nano-curcumin via anti-solvent supercritical method for sustained release. *J. Supercrit. Fluids* **2014**, *89*, 99–105. [CrossRef]
101. Huang, X.; Zhang, Y.; Yin, G.; Pu, X.; Liao, X.; Huang, Z.; Chen, X.; Yao, Y. Tumor-targeted paclitaxel-loaded folate conjugated poly(ethylene glycol)-poly(L-lactide) microparticles produced by supercritical fluid technology. *J. Mater. Sci. Mater. Med.* **2015**, *26*, 95. [CrossRef]
102. Yoshida, V.M.H.; Balcao, V.M.; Vila, M.M.; Oliveira Junior, J.M.; Aranha, N.; Chaud, M.V.; Gremiao, M.P. Zidovudine-poly(L-lactic acid) solid dispersions with improved intestinal permeability prepared by supercritical antisolvent process. *J. Pharm. Sci.* **2015**, *104*, 1691–1700. [CrossRef]
103. Chen, A.-Z.; Tang, N.; Wang, S.-B.; Kang, Y.-Q.; Song, H.-F. Insulin-loaded poly-L-lactide porous microspheres prepared in supercritical CO2 for pulmonary drug delivery. *J. Supercrit. Fluids* **2015**, *101*, 117–123. [CrossRef]

104. Sacchetin, P.S.C.; Setti, R.F.; e Rosa, P.D.; Moraes, Â.M. Properties of PLA/PCL particles as vehicles for oral delivery of the androgen hormone 17alpha-methyltestosterone. *Mater. Sci. Eng. C* **2016**, *58*, 870–881. [CrossRef]
105. Campardelli, R.; Oleandro, E.; Reverchon, E. Supercritical assisted injection in a liquid antisolvent for PLGA and PLA microparticle production. *Powder Technol.* **2016**, *287*, 12–19. [CrossRef]
106. Songtipya, L.; Thies, M.C.; Sane, A. Effect of rapid expansion of subcritical solutions processing conditions on loading capacity of tetrahydrocurcumin encapsulated in poly(L-lactide) particles. *J. Supercrit. Fluids* **2016**, *113*, 119–127. [CrossRef]
107. Alias, D.; Yunus, R.; Chong, G.H.; Abdullah, C.A.C. Single step encapsulation process of tamoxifen in biodegradable polymer using supercritical anti-solvent (SAS) process. *Powder Technol.* **2017**, *309*, 89–94. [CrossRef]
108. Campardelli, R.; Reverchon, E. Instantaneous coprecipitation of polymer/drug microparticles using the supercritical assisted injection in a liquid antisolvent. *J. Supercrit. Fluids* **2017**, *120*, 151–160. [CrossRef]
109. Lin, Q.; Liu, G.; Zhao, Z.; Wei, D.; Pang, J.; Jiang, Y. Design of gefitinib-loaded poly (l-lactic acid) microspheres via a supercritical anti-solvent process for dry powder inhalation. *Int. J. Pharm.* **2017**, *532*, 573–580. [CrossRef] [PubMed]
110. Lin, X.-F.; Kankala, R.K.; Tang, N.; Xu, P.-Y.; Hao, L.-Z.; Yang, D.-Y.; Wang, S.-B.; Zhang, Y.S.; Chen, A.-Z. Supercritical Fluid-Assisted Porous Microspheres for Efficient Delivery of Insulin and Inhalation Therapy of Diabetes. *Adv. Healthc. Mater.* **2019**, *8*, 1800910. [CrossRef] [PubMed]
111. Cuadra, I.A.; Zahran, F.; Martín, D.; Cabañas, A.; Pando, C. Preparation of 5-fluorouracil microparticles and 5-fluorouracil/poly(L-lactide) composites by a supercritical CO_2 antisolvent process. *J. Supercrit. Fluids* **2019**, *143*, 64–71. [CrossRef]
112. Lin, C.; Ng, K.M.; Wibowo, C. Producing nanoparticles using precipitation with compressed antisolvent. *Ind. Eng. Chem. Res.* **2007**, *46*, 3580–3589. [CrossRef]
113. Gimenez-Rota, C.; Palazzo, I.; Scognamiglio, M.R.; Mainar, A.; Reverchon, E.; Della Porta, G. β-Carotene, α-tocoferol and rosmarinic acid encapsulated within PLA/PLGA microcarriers by supercritical emulsion extraction: Encapsulation efficiency, drugs shelf-life and antioxidant activity. *J. Supercrit. Fluids* **2019**, *146*, 199–207. [CrossRef]
114. Kluge, J.; Fusaro, F.; Mazzotti, M.; Muhrer, G. Production of PLGA micro- and nanocomposites by supercritical fluid extraction of emulsions: I. Encapsulation of lysozyme. *J. Supercrit. Fluids* **2009**, *50*, 327–335. [CrossRef]
115. Kluge, J.; Fusaro, F.; Mazzotti, M.; Muhrer, G. Production of PLGA micro- and nanocomposites by supercritical fluid extraction of emulsions: II. Encapsulation of Ketoprofen. *J. Supercrit. Fluids* **2009**, *50*, 336–343. [CrossRef]
116. Della Porta, G.; Falco, N.; Reverchon, E. NSAID drugs release from injectable microspheres produced by supercritical fluid emulsion extraction. *J. Pharm. Sci.* **2010**, *99*, 1484–1499. [CrossRef] [PubMed]
117. Della Porta, G.; Campardelli, R.; Falco, N.; Reverchon, E. PLGA microdevices for retinoids sustained release produced by supercritical emulsion extraction: Continuous versus batch operation layouts. *J. Pharm. Sci.* **2011**, *100*, 4357–4367. [CrossRef] [PubMed]
118. Della Porta, G.; Campardelli, R.; Reverchon, E. Monodisperse biopolymer nanoparticles by continuous supercritical emulsion extraction. *J. Supercrit. Fluids* **2013**, *76*, 67–73. [CrossRef]
119. Dhanda, D.S.; Tyagi, P.; Mirvish, S.S.; Kompella, U.B. Supercritical fluid technology based large porous celecoxib–PLGA microparticles do not induce pulmonary fibrosis and sustain drug delivery and efficacy for several weeks following a single dose. *J. Control. Release* **2013**, *168*, 239–250. [CrossRef]
120. Falco, N.; Reverchon, E.; Porta, G.D. Injectable PLGA/hydrocortisone formulation produced by continuous supercritical emulsion extraction. *Int. J. Pharm.* **2013**, *441*, 589–597. [CrossRef] [PubMed]
121. Perrut, M.; Clavier, J.-Y. Supercritical fluid formulation: Process choice and scale-up. *Ind. Eng. Chem. Res.* **2003**, *42*, 6375–6383. [CrossRef]
122. Corazza, M.L.; Cardozo Filho, L.; Dariva, C. Modeling and simulation of rapid expansion of supercritical solutions. *Braz. J. Chem. Eng.* **2006**, *23*, 417–425. [CrossRef]
123. Sievers, R.E.; Karst, U. Methods for Fine Particle Formation. US Patents 5,639,441, 17 June 1997.
124. Shekunov, B.Y.; Chattopadhyay, P.; Huff, R.W. Method for Producing Solid-Lipid Composite Drug Particles. US Patents US8642091 B2, 4 February 2014.

125. Tabernero, A.; del Valle, E.M.M.; Galán, M.A. Supercritical fluids for pharmaceutical particle engineering: Methods, basic fundamentals and modelling. *Chem. Eng. Process.* **2012**, *60*, 9–25. [CrossRef]
126. Chakravarty, P.; Famili, A.; Nagapudi, K.; Al-Sayah, M.A. Using Supercritical Fluid Technology as a Green Alternative During the Preparation of Drug Delivery Systems. *Pharmaceutics* **2019**, *11*, 629. [CrossRef]

2

Development and Evaluation of Multifunctional Poly(Lactic-*co*-glycolic acid) Nanoparticles Embedded in Carboxymethyl β-Glucan Porous Microcapsules as a Novel Drug Delivery System for Gefitinib

Xiaonan Li [1,2], Jinglei Wang [2], Shang Li [1], Zhaorong Liu [2], Zhiru Zheng [2] and Yanzhuo Zhang [1,2,*]

1 Jiangsu Key Laboratory of New Drug Research and Clinical Pharmacy, Xuzhou Medical University, Xuzhou 221004, China; xiaonanlike@126.com (X.L.); lishang95@126.com (S.L.)

2 Department of Pharmaceutics, School of Pharmacy, Xuzhou Medical University, Xuzhou 221004, China; jinglei94@126.com (J.W.); liuzhaorong123@126.com (Z.L.); xuyynt@126.com (Z.Z.)

* Correspondence: yanzhuozhang@126.com.

Abstract: In this study, a new kind of folic acid (FA)-conjugated and chitosan (CS)-coated poloxamer 407 (P407)/poly(lactic-*co*-glycolic acid) (PLGA) nanoparticles (NPs), FCPP NPs, were prepared, and further micro-encapsulated by carboxymethyl β-glucan microcapsules (MCs) to produce a multifunctional system of NPs embedded in MCs (NEMs) for potential lung tumor-targeted delivery of gefitinib. The prepared gefitinib-loaded FCPP (GFB/FCPP) NPs showed a hydrodynamic diameter of 255.4 ± 14.5 nm and existed in an amorphous state. After encapsulation in carboxymethyl β-glucan MCs, the GFB/FCPP-based NEMs (GFB/FCPP-NEMs) also exhibited a spherical morphology with a median diameter (d_{50}) of around 2.2 μm. After hydration, GFB/FCPP- NEMs can quickly dissociate into its primary particles, GFB/FCPP NPs. Our in vitro drug release study revealed that these GFB/FCPP-NEMs exhibited a pH-responsive prolonged release property. In addition, the cellular uptake study demonstrated that FCPP-NEMs serve as an efficient carrier to enhance the delivery of the entrapped drug into the target lung tumor cells. Moreover, the GFB/FCPP-NEMs induced a superior cytotoxic effect compared with free gefitinib. The inhibitory concentration to achieve 50% cell death (IC_{50}) of GFB/FCPP-NEMs in A549 cells was 3.82-fold lower than that of free gefitinib. According to these results, FCPP-NEMs hold a great potential as a multifunctional and high-performance biomaterial for lung tumor targeting delivery, pH-responsive sustained release, facilitated cellular uptake, and enhanced antitumor effect of antitumor drugs, like gefitinib.

Keywords: nanocomposites; controlled delivery; dual-particulate; cellular uptake; carboxymethyl β-glucan; chemotherapeutic drugs

---

1. Introduction

According to the 2018 report of the World Health Organization (WHO), lung cancer, particularly non-small cell lung cancer (NSCLC), is the leading cause of cancer-related human death worldwide. Until now, depending on the cancer cell type and stage, lung cancer has been treated primarily by chemotherapy, radiotherapy, surgery or a combination of them [1,2]. However, due to the high toxicity of most anticancer drugs, undesirable tissue distribution, inadequate penetration, and rapid clearance from blood circulation, chemotherapy often has in low efficacy, severe systemic toxicity and adverse effects [3,4].

Gefitinib is a tyrosine kinase inhibitor that targets the epidermal growth factor receptor (EGFR), which is overexpressed in lung, colon, breast, brain, and ovarian tumors. Due to the dramatic clinical response to gefitinib in NSCLC, gefitinib was approved by the United States (US) Food and Drug Administration (FDA) in 2015 as the first-line treatment for patients with NSCLC [3]. However, a high dose (250 mg/day) of gefitinib is required for its commercial tablets due to its low aqueous solubility, high P-glycoprotein efflux, as well as first-pass metabolism [5,6]. Consequently, oral gefitinib treatment leads to dose-related adverse effects, such as gastrointestinal disorders, nutritional as well as metabolism imbalances, and even, interstitial lung disease, which is fatal in some patients [7]. All the above-mentioned issues indicate that there is a need to design a novel approach or more effective and safer formulation, for the delivery of gefitinib, preferably as a pulmonary inhalant. Pulmonary inhalant would target delivery of therapeutics to the lungs with effective drug concentrations, and afford rapid onset of therapeutic action as well as minimal systemic side effects [8].

Over the last decade, the biodegradable and body-friendly polymeric micro/nanoparticles (NPs) have played an important role in cancer treatment. Among the various polymeric materials, poly(lactic-*co*-glycolic acid) (PLGA), a pharmaceutical excipient in the US Pharmacopeia and National Formulary (USP/NF) monograph, has become very popular in drug delivery systems due to its modified particle sizes, stable solid structure, facile surface functionalization, and excellent biocompatibility and biodegradability [9,10]. As a result of their stable micro/nanoscale solid structure, PLGA NPs exhibit an excellent ability to control release of their incorporated drug, which may be of value to prolong the systemic circulation time. More importantly, surface modification of PLGA NPs with functional polymers can confer them additional favorable characteristics. It is well established that chitosan (CS)-coated PLGA NPs have enhanced muco-adhesiveness and enabled sustained delivery of peptides to lungs [11]. Recently, Vasudev et al. prepared trimethyl CS chloride- modified PLGA NPs and demonstrated that these NPs combine the controlled release property of PLGA NPs with the muco-adhesive property of trimethyl CS chloride for oral insulin delivery [12]. In addition, Dhas et al. used FA-conjugated CS-coated PLGA NPs for delivery of bicalutamide in prostate cancer [13]. Unlike the above-mentioned surface modification, some reports have described the incorporation of a functional polymer into PLGA NPs. For example, Zhu et al. used a co-matrix of PLGA and D-tocopherol polyethylene glycol (1000) succinate (TPGS) to control the release rate, enhance encapsulation efficiency, and the antitumor effect of docetaxel [14]. Together, these findings suggest that the combination of PLGA and functional polymers may be a suitable strategy to achieve efficient delivery of antitumor drugs.

Therefore, the design and fabrication of a novel FA-conjugated and CS-coated poloxamer 407 (P407)/PLGA NPs (FCCP NPs) co-matrix nanocarrier for gefitinib delivery is highly desirable. This hybridized nanocarrier, FCPP NPs, would combine the unique benefits of FA, CS, PLGA NPs, and P407 into a single carrier system. On the one hand, the FA-conjugated CS affords the FA receptor (overexpressed on the cell surface of many human epithelial tumor cells) targeted feature, muco-adhesive property and pH-triggered release control capacity [15,16]. On the other hand, P407, as a co-matrix agent, can enhance drug permeability by reducing the P-glycoprotein efflux of tumor cell membranes, and thus suppresses the multidrug resistance of the tumor cells [17].

However, despite the multiple attractive advantages of FCPP NPs, nanoscale particles are not suitable for efficient pulmonary inhalation delivery [8,18]. To address this issue, it is necessary to encapsulate these FCPP NPs into soluble and biodegradable porous microcapsules (MCs, specifically 1–5 μm) that can effectively deposit in the lungs, and then dissociate to their primary particles (FCPP NPs) for tumor-targeted delivery. Among the various available MC materials, carboxymethyl β- glucan (a water-soluble β-glucan derivative) may be an excellent candidate due to its high biocompatibility, biodegradability, and bioadhesion [19]. More importantly, carboxymethyl β-glucan is a polysaccharide, which has well-known immunomodulatory properties, including direct activation of NK cells and cytokine release by specialized phagocytes that stimulate phagocytosis [20]. Quite recently, a new approach using resveratrol and carboxymethyl β-glucan has been developed to treat respiratory diseases [21]. Accordingly, these findings make it very tempting to undertake the fabrication of a multifunctional biocompatible and stable NEM system for lung- targeted antitumor drug delivery via the encapsulation of these FCPP NPs into carboxymethyl β-glucan MCs, which, to the best of our knowledge, has not been reported to date.

Therefore, in this study, we sought to develop such a novel type of FCPP-NEM carrier system to achieve effective lung tumor-targeted delivery, pH-responsive sustained release, facilitated cellular uptake, and enhanced antitumor effects of the antitumor drugs, like gefitinib. To achieve this goal, we systematically evaluated the physicochemical properties of the newly developed GFB/FCPP-NEMs, including morphology, particle size distribution (PSD), crystalline state, drug loading amount, Fourier transform infrared (FT-IR) spectrum, drug release profiles, and release mechanism. In addition, besides studying the cellular uptake of FCPP NPs (the primary particles of FCPP-NEMs), the cytotoxicity of GFB/FCPP-NEMs was evaluated in the lung cancer cell lines A549 and PC-9. Additionally, an accelerated stability study was conducted to determine the physicochemical stability of GFB/FCPP-NEMs.

2. Materials and Methods

2.1. Materials

P407 was obtained from BASF SE (Ludwigshafen, Germany). Carboxymethyl β-glucan was purchased from Yuancheng Chemical Co., Ltd. (Suzhou, China). PLGA (Mw = 24,000–38,000, lactide/glicolide = 50/50) was provided by Daigang Biomaterials (Jinan, China). USP grade gefitinib (purity ≥99%) was obtained from Yadong Pharma Ltd. (Nanjing, China). FA, polyvinyl alcohol (PVA), and CS (Mw = 8000 Da, degree of deacetylation ≥75%) were purchased from Aladdin Reagent Co., Ltd. (Shanghai, China). High-performance liquid chromatography (HPLC) grade acetonitrile and methanol were purchased from Sinopharm Chemical Reagent Co., Ltd. (Shanghai, China). The other chemicals and reagents were of analytical grade.

2.2. Cell Culture

The human NSCLC cell lines A549 and PC-9 were obtained from the Chinese Academy of Sciences (Shanghai, China). A549 and PC-9 cells were cultured in high glucose Dulbecco's modified Eagle's medium (DMEM) and Roswell Park Memorial Institute (RPMI)-1640 medium, respectively. Both culture media were supplemented with antibiotic (100 U/mL penicillin and 100 μg/mL streptomycin) and 10% fetal bovine serum. The cells were cultured under humidified conditions at 37 °C and 5% CO_2.

2.3. Fabrication of GFB/FCPP NPs

The monodispersed GFB/FCPP NPs were prepared by a two-step process: First, the gefitinib-loaded P407/PLGA (GFB/P407/PLGA) NPs were fabricated by a double emulsion–solvent evaporation method (Step 1 in Figure 1) [22]. Briefly, 20 mg of P407, 10 mg of gefitinib, and 80 mg of PLGA were dissolved in 7 mL of dichloromethane (DCM) to obtain the organic phase. Subsequently, 2 mL of distilled water, used as the aqueous phase, was poured into the above organic phase, and mixed by stirring at 12,000 rpm for 6 min to obtain a coarse emulsion. Then, the coarse emulsion was sonicated with an ultrasonic probe for 6 min (pulsing mode 3 s on and 2 s off, 300 Walt) in an ice water bath. Next, the resulting emulsion was poured into 30 mL of a 1% PVA aqueous solution and the mixture was further sonicated for 6 min in an ice water bath. After sonication, the resulting double emulsion was stirred overnight using a propeller-type agitator at 200 rpm to remove the DCM. Afterwards, the suspension was centrifugated at 9000 rpm for 15 min, washed with distilled water and the GFB/P407/PLGA NPs were collected.

In the subsequent step, the obtained GFB/P407/PLGA NPs were coated with FA-conjugated CS and then lyophilized to form the GFB/FCPP NPs (Step 2 in Figure 1). Briefly, FA conjugated CS was prepared based on a carbodiimide reaction as previously reported (Supplementary Materials) [23]. Then, 0.5 g of GFB/P407/PLGA NPs was resuspended in 10 mL of the FA-conjugated CS solution (1%, in 1% acetic acid solution). Next, the resulting mixture was vortexed for 5 min and stirred for

3 h. After centrifugation at 9000 rpm for 20 min, the collected GFB/FCPP NPs were washed with distilled water, and lyophilized at −55 °C for 10 h using a laboratory-scale freeze-drying device (Evela Instruments, Tokyo, Japan) at a pressure below 10 Pa. Ultimately, the lyophilized powder was passed through a 80-mesh sieve, and stored in a screw cap sealed glass bottle.

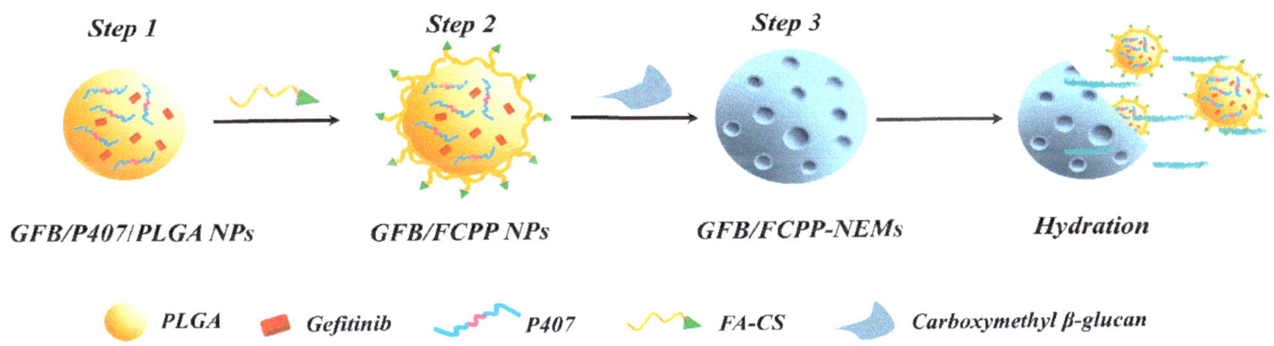

Figure 1. Schematic diagram of the preparation of gefitinib-loaded and folic acid (FA)-conjugated chitosan (CS)-coated poloxamer 407 (P407)/poly (lactic-co-glycolic acid) (PLGA) nanoparticles (NPs), namely GFB/FCPP NPs and GFB/FCPP NPs embedded in microcapsules (MCs), namely GFB/FCPP- NEMs.

2.4. *Fabrication of GFB/FCPP-NEMs*

The encapsulation of GFB/FCPP NPs in carboxymethyl β-glucan MCs was carried out by the well-known spray drying method (Step 3 in Figure 1). In a typical preparation, 1 g of carboxymethyl β-glucan was dissolved in 100 mL of purified water to form a 1% carboxymethyl β-glucan aqueous solution. Then, 0.4 g GFB/FCPP NPs was dispersed in the above solution under magnetic stirring until a uniform dispersion was formed. Eventually, the dispersion was pumped into an ADL-310 mini bench-top spray dryer (Nanjing, China) to obtain the GFB/FCPP-NEMs. The inlet and outlet temperatures of the drying chamber were set to 170 and 60 °C, respectively. The atomization pressure was set to 170 kPa. The drying air flow rate and feed rate were 0.6 m^3/min and 5.0 mL/min, respectively. The GFB/FCPP NPs dispersion was continuously stirred during the drying process. Finally, the resulting dry powder was stored in a screw cap sealed glass bottle.

2.5. *Characterization of the GFB/FCPP NPs and GFB/FCPP-NEMs*

2.5.1. Morphological Analysis

Particle shape and surface morphology of the powdered GFB/P407/PLGA NPs, GFB/FCPP NPs, and GFB/FCPP-NEMs were examined by scanning electron microscopy (SEM) using a Teneo VS™ scanning electron microscope (FEI Co., Hillsboro, OR, USA). Before SEM analysis, a small section of each sample was sputtered with a thin gold/palladium layer for conductivity.

2.5.2. Particle Size Distribution and Zeta Potential Measurements

For the prepared GFB/P407/PLGA NPs and GFB/FCPP NPs, the mean hydrodynamic diameter, polydispersity index, and surface charge were measured using a Nicomp™ 380 ZLS zeta potential/size analyzer (Particle Sizing Systems, Santa Barbara, CA, USA). Prior to measurements, each sample was appropriately diluted and highly dispersed in distilled water. For the prepared GFB/FCPP-NEMs powder, laser diffraction was used to determine the particle size distribution using a WJL-612 laser diffraction particle size analyzer (Rise Instruments Co., Ltd., Nanjing, China). The particle size was expressed as the median diameter (d_{50}). The span values = $[d_{90}-d_{10}]/d_{50}$, where d_{90}, d_{50} and d_{10} indicate the equivalent volume diameters corresponding to the 90%, 50%, and 10% points of the cumulative distribution curve, respectively. All the measurements were performed in triplicate for each sample.

2.5.3. Solid-State Test

The thermal behavior of crude gefitinib, GFB/P407/PLGA NPs, physical mixture of gefitinib and P407/PLGA NPs, GFB/FCPP NPs, carboxymethyl β-glucan, and GFB/FCPP-NEMs was analyzed by differential scanning calorimetry (DSC) using an NY-101B, differential scanning calorimeter (Netzyu Electronics Technology Co., Ltd., Shanghai, China). Powder samples (approximately 10–16 mg) were accurately weighed, placed in ceramic crucibles with a lid under a constant purge of nitrogen at 40 mL/min. Each sample was scanned from 40 to 300 °C (at a ramp rate of 10 °C/min).

2.5.4. FT-IR Spectroscopy Analysis

FT-IR spectra of the FA conjugated CS, crude gefitinib, P407/PLGA NPs, physical mixture of gefitinib and P407/PLGA NPs, GFB/FCPP NPs, and GFB/FCPP-NEMs were recorded using a Bruker IFS 55 FT-IR spectrometer (Bruker Optics GmbH, Ettlingen, Germany). Before measurement, each sample was ground and pressed into potassium bromide discs.

2.5.5. Drug Loading Amount Measurements

Gefitinib content was determined by HPLC analysis using the Agilent 1200 series HPLC system (Agilent Technologies, Santa Clara, CA, USA), which consisted of a tunable UV detector, an autosampler, and a column heater (set at 35 °C). The stationary phase was a reverse phase Agilent Zorbax Eclipse Plus C18 column, while the mobile phase was a mixture of acetonitrile and 10 mM ammonium dihydrogen phosphate buffer (51:49, *v*/*v*). To determine the drug loading amount and entrapment efficiency (EE) of each gefitinib formulation, a predetermined amount of GFB/FCPP NPs or GFB/FCPP-NEMs powder was added in 4 mL of a mixture solution (DCM: acetonitrile, 50/50), and continuously vortexed for 10 min to ensure complete release of the encapsulated gefitinib. Subsequently, the solvent was evaporated under nitrogen. Then, 4 mL of acetonitrile was added to the extract and vortex mixed for 2 min followed by agitation overnight to dissolve the gefitinib. After centrifugation at 9000 rpm for 5 min, the supernatant was collected for HPLC analysis. The EE was defined as: the amount of gefitinib in the samples ×100%/total amount of gefitinib added during the fabrication of the samples. The drug loading amount was expressed as: total amount of gefitinib in the samples ×100%/the amount of the samples.

2.5.6. In Vitro Drug Release Test

A dialysis bag diffusion method was used to examine the drug release behaviors of GFB/FCPP NPs, and GFB/FCPP-NEMs under two different pH values. Briefly, raw gefitinib, GFB/FCPP NPs, or GFB/FCPP-NEMs with equal amount of gefitinib (4 mg) were individually suspended in 2 mL of phosphate-buffered solution (PBS, pH 7.4) containing 1% Tween 80 and sealed in a pre-swelled cellulose acetate dialysis bag. Then, the dialysis bag was immersed in another 100 mL of PBS and shaken horizontally at 100 rpm and 37 °C for 48 h. Tween 80 was used to maintain the sink conditions. At the scheduled time intervals, samples of approximately 4.0 mL were collected from the release medium and replaced with fresh PBS. Each sample was filtered (through a 0.45-μm membrane), transferred into a vial and the released amount of drug was determined by HPLC analysis. Additionally, to evaluate the pH-responsive controlled release property of GFB/FCPP NPs and GFB/FCPP-NEMs, the above-mentioned analysis was performed with pH 5.0 PBS as another release medium. Different kinetic models of zero-order, first-order, Higuchi, and Korsmeyer–Peppas were used to investigate potential release mechanisms of GFB/FCPP-NEMs [24].

2.6. Cellular Uptake Study

The primary particles of FCPP-NEMs, namely FCPP NPs, taken up by A549 cells were determined by fluorescence microscopy analysis. Coumarin-6 was used to visualize FCPP NPs. The preparation method for coumarin-6-loaded FCPP NPs was the same as that used for GFB/FCPP NPs except that gefitinib was replaced with coumarin-6. For cellular uptake experiments, A549 cells were seeded on cover slips at a density of 1×10^5 cells/well in 12-well plates and incubated for 24 h. After removal of the culture medium, A549 cells were incubated with 1 mL DMEM containing coumarin- 6-loaded FCPP or coumarin-6-loaded P407/PLGA samples. Following incubation for 4 h, the A549 cells on the cover slips were washed with PBS, fixed with 4% paraformaldehyde for 10 min at room temperature, and then washed again with PBS. After staining with Hoechst 33,342, the A549 cells were washed with PBS. Then, the cover slip containing A549 cells was covered with 50% glycerol and visualized by fluorescence microscopy using an Olympus IX73 fluorescence microscope (Olympus Corp., Tokyo, Japan).

2.7. Cytotoxicity Evaluation of GFB/FCPP-NEMs

The in vitro anticancer activity of GFB/FCPP-NEMs was evaluated in two lung cancer cell lines (A549 and PC-9 cells) by the colorimetric MTT (3-(4,5-dimethylthiazol-2-yl)-2,5-diphenyltetrazolium bromide) assay. Briefly, A549 and PC-9 cells were seeded in 96-well plates at the density of 1×10^4 cells/well in 100 μL of normal culture medium, and cultured overnight. Afterwards, the culture medium was replaced with 100 μL of DMEM or RPMI-1640 containing serial concentrations of gefitinib or GFB/FCPP-NEMs. The graded concentration of gefitinib ranged from 0.2 to 20 μg/mL. After incubation at 37 °C for 48 h, the treatment medium was aspirated from the wells, and replaced with 100 μL of fresh culture medium containing the MTT solution (20 μL, 5 mg/mL). After incubation for 4 h, the MTT solution was aspirated, and the formed formazan crystals were solubilized with 100 μL of dimethyl sulfoxide. Next, the absorbance of the resulting solution was detected at 490 nm using a microplate reader (BioTek, Winooski, VT, USA). Cells treated with normal medium served as the control cells. The cell viability was calculated as follows: optical density (OD) of test cells ×100%/OD of control cells. Additionally, empty FCPP-NEMs were also tested by this procedure.

2.8. Physicochemical Stability

To evaluate the physicochemical stability of GFB/FCPP-NEMs, an accelerated stability analysis was performed under the accelerated conditions currently recommended by the International Conference on Harmonization guideline. The GFB/FCPP-NEMs were stored in a screw cap sealed glass bottles in a humidity chamber (75% RH) at constant temperature (40 °C). At the specified time points (1, 2, and 3 months), their particle size, physical state, drug content and related substances of gefitinib were determined.

2.9. Statistical Analysis

All results were expressed as the mean ± standard deviation (SD) of three independent experiments. All statistical analyses were performed using the SPSS, predictive analysis software (PASW), Statistic Software (SPSS/IBM Corp., Armonk, NY, USA). Comparison between groups was performed by Student's *t*-tests. *P*-values <0.05 were considered statistically significant [15].

3. Results and Discussion

3.1. Preparation and Characterization of GFB/FCPP NPs and GFB/FCPP-NEMs

The processes for the fabrication of monodispersed GFB/FCPP NPs and GFB/FCPP-NEMs are depicted in Figure 1. In the first process, the GFB/FCPP NPs, which serve as nanoscale drug reservoirs, were prepared by an emulsion–diffusion solvent evaporation process followed by coating with FA-conjugated CS. As shown in Figure S1, the gefitinib crystals consisted of irregularly shaped and dozens of micrometer-sized particles. Unlike gefitinib crystals, the prepared GFB/P407/PLGA samples consisted of a large number of regular spherical NPs with smooth surface without any noticeable cracks (Figure 2A). Moreover, hardly any gefitinib crystals was visible in the GFB/P407/PLGA sample, suggesting that most gefitinib molecules were encapsulated in the P407/PLGA NPs, which was critical for attaining sustained deliver, enhanced cellular uptake, and thereby improving the cytotoxicity of the encapsulated gefitinib molecules [9,24,25]. As shown in Figure 2B, after the FA-conjugated CS coating (Step 2 in Figure 1), the degree of sphericity of the GFB/FCPP NPs was reduced and their surface was relatively coarse compared with that of the GFB/P407/PLGA NPs. The hydrodynamic diameter, surface charge and drug loading amount of the prepared NPs are listed in Table 1. Based on the dynamic light scattering results, the GFB/FCPP NPs had a mean size of 255.4 ± 14.5 nm with a low polydispersity index, suggesting that the GFB/FCPP NPs were monodispersed. The drug loading amount and EE for GFB/FCPP NPs were 7.68 ± 0.36% and 95.57 ± 1.33%, respectively. GFB/FCPP NPs exhibited nanoscale sizes and a narrow size distribution, but nanoscale particles are not suitable for efficient pulmonary delivery. In order to achieve an effective deposition of the gefitinib formulation in deep lung regions (with huge inner surface area), the diameter of the powder particles is required to range from 1 to 5 μm [18]. Thus, the biodegradable and biocompatible polymer excipient, carboxymethyl β-glucan, was used as the MC material and the commonly used spray-drying technique was used for the encapsulation of GFB/FCPP NPs in carboxymethyl β-glucan MCs (Step 3 in Figure 1). Remarkably, as shown in Figure 2C, the formed GFB/FCPP-NEMs were nearly spherical capsules with a highly porous and sunken surface (their pore size was around 20 nm, inset of Figure 2C). The median diameter (d_{50}), d_{10}, d_{90} and span of GFB/FCPP-NEMs were about 2.2 ± 0.1 μm, 1.2 ± 0.1 μm, 4.6 ± 0.3 μm and 1.6 ± 0.2 μm, respectively. Due to their highly porous surface, GFB/FCPP-NEMs can quickly dissociate into its primary particles (GFB/FCPP NPs) for FA-mediated tumor-targeted drug delivery after hydration, as shown in Figure 2D.

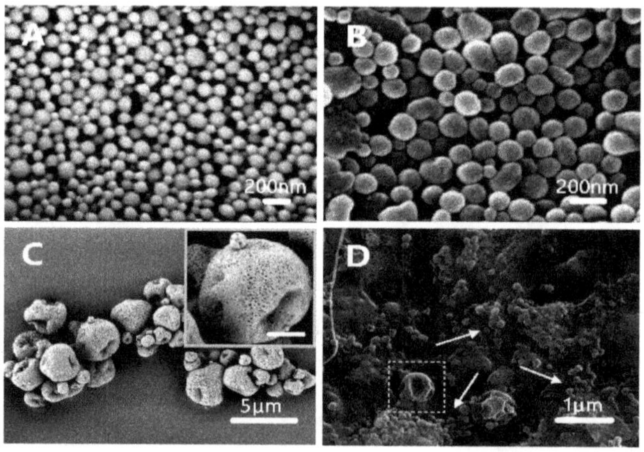

Figure 2. Scanning electron microscopy (SEM) photomicrographs of (**A**) GFB/P407/PLGA NPs, (**B**) GFB/FCPP NPs, (**C**) GFB/FCPP-NEMs (inset, high magnification image, scale bar =1 μm), and (**D**) GFB/FCPP-NEMs after exposure to PBS (pH 7.4). The arrow is pointing to the GFB/FCPP NPs, while the square frame contains a GFB/FCPP-NEM.

Table 1. Characterization of different samples (n = 3).

Formulations	Particle Size (nm)	Polydispersity Index	Zeta Potential (mV)	[1] EE (%)	Drug Loading (%)
P407/PLGA NPs	175.8 ± 11.2	0.08 ± 0.01	−11.74 ± 1.24	——	——
GFB/P407/PLGA NPs	180.0 ± 12.3	0.16 ± 0.05	−12.54 ± 2.30	90.42 ± 0.89	12.96 ± 0.41
GFB/FCPP NPs	255.4 ± 14.5	0.24 ± 0.09	+3.75 ± 1.85	95.57 ± 1.33	7.68 ± 0.36

[1] EE, entrapment efficiency.

3.2. *Solid-State Characterization*

Thermal analysis has been widely used for determination of the physical state of drugs in the NPs or MCs. Thus, DSC analysis of pure gefitinib, GFB/P407/PLGA, the physical mixture of gefitinib and P407/PLGA NPs, GFB/FCPP NPs, and GFB/FCPP-NEMs was conducted and the obtained DSC thermograms are presented in Figure 3. As shown in Figure 3a, pure gefitinib crystals show an endothermic peak at around 195 °C (with an enthalpy of 390 J/g), which corresponds to its melting temperature. The DSC curve of the physical mixture (gefitinib and P407/PLGA NPs) shown in Figure 3b also exhibited the sharp peak associated with gefitinib, indicating that gefitinib was still present in a crystalline state. However, after loading gefitinib into P407/PLGA NPs, the endothermic peak of gefitinib is not observed in the DSC thermograms of GFB/P407/PLGA NPs (Figure 3c). The absence of the endothermic peak corresponding to crystalline gefitinib in the thermograms indicated that the gefitinib entrapped in the P407/PLGA NPs had mostly lost its crystallinity [26]. Similarly, the endothermic peak of crystalline gefitinib also disappeared for both the GFB/FCPP NPs and GFB/FCPP-NEMs samples (Figure 3e,g). According to the DSC measurements, the encapsulated gefitinib was mostly in an amorphous state in the GFB/FCPP-NEMs delivery system.

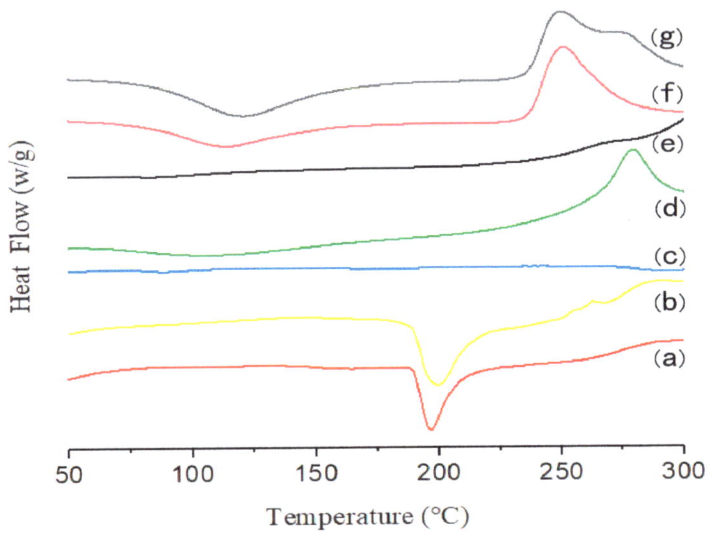

Figure 3. Differential scanning calorimetry (DSC) thermograms of (**a**) gefitinib crystals, (**b**) physical mixture of gefitinib and P407/PLGA NPs, (**c**) GFB/P407/PLGA NPs, (**d**) FA-conjugated CS, (**e**) GFB/FCPP NPs, (**f**) carboxymethyl β-glucan, and (**g**) GFB/FCPP-NEMs.

3.3. FT-IR Characterization

The FT-IR spectra of CS, FA, and FA-conjugated CS samples are displayed in Figure S2. For the FA sample, the typical band at 1694 cm^{-1} is attributed to the C=O stretching vibration, while the band at 1606 cm^{-1} is the characteristic peak of the amino group in the pteridine ring. In addition, the peak at 1484 cm^{-1} corresponds to the vibration of the benzene ring [23]. For the CS sample, the characteristic absorption peaks around 1619 and 1092 cm^{-1} belong to the N–H and C–O stretching vibrations, respectively. After conjugation of FA with CS, the absorption peak at 1514 cm^{-1} was weakened as a result of the reaction of the amino group of CS with the carboxylate group of FA. In addition, the appearance of a new peak at 1606 cm^{-1}, which corresponds to the amino group in the pteridine ring of FA, also confirmed that FA was conjugated with CS.

The FT-IR spectra of pure gefitinib, GFB/P407/PLGA, the physical mixture of gefitinib and P407/PLGA NPs, GFB/FCPP NPs, and GFB/FCPP-NEMs are presented in Figure 4. Pure gefitinib displays several absorption peaks. The FT-IR spectrum of gefitinib shown in Figure 4a reveals a characteristic absorption peak at 1625 cm^{-1} that was attributed to C = N stretching vibrations, while the peaks at 1110 cm^{-1} and 1028 cm^{-1} corresponded to the C–O and C–F stretching vibrations, respectively [27]. As anticipated, these gefitinib absorption peaks are also present in the spectrum of the physical mixture of gefitinib and P407/PLGA NPs (Figure 4c). Compared with the physical mixture, most of the gefitinib characteristic absorption bands were weakened in the FT-IR spectrum of the GFB/P407/PLGA sample (Figure 4d), suggesting that gefitinib was entrapped in the P407/PLGA NPs.

After FA-conjugated CS coating, the absorption peaks at 1694, 1606, and 1484 cm^{-1} corresponding to the FA-conjugated CS can be observed in the FTIR spectrum of the GFB/FCPP NPs (Figure 4e). Moreover, the absorption peaks of GFB/FCPP-NEMs (Figure 4g) were similar to those of the blank carboxymethyl β-glucan MCs, except for the intense peak at 1752 cm^{-1} corresponding to the C=O bond of the ester group from PLGA. Combine with the SEM analysis, these results clearly suggest that GFB/FCPP NPs and GFB/FCPP-NEMs were successfully prepared.

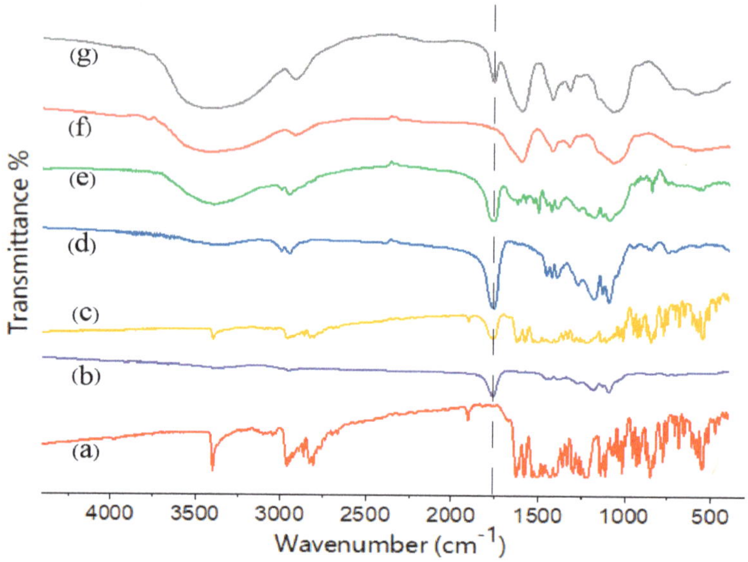

Figure 4. Fourier transform infrared (FT-IR) spectra of (**a**) gefitinib crystals, (**b**) P407/PLGA NPs, (**c**) physical mixture of gefitinib and P407/PLGA NPs, (**d**) GFB/P407/PLGA NPs, (**e**) GFB/FCPP NPs, (**f**) carboxymethyl β-glucan, and (**g**) GFB/FCPP-NEMs.

3.4. Drug Release Profiles

In vitro drug release tests were conducted at two different pH values (pH 7.4 and pH 5.0) to simulate the systemic circulation conditions and weakly acidic environments inside the tumor sites, respectively. The results revealed that the release rate of gefitinib from the gefitinib suspension was fast in both media. Even at pH 7.4 (mimic physiological conditions), approximately 60% of gefitinib was released from the gefitinib suspension within 4 h (Figure 5A). Unlike the rapid release pattern of the gefitinib suspension, the release profiles of gefitinib from GFB/FCPP NPs exhibited a slow and prolonged drug release behavior. Only about 13% of gefitinib was released in the initial 4 h, and the cumulative release rate of gefitinib from GFB/FCPP NPs was no more than 60% after 48 h. Compared with gefitinib suspension, the sustained-release behavior of GFB/FCPP NPs can be attributed to the encapsulation of gefitinib into FCPP NPs, which can lessen the damage of gefitinib to normal cells in the human body [28,29]. In addition, it is worth noting that the release of gefitinib from GFB/FCPP- NEMs was slower than that of GFB/FCPP NPs. As shown in Figure S3, after hydration of carboxymethyl β-glucan MCs, a hydrophilic gel of carboxymethyl β-glucan was formed and surrounded the GFB/FCPP NPs, which contributed to the decreased release rate of gefitinib from GFB/FCPP-NEMs. As expected, the release rate of gefitinib from the GFB/FCPP NPs or GFB/FCPP-NEMs at pH 5.0 was significantly fast compared with that at pH 7.4, as shown in Figure 5B. For the GFB/FCPP NPs, the amount of released gefitinib from at the sampling time of 2 h reached approximately 45% and was almost 60% within 4 h at pH 5.0. In addition, nearly 70% of gefitinib was released after 48 h. The enhanced drug release rate of GFB/FCPP NPs can be attributed to the pH-dependent FA-conjugated CS coating. As is well known, CS can be dissolved under acidic conditions. Since tumor microenvironment is weakly acidic, with pH values down to 5.0, the enhanced drug release efficiency of GFB/FCPP NPs at acidic pH would be beneficial in improving the cytotoxic and antitumor effects of the entrapped drug [30,31]. More importantly, GFB/FCPP NPs can release many more drug molecules at tumor sites than at normal tissues and thereby avoid side effects due to universal cytotoxicity. The above results indicated that the prepared FCPP-NEMs are likely an ideal drug delivery system for pH-dependent sustained drug release. Additionally, the probable release mechanism was investigated using different kinetic models of zero-order, first- order, Higuchi, and Korsmeyer–Peppas to fit the drug release curves of GFB/FCPP NPs and GFB/FCPP-NEMs, and their model parameters are summarized in Tables S1 and S2. The results revealed that the gefitinib release from both GFB/FCPP NPs and GFB/FCPP-NEMs was best fitted with the first-order model (with the highest value of regression coefficients, $r^2 \geq 0.96$) suggesting diffusion-controlled drug release kinetics. In addition, based on the Korsmeyer–Peppas model, the release exponent (n) for the tested GFB/FCPP NPs (at pH 5.0 and 7.4) or GFB/FCPP-NEMs (at pH 5.0) below 0.45, suggesting that the release of gefitinib from the test samples mainly follows the Fickian diffusion mechanism [32,33]. In contrast, the release exponent (n) for the tested GFB/FCPP-NEMs at pH 7.4 up to 0.69, indicated that gefitinib release from GFB/FCPP-NEMs was based on a combined diffusion/erosion process [34].

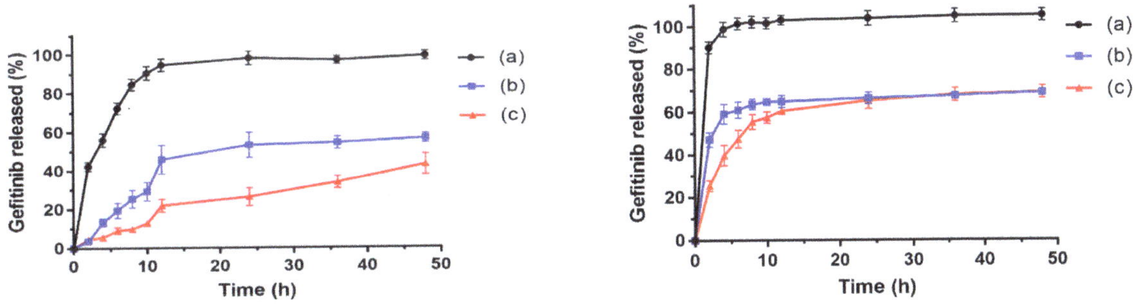

(A) (B)

Figure 5. Drug release of different gefitinib formulations at (**A**) pH 7.4 and (**B**) pH 5.0. (**a**) gefitinib suspension, (**b**) GFB/FCPP NPs, and (**c**) GFB/FCPP-NEMs. Each data point represents the mean ± SD (n = 3).

3.5. Cell Uptake and Intracellular Localization

To confirm the cell uptake of the primary particles of FCPP-NEMs, namely FCPP NPs, a fluorescence imaging analysis was carried out. The fluorescence microscopy images of A549 cells after 4 h incubation with coumarin-6-loaded FCPP NPs are shown in Figure 6. For comparison purposes, the cellular uptake behavior of coumarin-6-loaded P407/PLGA NPs was also studied. As shown in Figure 6A,B, the nucleus of the cells was stained blue with the Hoechst 33,342 dye. Also, obvious green fluorescence can be observed in the cytoplasmic region of cells with both coumarin- 6- loaded NPs tested, indicating that both coumarin-6-loaded FCPP NPs and coumarin- 6- loaded P407/PLGA NPs can be internalized by the A549 cells. Moreover, a significant enhancement in the green fluorescence intensity in the cytoplasmic region was observed with the increase of the dose of each carrier, suggesting that the uptake of both carriers was dose-dependent. As anticipated, compared with coumarin-6-loaded P407/PLGA NPs, cells exposed to coumarin- 6- loaded FCPP NPs had a slightly stronger green fluorescence at concentrations from 50 to 500 μg/mL. Such enhanced uptake can be attributed to the introduction of FA on the surface of the FCPP NPs. As is well known, FA has a high binding affinity for the FA receptor which is frequently overexpressed in human cancer cells. Several studies in the literature confirm that FA modified NPs can improve the chemotherapeutic efficacy of drugs due to their efficient cellular internalization through FA-mediated endocytosis [35]. Together, the results of the cell uptake study indicated that FCPP-NEMs can serve as an efficient carrier for enhanced delivery of a drug to tumor cells, thereby improving the antitumor effects of the encapsulated chemotherapeutic drug.

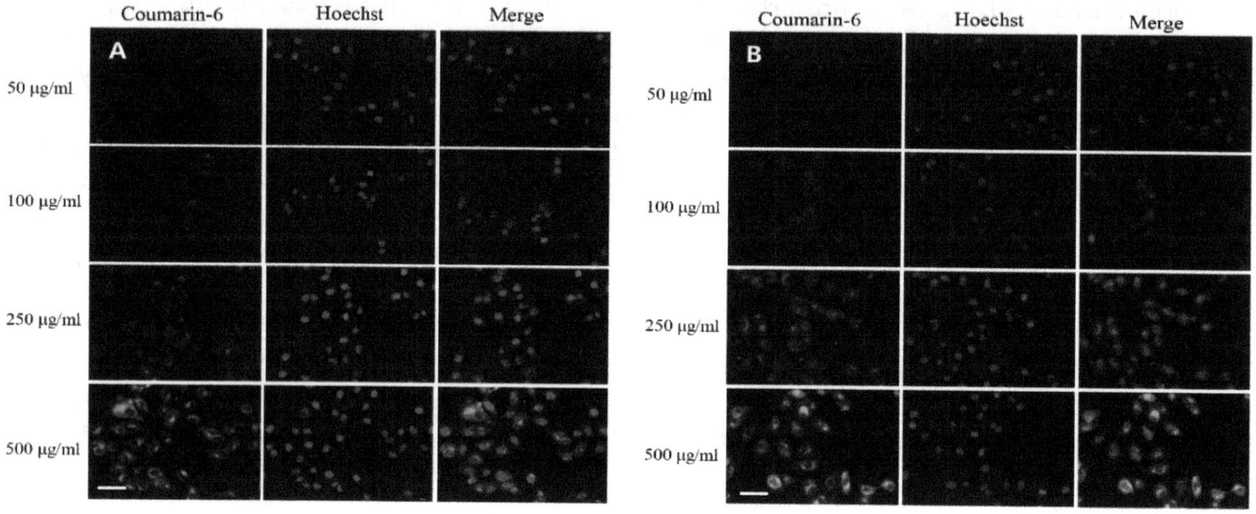

(**A**) (**B**)

Figure 6. Fluorescence images of A549 cells after incubation with coumarin-6-loaded P407/PLGA NPs (**A**) and coumarin-6-loaded FCPP NPs (**B**). Scale bar = 20 μm.

3.6. Cytotoxicity

After the drug release and cell uptake evaluation, the GFB/FCPP-NEMs may be assumed to display a more enhanced cytotoxic effect than gefitinib crystals. In order to confirm such an assumption, A549 and PC-9 cells were treated with blank FCPP-NEMs, gefitinib crystals, and GFB/FCPP-NEMs at various concentrations for 48 h, and their cytotoxicity was assessed by the MTT colorimetric assay. The results presented in Figure 7 reveal that blank FCPP-NEMs had no apparent inhibitory effect on the proliferation of both A549 and PC-9 cells at the tested concentrations. More than 90% of the cells were viable at concentrations as high as 1000 μg/mL, which indicated that the FCPP-NEMs had little cytotoxic effect on both A549 and PC-9 cells. Since CS, P407, PLGA and β- glucan are FDA-approved biodegradable and biocompatible polymers, FCPP-NEMs could be safely used as a drug delivery system for targeted treatment of lung tumors with chemotherapeutic agents. On the other hand, both free gefitinib and GFB/FCPP-NEMs showed a significant dose- dependent cytotoxicity against A549 cells after incubation for 48 h (Figure 8A). The 50% inhibitory concentrations (IC_{50}) for free gefitinib was 8.69 μg/mL, while that for GFB/FCPP-NEMs was decreased by 3.82-fold to 2.27 μg/mL, compared to that of free gefitinib. After encapsulation of gefitinib into FCPP-NEMs, the enhanced cytotoxicity of gefitinib can be mainly attributed to their efficient cellular internalization and pH-dependent prolonged release effect resulting from the encapsulation by FCPP-NEMs. As previously reported, encapsulation of chemotherapeutic agents into NPs or MCs is an effective approach to improve their intracellular delivery, and thereby, enhance their antitumor efficacy [14,16]. For example, Cosco et al. reported that CS-coated PLGA complexes increased the tumor cells uptake of miR-34a, which led to a significant decrease in tumor cell viability [36]. Similarly, GFB/FCPP-NEMs showed an enhanced cytotoxicity to PC-9 cells at the tested concentrations compared with free gefitinib (Figure 8B). The IC_{50} for free gefitinib and GFB/FCPP- NEMs was 10.09 μg/mL and 4.52 μg/mL, respectively. Thus, the prepared FCPP-NEMs system is a promising multifunctional carrier system for improving the antitumor effects of the chemotherapeutic agent gefitinib.

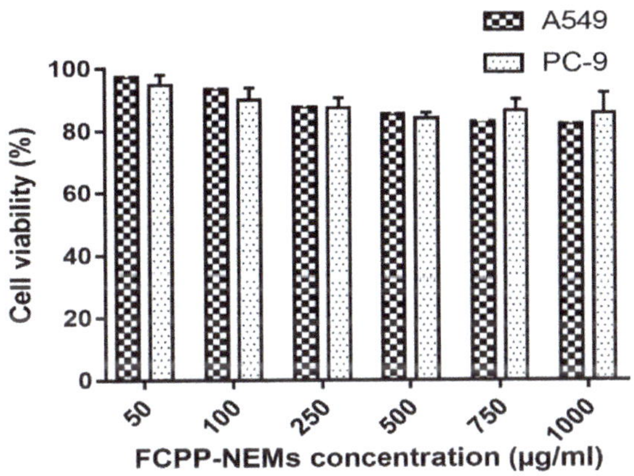

Figure 7. Effect of FCPP-NEMs on A549 and PC-9 cells at various concentrations ($n = 6$).

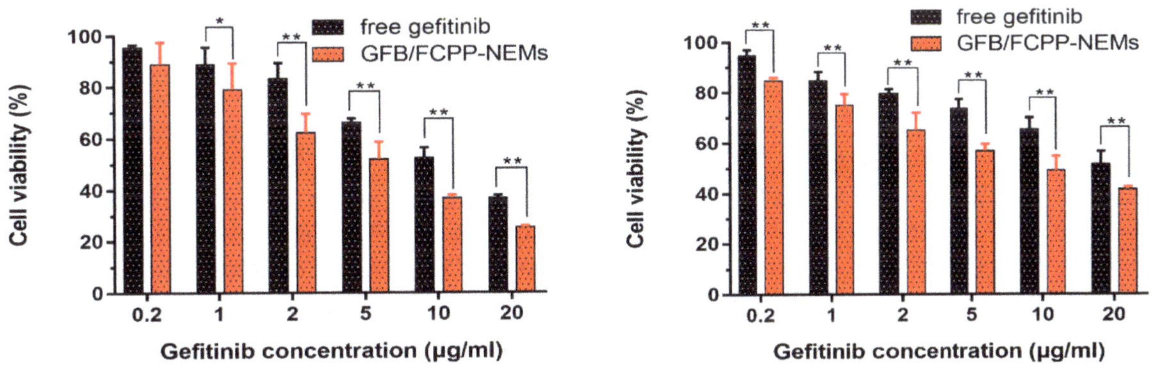

(A) (B)

Figure 8. Effect of free gefitinib and GFB/FCPP-NEMs on A549 cells (**A**) and PC-9 cells (**B**) viability at various concentrations ($n = 6$), * $p < 0.05$, ** $p < 0.01$.

3.7. Physicochemical Stability

The particle size, crystallinity, drug content, and related substance of gefitinib were used to evaluate the physicochemical stability of GFB/FCPP-NEMs after storage for 3 months. As shown in Table S3, there were no obvious differences in particle size, drug content, and related substances of gefitinib for the sample of GFB/FCPP-NEMs before and after storage. In addition, the endothermic peak of crystalline gefitinib also cannot be observed in the DSC thermogram of GFB/FCPP-NEMs, suggesting that the prepared GFB/FCPP-NEMs also existed in an amorphous state after storage (Figure S4). Taken together, the GFB/FCPP-NEMs showed an excellent physicochemical stability.

4. Conclusions

In this study, a novel FCPP-NEMs-based chemotherapeutic drug delivery system for targeted treatment of lung tumors was designed to afford an FA receptor-mediated tumor targeting property, facilitated intracellular accumulation, pH-triggered sustained release, and enhanced cytotoxicity of the chemotherapeutic agent gefitinib. The prepared GFB/FCPP-NEMs were nearly spherical capsules with a median diameter of around 2.2 μm and a highly porous surface. GFB/FCPP-NEMs can quickly dissociate into their primary particles, GFB/FCPP NPs, after hydration. Besides providing pH-triggered prolonged gefitinib release, the GFB/FCPP-NEMs can facilitate the uptake of the encapsulated cargo by tumor cells. Therefore, the use of GFB/FCPP-NEMs results in a significant improvement in the cytotoxicity of gefitinib compared with the free drug. This study suggests that the developed FCPP-NEMs is a promising carrier system for potential lung tumor-targeted delivery of gefitinib, which is anticipated to improve the antitumor effects of gefitinib and reduce its systemic side effects.

Supplementary Materials:
Figure S1: SEM photograph of gefitinib crystals, Figure S2: FT-IR spectra of (**a**) FA-conjugated CS, (**b**) FA, and (**c**) CS, Figure S3: SEM photograph of GFB/FCPP-NEMs after drug release for 2 h, Figure S4: DSC thermogram of GFB/FCPP-NEMs after storage for 3 months, Table S1: Model parameters of the tested samples at pH 5.0, Table S2: Model parameters of the tested samples at pH 7.4, Table S3: Median diameter, span, related substances of gefitinib, and drug content of GFB/FCPP-NEMs before and after storage for 3 months ($n = 3$).

Author Contributions: Conceptualization, X.L. and Y.Z.; methodology, X.L. and Y.Z.; software, X.L. and Z.L.; validation, X.L. and Y.Z.; formal analysis, X.L., J.W., S.L. and Z.Z.; writing—original draft preparation, X.L.; writing—review and editing, X.L. and Y.Z.

Acknowledgments: The authors would like to thank the pharmacy students Hongtao Wang, Chan Wang, and Fang Wang who helped in the cell uptake and drug release experiments. The authors would also like to thank the Jiangsu Key Laboratory of New Drug Research and Clinical Pharmacy and the Resource Sharing Platform for Large-scale Instrument and Equipment at Xuzhou Medical University for use of its resources.

References

1. He, J.; Hu, Y.; Hu, M.; Li, B. Development of PD-1/PD-L1 pathway in tumor immune microenvironment and treatment for non-small-cell lung cancer. *Sci. Rep.* **2015**, *5*, 13110. [CrossRef] [PubMed]
2. Brahmer, J.; Reckamp, K.L.; Baas, P.; Crino, L.; Eberhardt, W.E.; Poddubskaya, E.; Antonia, S.; Pluzanski, A.; Vokes, E.E.; Holgado, E.; et al. Nivolumab versus docetaxel in advanced squamous-cell non-small-cell lung cancer. *N. Engl. J. Med.* **2015**, *373*, 123–135. [CrossRef] [PubMed]
3. Herbst, R.S.; Giaccone, G.; Schiller, J.H.; Natale, R.B.; Miller, V.; Manegold, C.; Scagliotti, G.; Rosell, R.; Oliff, I.; Revves, A.J.; et al. Gefitinib in combination with paclitaxel and carboplatin in advanced non-small-cell lung cancer: A phase III trial—INTACT 2. *J. Clin. Oncol.* **2004**, *22*, 785–794. [CrossRef] [PubMed]
4. Blanco, E.; Shen, H.; Ferrari, M. Principles of nanoparticle design for overcoming biological barriers to drug delivery. *Nat. Biotechnol.* **2015**, *33*, 941–951. [CrossRef] [PubMed]
5. Sordella, R.; Bell, D.W.; Haber, D.A.; Settleman, J. Gefitinib-sensitizing EGFR mutations in lung cancer activate anti-apoptotic pathways. *Science* **2004**, *305*, 1163–1167. [CrossRef] [PubMed]
6. Stuurman, F.E.; Nuijen, B.; Beijnen, J.H.; Schellens, J.H. Oral anticancer drugs: Mechanisms of low bioavailability and strategies for improvement. *Clin. Pharmacokinet.* **2013**, *52*, 399–414. [CrossRef] [PubMed]
7. Inoue, A.; Saijo, Y.; Maemondo, M.; Gomi, K.; Tokue, Y.; Kimura, Y.; Ebina, M.; Kikuchi, T.; Moriya, T.; Nukiwa, T. Severe acute interstitial pneumonia and gefitinib. *Lancet* **2003**, *361*, 137–139. [CrossRef]
8. Yang, Y.; Bajaj, N.; Xu, P.; Ohn, K.; Tsifansky, M.D.; Yeo, Y. Development of highly porous large PLGA microparticles for pulmonary drug delivery. *Biomaterials* **2009**, *30*, 1947–1953. [CrossRef] [PubMed]
9. Hamdy, S.; Haddadi, A.; Hung, R.W.; Lavasanifar, A. Targeting dendritic cells with nano-particulate PLGA cancer vaccine formulations. *Adv. Drug Deliv. Rev.* **2011**, *63*, 943–955. [CrossRef]
10. Bowerman, C.J.; Byrne, J.D.; Chu, K.S.; Schorzman, A.N.; Keeler, A.W.; Sherwood, C.A.; Perry, J.L.; Luft, J.C.; Darr, D.B.; Deal, A.M.; et al. Docetaxel-loaded PLGA nanoparticles improve efficacy in taxane-resistant triple-negative breast cancer. *Nano Lett.* **2017**, *17*, 242–248. [CrossRef]
11. Yamamoto, H.; Kuno, Y.; Sugimoto, S.; Takeuchi, H.; Kawashima, Y. Surface-modified PLGA nanosphere with chitosan improved pulmonary delivery of calcitonin by mucoadhesion and opening of the intercellular tight junctions. *J. Control. Release* **2005**, *102*, 373–381. [CrossRef] [PubMed]
12. Sheng, J.; Han, L.; Qin, J.; Ru, G.; Li, R.; Wu, L.; Cui, D.; Yang, P.; He, Y.; Wang, J. *N*-trimethyl chitosan chloride-coated PLGA nanoparticles overcoming multiple barriers to oral insulin absorption. *ACS Appl. Mater. Interfaces* **2015**, *7*, 15430–15441. [CrossRef] [PubMed]
13. Dhas, N.L.; Ige, P.P.; Kudarha, R.R. Design, optimization and in-vitro study of folic acid conjugated-chitosan functionalized PLGA nanoparticle for delivery of bicalutamide in prostate cancer. *Powder Technol.* **2015**, *283*, 234–245. [CrossRef]
14. Zhu, H.; Chen, H.; Zeng, X.; Wang, Z.; Zhang, X.; Wu, Y.; Gao, Y.; Zhang, J.; Liu, K.; Liu, R.; et al. Co-delivery of chemotherapeutic drugs with vitamin E TPGS by porous PLGA nanoparticles for enhanced chemotherapy against multi-drug resistance. *Biomaterials* **2014**, *35*, 2391–2400. [CrossRef] [PubMed]
15. Cheng, W.; Nie, J.; Xu, L.; Liang, C.; Peng, Y.; Liu, G.; Wang, T.; Mei, L.; Huang, L.; Zeng, X. pH-Sensitive delivery vehicle based on folic acid-conjugated polydopamine- modified mesoporous silica nanoparticles for targeted cancer therapy. *ACS Appl. Mater. Interfaces* **2017**, *9*, 18462–18473. [CrossRef] [PubMed]

16. Brannon-Peppas, L.; Blanchette, J.O. Nanoparticle and targeted systems for cancer therapy. *Adv. Drug Deliv. Rev.* **2012**, *64*, 206–212. [CrossRef]
17. Batrakova, E.V.; Kabanov, A.V. Pluronic block copolymers: Evolution of drug delivery concept from inert nanocarriers to biological response modifiers. *J. Control. Release* **2008**, *130*, 98–106. [CrossRef] [PubMed]
18. Shiehzadeh, F.; Tafaghodi, M. Dry powder form of polymeric nanoparticles for pulmonary drug delivery. *Curr. Pharm. Des.* **2016**, *22*, 2549–2560. [CrossRef] [PubMed]
19. Jesenak, M.; Urbancikova, I.; Banovcin, P. Respiratory tract infections and the role of biologically active polysaccharides in their management and prevention. *Nutrients* **2017**, *9*, 779. [CrossRef] [PubMed]
20. Roudi, R.; Mohammadi, S.R.; Roudbary, M.; Mohsenzadegan, M. Lung cancer and beta-glucans: Review of potential therapeutic applications. *Investig. New Drugs* **2017**, *35*, 509–517. [CrossRef] [PubMed]
21. Francioso, A.; Cossi, R.; Fanelli, S.; Mastromarino, P.; Mosca, L. Studies on trans-resveratrol/carboxymethylated (1,3/1,6)-beta-d-glucan association for aerosol pharmaceutical applications. *Int. J. Mol. Sci.* **2017**, *18*, 967. [CrossRef] [PubMed]
22. Yang, Y.Y.; Chia, H.H.; Chung, T.S. Effect of preparation temperature on the characteristics and release profiles of PLGA microspheres containing protein fabricated by double-emulsion solvent extraction/evaporation method. *J. Control. Release* **2000**, *69*, 81–96. [CrossRef]
23. Depan, D.; Shah, J.; Misra, R.D.K. Controlled release of drug from folate-decorated and graphene mediated drug delivery system: Synthesis, loading efficiency, and drug release response. *Mater. Sci. Eng.* **2011**, *31*, 1305–1312. [CrossRef]
24. Siepmann, J.; Siepmann, F. Mathematical modeling of drug delivery. *Int. J. Pharm.* **2008**, *364*, 328–343. [CrossRef] [PubMed]
25. Pakulska, M.M.; Donaghue, I.E.; Obermeyer, J.M.; Tuladhar, A.; McLaughlin, C.K.; Shendruk, T.N.; Shoichet, M.S. Encapsulation-free controlled release: Electrostaticadsorption eliminates the need for protein encapsulation in PLGA nanoparticles. *Sci. Adv.* **2016**, *2*, e1600519. [CrossRef] [PubMed]
26. Zhang, Y.; Dong, K.; Wang, F.; Wang, H.; Wang, J.; Jiang, Z.; Diao, S. Three dimensional macroporous hydroxyapatite/chitosan foam-supported polymer micelles for enhanced oral delivery of poorly soluble drugs. *Colloids Surf. B* **2018**, *170*, 497–504. [CrossRef] [PubMed]
27. Liu, G.; Lin, Q.; Huang, Y.; Guan, G.; Jiang, Y. Tailoring the particle microstructures of gefitinib by supercritical CO_2 anti-solvent process. *J. CO2 Util.* **2017**, *20*, 43–51. [CrossRef]
28. Peer, D.; Karp, J.M.; Hong, S.; Farokhzad, O.C.; Margalit, R.; Langer, R. Nanocarriers as an emerging platform for cancer therapy. *Nat. Nanotechnol.* **2007**, *2*, 751–760. [CrossRef] [PubMed]
29. Park, J.H.; Saravanakumar, G.; Kim, K.; Kwon, I.C. Targeted delivery of low molecular drugs using chitosan and its derivatives. *Adv. Drug Deliv. Rev.* **2010**, *62*, 28–41. [CrossRef] [PubMed]
30. Zhao, Y.; Luo, Z.; Li, M.; Qu, Q.; Ma, X.; Yu, S.H.; Zhao, Y. A preloaded amorphous calcium carbonate/doxorubicin@silica nanoreactor for pH-responsive delivery of an anticancer drug. *Angew. Chem. Int. Ed. Engl.* **2015**, *54*, 919–922. [CrossRef] [PubMed]
31. Liu, J.; Luo, Z.; Zhang, J.; Luo, T.; Zhou, J.; Zhao, X.; Cai, K. Hollow mesoporous silica nanoparticles facilitated drug delivery via cascade pH stimuli in tumor microenvironment for tumor therapy. *Biomaterials* **2016**, *83*, 51–65. [CrossRef] [PubMed]
32. Cannavà, C.; Tommasini, S.; Stancanelli, R.; Cardile, V.; Cilurzo, F.; Giannone, I.; Puglisi, G.; Ventura, C.A. Celecoxib-loaded PLGA/cyclodextrin microspheres: Characterization and evaluation of anti-inflammatory activity on human chondrocyte cultures. *Colloids Surf. B* **2013**, *111*, 289–296. [CrossRef] [PubMed]
33. Ford Versypt, A.N.; Pack, D.W.; Braatz, R.D. Mathematical modeling of drug delivery from autocatalytically degradable PLGA microspheres—A review. *J. Control. Release* **2013**, *165*, 29–37. [CrossRef] [PubMed]
34. Panda, A.; Meena, J.; Katara, R.; Majumdar, D.K. Formulation and characterization of clozapine and risperidone co-entrapped spray-dried PLGA nanoparticles. *Pharm. Dev. Technol.* **2014**, *21*, 43–53. [CrossRef] [PubMed]
35. Dong, S.; Cho, H.J.; Lee, Y.W.; Roman, M. Synthesis and cellular uptake of folic acid-conjugated cellulose nanocrystals for cancer targeting. *Biomacromolecules* **2014**, *15*, 1560–1567. [CrossRef] [PubMed]
36. Cosco, D.; Cilurzo, F.; Maiuolo, J.; Federico, C.; Di Martino, M.T.; Cristiano, M.C.; Tassone, P.; Fresta, M.; Paolino, D. Delivery of miR-34a by chitosan/PLGA nanoplexes for the anticancer treatment of multiple myeloma. *Sci. Rep.* **2015**, *5*, 17579. [CrossRef] [PubMed]

3

Recent Progress in the Development of Poly(lactic-*co*-glycolic acid) Based Nanostructures for Cancer Imaging and Therapy

Ki-Taek Kim [1,†], Jae-Young Lee [2,†], Dae-Duk Kim [3], In-Soo Yoon [4,*] and Hyun-Jong Cho [5,*]

1 College of Pharmacy and Natural Medicine Research Institute, Mokpo National University, Muan-gun, Jeonnam 58554, Korea; ktkim0628@mokpo.ac.kr
2 College of Pharmacy, Chungnam National University, Daejeon 34134, Korea; jaeyoung@cnu.ac.kr
3 College of Pharmacy and Research Institute of Pharmaceutical Sciences, Seoul National University, Seoul 08826, Korea; ddkim@snu.ac.kr
4 Department of Manufacturing Pharmacy, College of Pharmacy, Pusan National University, Busan 46241, Korea
5 College of Pharmacy, Kangwon National University, Chuncheon 24341, Korea
* Correspondence: insoo.yoon@pusan.ac.kr (I.-S.Y.); hjcho@kangwon.ac.kr (H.-J.C.)
† These authors are equally contributed to this work.

Abstract: Diverse nanosystems for use in cancer imaging and therapy have been designed and their clinical applications have been assessed. Among a variety of materials available to fabricate nanosystems, poly(lactic-*co*-glycolic acid) (PLGA) has been widely used due to its biocompatibility and biodegradability. In order to provide tumor-targeting and diagnostic properties, PLGA or PLGA nanoparticles (NPs) can be modified with other functional materials. Hydrophobic or hydrophilic therapeutic cargos can be placed in the internal space or adsorbed onto the surface of PLGA NPs. Protocols for the fabrication of PLGA-based NPs for cancer imaging and therapy are already well established. Moreover, the biocompatibility and biodegradability of PLGA may elevate its feasibility for clinical application in injection formulations. Size-controlled NP's properties and ligand–receptor interactions may provide passive and active tumor-targeting abilities, respectively, after intravenous administration. Additionally, the introduction of several imaging modalities to PLGA-based NPs can enable drug delivery guided by in vivo imaging. Versatile platform technology of PLGA-based NPs can be applied to the delivery of small chemicals, peptides, proteins, and nucleic acids for use in cancer therapy. This review describes recent findings and insights into the development of tumor-targeted PLGA-based NPs for use of cancer imaging and therapy.

Keywords: cancer; diagnosis; nanoparticle; PLGA; targeting; therapy

---

1. Introduction

There has been much progress in the development of nanomedicines for use cancer imaging and therapy [1–20]. To increase the potential for clinical application, nanomedicines with increased precision and safety have recently been designed and evaluated. Following intravenous administration, particles with a certain size range can localize to the tumor region through an "enhanced permeability and retention (EPR) effect" [21–23]. Molecules or particles with a size of >40 kDa (renal clearance threshold) may be present in the systemic circulation for a prolonged period [22,23]. Leaky tumor vasculature and insufficient lymphatic drainage of tumor tissue can increase the permeability and accumulation of particles [24]. Although the EPR effect has been proved in many animal studies, its usefulness for clinical application is still controversial [21]. The pathophysiological states are different according to the animal species (rodent versus human), tumor types originated from same source, and primary versus metastatic tumors in the same patient [21]. Consideration of the heterogeneity of EPR effect is necessary for the successful translation of nanomedicines to the clinical situation [21]. As drug delivery via EPR does not usually occur in normal tissues, it can be used as a passive tumor-targeting strategy [25]. However, the heterogeneity of tumor tissue, including highly hypovascular areas and necrotic tissues, frequently observed in large tumors may limit the efficiency of particle delivery. In addition to various factors that modulate the EFR effect [26] (e.g., bradykinin, nitric oxide derivatives, prostaglandins, angiotensin-converting enzyme inhibitors, and vascular endothelial growth factor [VEGF]), ligand–receptor interactions have been introduced as an active tumor-targeting strategy [27]. Ligands can be selected to bind receptors that are overexpressed in cancer cells compared with normal cells [27]. Receptors in tumor cells (e.g., transferrin [Tf] receptor, folate receptor, lectins, and epidermal growth factor receptor [EGFR]) or on the tumoral endothelium (e.g., VEGF receptors, $\alpha_v\beta_3$ integrin, vascular cell adhesion molecule-1 [VCAM-1] and matrix metalloproteinases [MMPs]) can be targets of ligand-tethered nanosystems [27]. Recently, internal (e.g., pH, enzyme, and redox state) and external (e.g., temperature, magnetism, and ultrasound) stimuli-sensitive smart nanosystems have been designed to provide more sophisticated drug-release patterns and selective uptake in cancer cells [27]. Additive properties, such as tumor penetration, the induction of apoptosis, and inhibition of metastasis, have been built in nanosystems for use in cancer imaging and therapy [28–38].

To reduce toxicity in the development of tumor-targeted nanomedicines, biocompatibility and biodegradability are considered principal issues in the selection of materials for nanosystems. Various types of synthetic polymers (e.g., poly(lactic-*co*-glycolic acid) [PLGA]), natural polymers (e.g., chitosan [CS], chondroitin sulfate [CD], and hyaluronic acid [HA]), lipids (e.g., phospholipid and cholesterol), nucleic acids (e.g., DNA), peptides/proteins (e.g., albumin and lysozyme), and inorganic materials (e.g., gold, iron, silver, and zinc) have been used to prepare nanoformulations for cancer therapy [39–58]. Among these diverse materials, PLGA is a favored substance for the fabrication of nanoparticles (NPs) aimed at drug delivery [59–61]. PLGA can be degraded into lactic acid (LA) and glycolic acid (GA), which can enter metabolic pathways. Therefore, it can be safely applied to the preparation of injection formulations. PLGA has received approval from the United States Food and Drug Administration and the European Medicine Agency for its application in injectable formulations [62]. It can be chemically modified to give biofunctionality (i.e., tumor-targeting capability), and the outer surface of PLGA-based NPs can be transformed to provide a prolonged circulation time and tumor targetability [63–66]. Small chemicals, peptides, proteins, and nucleic acids with diverse physicochemical properties can be entrapped in PLGA or PLGA derivative-based NPs or adsorbed onto the outer surface of NPs [61,67–70]. Convenient modification and reliability in the fabrication of NPs, as well as their favorable biosafety, may elevate the feasibility of applying PLGA-based NPs in the clinic.

Several articles have reviewed the application of PLGA nanomedicines to drug delivery [59,61,62, 67]. Herein, we introduce recent progress in the development and evaluation of PLGA-based NPs for cancer imaging and therapy. Information regarding the preparation, cellular uptake and distribution, in vivo tumor targeting, in vivo cancer therapy, and in vivo pharmacokinetics of PLGA-based NPs will be provided.

2. Preparation and Modification of PLGA-Based NPs

2.1. *Preparation of PLGA NPs*

The fabrication method of PLGA NPs may affect their physicochemical properties, such as particle size, particle size distribution, particle shape, drug encapsulation efficiency, and particle stability [71]. The most common methods for the preparation of PLGA NPs, such as emulsification, nanoprecipitation, spray-drying, and microfluidics, are described in following sections.

2.1.1. Emulsification-Evaporation Method

Emulsification is the most frequently used method. This method can be subdivided based on the emulsion (single; e.g., oil in water [O/W] emulsion and double or multiple; e.g., water in oil in water [W/O/W] emulsion) and acquisition of the NPs (i.e., solvent evaporation and dialysis). PLGA polymers and hydrophobic drugs can be dissolved in water-immiscible organic solvents, such as chloroform or dichloromethane, followed by addition to the aqueous phase containing a surfactant such as poly(vinyl alcohol) (PVA) to obtain an O/W emulsion. This emulsification can be prepared using a homogenizer or ultrasonic probe, which can provide high shear energy. Then, the organic solvent can be evaporated with simple stirring, under a gentle nitrogen gas stream, or in a vacuum state. The hardened NPs can be obtained by centrifugation, washed to remove remaining surfactants, and lyophilized for further storage. The organic solvent in the oil phase of emulsion systems can also be diffused by dialysis against a large amount of water. Solidified particles containing PLGA polymer and drugs may be precipitated and acquired [60,62].

The double or multiple emulsion method can be used to encapsulate further hydrophilic drugs. An aqueous solution containing hydrophilic drugs is added to the PLGA-dissolved organic phase under vigorous stirring to obtain a W/O emulsion. This emulsion is added to the second aqueous solution containing a surfactant under high-shear energy to form a W/O/W emulsion. Then, the hardened NPs can be obtained by solvent evaporation [72].

The emulsification method can be used to encapsulate both hydrophobic and hydrophilic drugs. Furthermore, it can be used to prepare particles, varying from nano to micron size by adjusting the stirring speed and input rate [71]. Nonetheless, there are some problems with this method, such as the requirement for heat or a vacuum for solvent evaporation and the imperfect elimination of stabilizer [72]. Recently, membrane extrusion has been used to prepare NPs with a narrow size distribution after the emulsification process. Membrane extrusion is performed using a polycarbonate membrane under high pressure [60].

2.1.2. Nanoprecipitation Method

PLGA and hydrophobic drugs can be dissolved in a water-miscible solvent such as dimethyl sulfoxide (DMSO), acetone, and ethanol. This organic solution is usually injected into an aqueous solution containing surfactant at a controlled speed with an auto-injector. NPs can be formed by the rapid diffusion of polymers and drugs out of organic phase. Then, they can be obtained by solvent elimination [73].

Nanoprecipitation is used to load hydrophobic drugs into the NPs via a one-step procedure. This method can be useful to prepare PLGA NPs with a <100 nm particle size, which can be determined by the polymer concentration [60]. The advantages of this method include its easy scale-up, low energy requirement, high reproducibility, and single step process. The limitations include the low encapsulation efficiency of the hydrophilic drug and particle size variation, which is dependent on the mixing process [72].

2.1.3. Spray-Drying Method

The spray-drying method is a rapid process that can be used to encapsulate both hydrophobic and hydrophilic drugs. Aqueous solution containing hydrophilic drugs may be added to the PLGA-dissolved organic phase under vigorous stirring to obtain the W/O emulsion, and can be used to make multiple emulsion. Particles are obtained by spraying W/O emulsion or multiple emulsion with a stream of heated air [74]. However, the main limitation of this method is the adhesion of particles to the walls and cyclone part of the spray dryer, resulting in low productivity [68].

2.1.4. Microfluidics Method

The continuous-phase flow microfluidic system, including a flow-focusing system and co-flowing system, can be used to prepare nano-sized PLGA particles by forming single emulsions. In the flow-focusing system, the dispersed phase flows through a narrow capillary and the continuous phase flows from the two side channels with the vertical direction of the dispersed phase. In the co-flowing system, the dispersed phase flows inside the capillary and the continuous phase flows outside the capillary in the same direction [60].

The microfluidic method has several advantages for preparing PLGA NPs, such as a narrow size distribution, high reproducibility, and the prevention of an initial burst release. Moreover, the microfluidic system can be used to prepare various surface-modified PLGA NPs, such as PEGylated NPs and NPs carrying targeting moieties [72]. However, it also has limitations, including limited production scale (and scale-up), and problems associated with microchannel clogging and fouling [72].

2.2. Surface Modification of PLGA NPs for Tumor Targeting

2.2.1. Physicochemical and Biological Properties of PLGA

PLGA is a copolymer composed of LA and GA and those two units are linked via an ester bond. Therefore, PLGA can be degraded into LA and GA by hydrolysis in the body and can join in metabolic pathways [67,75]. The degradation of PLGA NPs may be influenced by the molecular weight (MW), molar ratio between LA and GA, crystalline degree, glass transition temperature, and the type of end cap (acid versus ester) [62,67]. Poly(lactic acid) (PLA) is more hydrophobic than poly(glycolic acid) (PGA); thus, a PLGA copolymer with a higher ratio of LA/GA may be degraded more slowly [62]. Additionally, PLGA with an ester end cap may have higher resistance to hydrolysis compared with PLGA with an acid end cap [62]. This biocompatibility and biodegradability can increase the feasibility of using PLGA NPs in clinical applications. By modulating the polymerization process, various types of PLGA in terms of MW, LA:GA ratio, end cap, and chirality, can be prepared. Those properties can affect polymer degradation, drug release from NPs, cellular uptake, and the in vivo fate of NPs [59–62,65–69]. Furthermore, several block or grafted copolymer types (e.g., linear, branched, and star-shaped) based on PLGA can be synthesized with CS, HA, poly(caprolactone) (PCL), poly(ethylene glycol) (PEG), polyethylenimine (PEI), poly-L-lysine (PLL), poly(styrene), and PVA [59,62,76–78]. Amphiphilic copolymers (e.g., PEG-PLGA and PLGA-PEG-PLGA) can form a micellar structure following dispersal in an aqueous environment, and present different particle characteristics [79,80]. In addition, reactive units (e.g., amine, maleimide, *N*-hydroxysuccinimide, and vinyl) can be attached to the terminal end of a PLGA copolymer. These functional groups can participate in further modifications with tumor-targeting ligands or drug cargos. These structural changes can modulate the physicochemical and biological properties of PLGA-based NPs [62,67,69].

2.2.2. Surface Engineering of PLGA-Based NPs

For active tumor-targeting strategies (i.e., ligand–receptor interaction) together with a passive tumor-targeting approach (i.e., EPR effect), the outer surface of PLGA-based NPs has been engineered with various functional groups. Two methods can be used to prepare surface-engineered PLGA NPs; 1) After synthesizing PLGA derivatives (linked to functional groups), they can then be used to fabricate NPs. 2) After fabricating PLGA NPs, the exposed functional groups (i.e., carboxylic acid and hydroxyl groups) of PLGA are chemically linked to targeting moieties, or the outer surface of PLGA NPs are coated with functional materials.

For prolonged circulation in the blood, hydrophilic molecules such as PEG, poloxamers, and Tween 80 are usually conjugated on the surface of PLGA NPs. These hydrophilic molecules on the NPs can infer stealth properties, leading to the evasion of phagocytic uptake by the reticuloendothelial system (RES), and a prolonged time in the systemic circulation [81]. Furthermore, PLGA NPs conjugated or coated with positively-charged molecules such as CS can be taken into the tumor cells more easily via adsorptive-mediated transcytosis [82].

Active targeting for tumor-specific delivery can be achieved by introducing targeting moieties to the surface of NPs, which are specifically recognized by receptors on the tumor cells or tumor vasculature, resulting in the increased penetration of tumor cells via receptor-mediated endocytosis [83]. The receptors or surface-bound antigens may be expressed exclusively or overexpressed on the tumor cells compared with normal cells. Various targeting moieties such as folic acid (FA), Tf, biotin, HA, peptides, aptamers, and antibodies (Abs) have been used on the surface of PLGA NPs to actively target tumor microenvironments (Table 1). However, the expression of receptors on the tumor cell or vasculature can be altered and alternative receptors can be upregulated [72]. Recently, NPs carrying multiple (e.g., dual or triple) ligands have been investigated to maximize tumor-targeting efficiency.

The development of multi-functional PLGA NPs modified with cell-penetration peptides, Pluronic® P85 (an inhibitor for drug efflux pump), or PEG are promising strategies for use in cancer therapy [84]. These PLGA NPs can passively target delivery to tumors via the EPR effect, and actively target delivery to tumors based on ligand–receptor interactions, and overcome drug resistance with inhibitors of efflux pumps, finally improving anti-tumor efficacies and reducing systemic toxicity in normal tissues and organs [85,86]. Surface-engineered PLGA NPs for passive and active tumor targeting are illustrated and summarized in Figure 1 and Table 1, respectively.

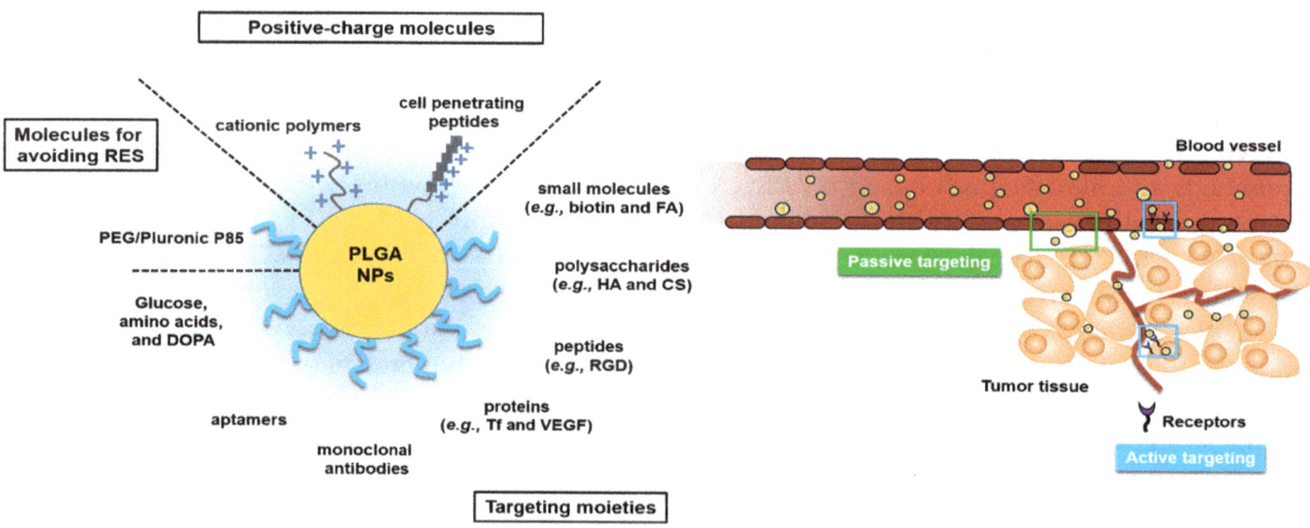

Figure 1. Various surface-engineered poly(lactic-*co*-glycolic acid) (PLGA) nanoparticles (NPs) for passive or active tumor targeting. Arg-Gly-Asp (RGD); chitosan (CS); dopamine (DOPA); folic acid (FA); hyaluronic acid (HA); poly(ethylene glycol) (PEG); reticuloendothelial system (RES); transferrin (Tf); vascular endothelial growth factor (VEGF).

Table 1. Surface modification methods of PLGA NPs for tumor targeting.

Formulation	Anticancer Agent	Target (Cell Line)	Surface Modification Method	Ref.
mPEG-PLGA NPs	Mitramycin	Pancreatic carcinoma (BxPC-3 and MIA Paca-2 cells)	Mitramycin was loaded onto mPEG-PLGA NPs by the single-emulsion solvent evaporation method using poloxamer 188 as a stabilizer	[87]
CS-modified PLGA NPs	PTX	Breast cancer (MDA-MB- 231 cells)	PTX-loaded PLGA NPs were prepared by the nanoprecipitation method using a high-gravity rotating packed bed. Then, PLGA NPs were modified with CS through electrostatic adherence	[88]
Pluronic® P85 or Tf-modified PLGA NPs	PTX	Glioma (C6 cells)	PTX-loaded PLGA NPs were prepared by the nanoprecipitation method. PLGA NPs were coated with Pluronic® P85 or conjugated with Tf	[89]
C_{24}-LMWP peptide-modified PLGA NPs	DOX	Drug-resistant lung cancer (A549/T cells) and drug-resistant breast cancer (MCF-7/ADR cells)	Desalted DOX-loaded PLGA NPs were prepared by the nanoprecipitation method. Then, a C_{24}-LMWP hybrid peptide was introduced to PLGA NPs by electrostatic interaction	[90]
HA-PEG- PLGA or CD-PEG-PLGA NPs	pDNA lipoplex	Glioblastoma (U87 cells)	HA or CD was conjugated to PLGA-PEG-NH_2 using a reducing agent and a catalyst. HA-PEG-PLGA or CD-PEG-PLGA NPs were prepared by the dialysis method	[91]
PLGA-PEG-biotin NPs	SN-38 (active metabolite of irinotecan)	Breast cancer (4T1 cells)	NHS-Biotin and H_2N-PEG-NH_2 were conjugated. Then, PEG-biotin was conjugated to PLGA-NHS to synthesize PLGA-PEG-biotin. PLGA-PEG-biotin NPs were prepared by the modified emulsification solvent evaporation method	[92]
PLGA-PLL-PEG-Tf NPs	DNR	Leukemia (K562 cells)	DNR-loaded PLGA-PLL-PEG NPs were prepared by the modified double-emulsion solvent evaporation/diffusion method. Tf was conjugated to the surface of NPs with CDI	[93]
Anti-EGFR mAb-PLGA-PEG NPs	PTX	Triple-negative breast cancer (MDA-MB-468 cells)	PTX-loaded PLGA-PEG NPs were prepared by the nanoprecipitation method. The anti-EGFR mAb was anchored on the surface of NPs by crosslinking with MBS	[94]
CS-RGD-modified PLGA NPs	PTX or CDDP	Lung cancer (H1299 and A549 cells)	Drug-loaded PLGA NPs were prepared by the emulsification solvent evaporation (PTX) or double emulsion (CDDP) method. CS-RGD was synthesized by conjugating the GRGDSP peptide to chitosan via maleimide-PEG-NHS. CS-RGD was physically adsorbed onto the PLGA NPs	[95]
Glucose-PLGA	DTX	Human laryngeal carcinoma (Hep-2 cells)	DTX-loaded glucose-PLGA NPs were prepared by the single-emulsion solvent evaporation method.	[70]
CD133 aptamer-PEG-PLGA	Salinomycin	CD133-positive osteosarcoma (Saos-2 cells) and cancer stem cells	Salinomycin was loaded into PLGA-PEG-COOH NPs by the single-emulsion solvent evaporation method. CD133 aptamers were conjugated to PLGA-PEG-COOH NPs by EDC/NHS coupling.	[96]

Arg-Gly-Asp (RGD); chitosan (CS); chondroitin sulfate (CD); *cis*-diamine platinum (CDDP); daunorubicin (DNR); dicyclohexylcarbodiimide (DCC); docetaxel (DTX); doxorubicin (DOX); epidermal growth factor receptor (EGFR); 1-Ethyl-3-(3-dimethylaminopropyl) carbodiimide (EDC); hyaluronic acid (HA); low-molecular-weight protamine (LMWP); methoxypolyethylene glycol (mPEG); *m*-maleimidobenzoyl-*N*-hydroxysuccinimide (MBS); monoclonal antibody (mAb); *N*-hydroxysuccinimide (NHS); *N,N*-carbonyldiimidazole (CDI); paclitaxel (PTX); polyethylene glycol (PEG); poly(lactic-*co*-glycolic acid) (PLGA); poly-L-lysine (PLL); transferrin (Tf).

3. Uptake of PLGA NPs into Cancer Cells

The uptake of surface-engineered PLGA NPs into tumor cells can be described through several endocytosis mechanisms, such as receptor-, carrier-, and adsorption-mediated endocytosis (Figure 2). Increased cellular uptake of NPs can be observed using those endocytosis mechanisms, and thereby regarded as tumor-specific drug delivery strategies through passive or active targeting. Particle size, particle shape, the surface charge of particles, hydrophilicity/hydrophobicity of particles, elasticity of particles, and cell type can affect and determine the endocytosis pathway and efficiency [46,97–101]. Particles with 10–100 nm are reported to be necessary for entering the endocytic vesicles and smaller particles are known to be beneficial for their rapid cellular entry [100]. In addition, polydispersity and surface charge of particles may affect the cellular entry [100].

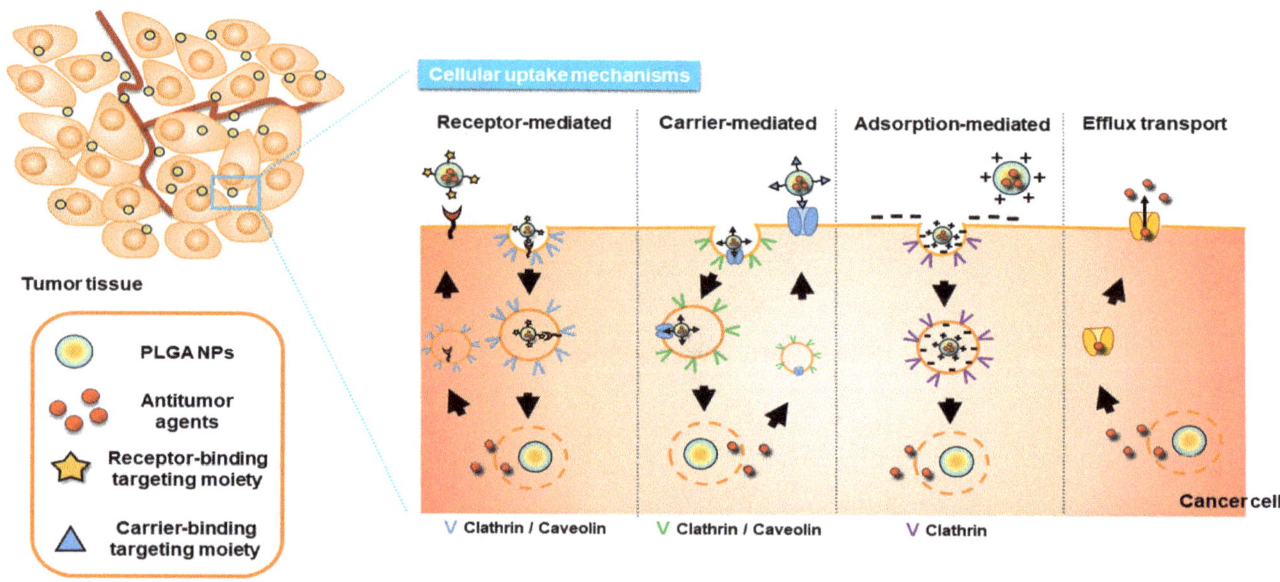

Figure 2. Cellular uptake mechanisms of surface-modified PLGA NPs.

3.1. Receptor-Mediated Endocytosis

Most NPs carrying anti-tumor agents, including PLGA NPs, can be internalized by endocytosis into the tumor cells. In receptor-mediated endocytosis, the NPs can be efficiently internalized into cells by the specific binding of targeting moieties anchored on the PLGA NPs and the corresponding receptors expressed on the tumor cell membrane or tumor vasculatures [102]. These specific ligand–receptor complexes include the biotin–biotin receptor, HA-CD44 receptor, anti-epidermal growth factor (EGF) antibody (Ab)-EGF receptor (EGFR), FA-folate receptor, Arg-Gly-Asp (RGD)-based peptide-integrin $\alpha_v\beta_3$, and Tf–Tf receptor (Table 1).

Clathrin and caveolin are endogenous molecules that exist in the cytosol and function in receptor-mediated endocytosis. When NPs conjugated to targeting moieties interact with the receptor, each clathrin or caveolin molecule migrates from the cytosol to the cell membrane, encompasses the ligand–receptor complexes, and contributes to the production of clathrin-coated vesicles or caveosomes containing the complexes [97,98]. Clathrin-dependent endocytosis is a representative route of entry into mammalian cells [100]. In clathrin-dependent endocytosis, coated clathrin may be peeled off prior to fusion with early endosomes and NP will reach lysosomes via the endo-lysosomal route [97]. Conversely, in caveolin-dependent endocytosis, NPs can be internalized as a form of caveosome, which can avoid fusion with lysosomes and prevent lysosomal degradation [97,103].

3.2. Carrier-Mediated Endocytosis

Some hydrophilic molecules, such as amino acids, peptides, monoamines, and glucose, which can be used as building blocks, neurotransmitters, and energy sources for cells are usually recognized selectively and transported actively via interaction with carrier proteins expressed on the cell membrane [104]. Tumor cells require high levels of energy and building blocks for their abnormal rapid growth, and thereby overexpress those carrier proteins, including hexose carriers and amino acid carriers. Thus, glucose can be used as a promising targeting moiety for the tumor-specific delivery of PLGA NPs. Glucose-included PLGA NPs can be specifically bound to glucose transporters such as GLUT-1 and GLUT-3 or sodium-glucose linked transporter (SGLT) -1 and -2 on certain tumor cells, followed by internalization into cells via carrier-mediated endocytosis [70].

For the treatment of brain tumors such as glioblastoma, therapeutic molecules should cross the blood-to-brain barrier (BBB), which is the most impermeable barrier in the human body [105]. Fortunately, for the purpose of transporting neurotransmitters (i.e., choline and L-dopa) and energy sources (i.e., glucose) into the brain, specific carriers, including choline transporter, L-system large neutral amino acid transporter, GLUT, and SGLT are present on the BBB [70,106]. Therefore, NPs loaded with anti-tumor agents for brain tumor-specific delivery could be modified with targeting moieties, which can be bound to those carriers on the BBB and receptors (i.e., CD44 receptor, folate receptor, and Tf receptor) on the tumor cells [27,51,89,91].

3.3. *Adsorption-Mediated Endocytosis*

As the surface of cell membranes at physiological pH carries a slight negative charge, electrostatic interactions between cationic NPs and tumor cell membranes can promote particle adsorption to the tumor cells [107]. Non-functionalized PLGA NPs have a negative surface charge due to the structure of PLGA polymer, resulting in lower penetration into the tumor cells due to the electrostatic repulsion. Therefore, NPs functionalized with a cationic polymer such as CS and cell-penetrating peptides (CPPs) (e.g., low-molecular-weight protamine [LMWP], transactivator of transcription [TAT], and penetratin) can easily penetrate tumor cells via adsorption-mediated endocytosis [90,95,108]. Although there are some exceptions, positively charged NPs may be dominantly internalized via a clathrin-mediated pathway [100]. For example, CS-coated PLGA NPs were found to be internalized via both macropinocytosis and clathrin-mediated endocytosis, while the uptake PLGA NPs involved caveolin-mediated endocytosis in MDCK cells [108]. The positively charged surface of NPs may be associated with some issues, such as reduced circulation time due to the enhanced opsonization and recognition by the RES. Recent progress regarding particle properties-dependent endocytosis types is summarized in Table 2.

Table 2. Type of endocytosis depending on the particle properties of PLGA-based NPs.

Surface Functionalities	Mean Diameter (nm)	Type of Endocytosis	Ref.
AS1411 aptamer	128	Receptor (nucleotin)-mediated endocytosis	[109]
CD44 antibodies	140	Receptor (CD44)-mediated endocytosis	[110]
L-carnitine	189	Carrier (OCTN2)-mediated endocytosis	[111]
Glutamate-polyoxyethylene stearate	152–181	Carrier (LAT1)-mediated endocytosis	[112]
CS	140–173	Adsorption-mediated endocytosis	[88]
PEG-HIV-TAT	97–176	Adsorption-mediated endocytosis	[113]
Arginine-rich peptide	156	Adsorption-mediated endocytosis	[114]

Organic cation/carnitine transporter 2 (OCTN2); large amino acid transporter 1 (LAT1); chitosan (CS); polyethylene glycol (PEG); human immunodeficiency virus (HIV); transactivator of transcription (TAT).

4. Visualization of Tumor Targeting by In Vivo Imaging

4.1. *Design of NPs with Imaging Modalities*

The tumor targeting ability of PLGA-based NPs can be demonstrated using in vivo imaging techniques. To monitor the in vivo fate of NPs, a corresponding imaging modality should be introduced to NPs (Figure 3). Imaging agents can be attached to the PLGA backbone (prior to NP fabrication) or to the outer surface of NPs (after NP fabrication) [59,115]. As commercial PLGA products possess a carboxylic acid or ester end group, they can be used to generate covalent bonding with the functional groups of imaging modalities [59]. For instance, amine or hydroxyl groups in the imaging agent can directly form an amide or ester linkage with the terminal carboxylic acid group of PLGA [99,116]. The imaging modality can be also attached to the functional groups (e.g., amine group) of PLGA derivatives or appropriate linkers (e.g., bifunctional PEG linker) can be used to connect the imaging modality and PLGA [65]. In addition, the outer surface of PLGA NPs can be modified with imaging agents [115]. Exposed functional groups of PLGA NPs can participate in the reaction with imaging modalities [117,118]. Covalent bonding between PLGA (or PLGA NPs) and an imaging agent can reduce the loss of imaging agent prior to the localization of NPs to the tumor region following injection. To acquire a sufficient resolution for in vivo imaging, it is important to optimize the degree of substitution by the imaging agent. Imaging agents can be physically introduced to PLGA-based NPs [115]. After PLGA NPs are fabricated, the outer surface of NPs can be coated with the imaging agent by adsorption. However, this may risk an initial burst of imaging agent release following injection into the blood stream, and reduce the efficiency of visualizing target sites. Together with the solubilization of PLGA in the organic phase, several imaging agents can be added to the organic solvents (e.g., acetone, chloroform, dichloromethane, DMSO, and ethanol) during the fabrication of NPs [33,119,120]. To encapsulate an imaging modality in PLGA NPs, drug encapsulation efficiency and release rate also should be evaluated prior to application for in vivo imaging.

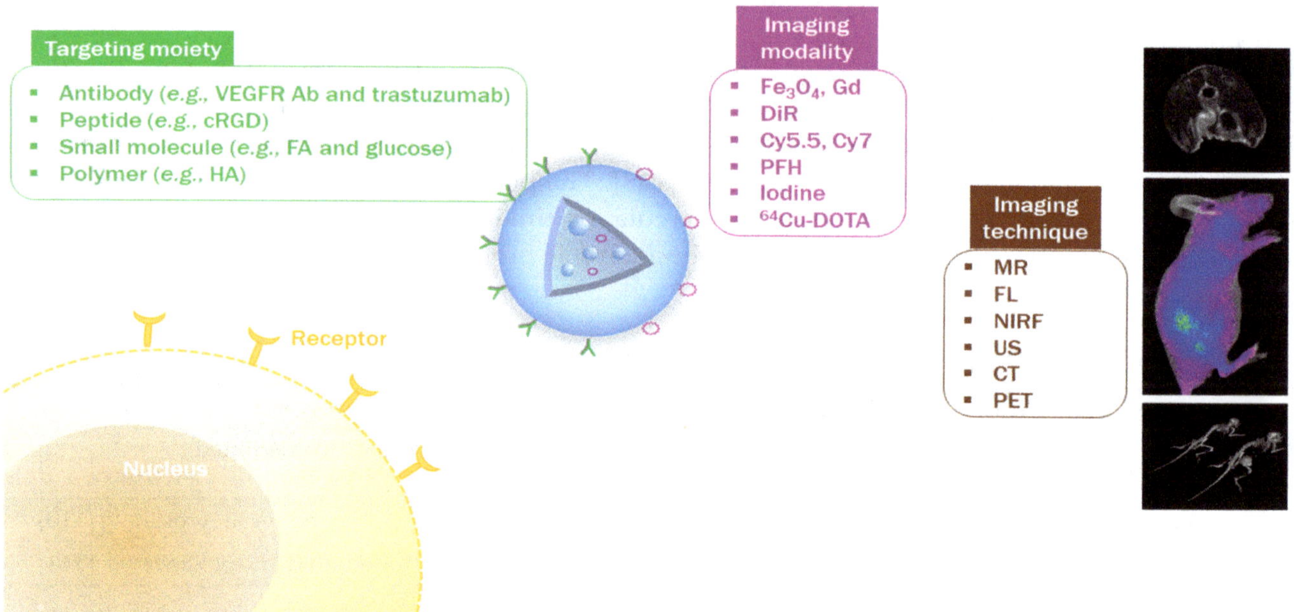

Figure 3. Evaluation of tumor-targeting efficiency by in vivo imaging techniques. Antibody (Ab); computed tomography (CT); cyclic Arg-Gly-Asp (cRGD); fluorescence (FL); folic acid (FA); gadolinium (Gd); hyaluronic acid (HA); magnetic resonance (MR); near-infrared fluorescence (NIRF); perfluorohexane (PFH); positron emission tomography (PET); 1,4,7,10-tetraazacyclododecane-*N*,*N′*,*N″*,*N‴*-tetraacetic acid (DOTA); ultrasound (US); vascular endothelial growth factor receptor (VEGFR).

For magnetic resonance (MR) imaging, T_1-or T_2-weighed contrast agents can be introduced to PLGA NPs. In general, gadolinium (Gd) derivatives or iron oxide (Fe_3O_4) NPs have been loaded to NPs to enhance the contrast in MR imaging [120–122]. 1,1′-Dioctadecyl-3,3,3′,3′-tetramethylindotricarbocyanineiodide (DIR) has been widely used for in vivo fluorescence imaging [123,124]. Recently, many attempts have been made using near-infrared fluorescence (NIRF) imaging during the development of nanoformulations due to its deeper tissue penetration and lower tissue scattering property than fluorescence imaging [125]. In NIRF imaging, several kinds of fluorescence molecules (e.g., Cy5.5, Cy7, protoporphyrin IX [PpIX], and indocyanine green [ICG]) can be introduced to PLGA NPs [33,126,127]. Derivatives of NIRF dyes can be covalently conjugated to PLGA or encapsulated in PLGA NPs. For ultrasound (US) diagnosis, bubble-generating agents (e.g., perfluorohexane [PFH]) can be incorporated into the PLGA NPs [128,129]. In computed tomography (CT) imaging, several contrast agents (e.g., iodine derivatives and gold nanostructures) can be entrapped in PLGA NPs or coated on the outer surface of PLGA NPs [115,130]. Prior to application in in vivo imaging, the appropriate dose for visualizing the tumor tissue should be determined. Additionally, chemical modification and physical loading of imaging modalities should not affect the intrinsic biofunctions of PLGA NPs, including drug release, cellular binding, and in vitro/in vivo anticancer activities, in cancer theranostics.

Detection of signals from imaging modality-contained PLGA-based NPs in the body can indicate their biodistribution. Unfortunately, advantages and disadvantages for cancer diagnosis have been reported for each imaging modality [115]. For instance, MR imaging has high spatial resolution and relatively low sensitivity. In contrast, positron emission tomography (PET) imaging exhibits high sensitivity and low spatial resolution. Therefore, the combination of PET/MR imaging can provide a high sensitivity and high spatial resolution in the diagnosis of diseases. Therefore, in vivo imaging methods with dual or triple modalities have been combined to exploit the benefits of each imaging technique [128,131]. Multiple imaging modalities can enable more accurate tracing of NPs and the diagnostic ability of the disease state following systemic administration.

4.2. Introduction of Tumor-Targeting Ligands to PLGA NPs

To increase the tumor-targeting efficiency by active tumor-targeting strategies, diverse kinds of ligands can be introduced to PLGA-based NPs (Figure 3). Together with the "EPR effect" as a passive tumor targeting strategy, ligand–receptor interactions can improve tumor-targeting efficiency in cancer imaging and therapy [25,27]. Small molecules, polymers, proteins, peptides, and Abs can be linked to the PLGA backbone or the functional groups of PLGA derivatives [132]. Amine-, aldehyde-, carboxyl-, maleimide-, succinimidyl ester-, or sulfhydryl-functionalized PEG-linked PLGA can be coupled with various kinds of tumor-targeting ligands [132]. Amine-functionalized folate-polyethylene glycol (PEG) was conjugated to PLGA-PEG-COOH via a carbodiimide reaction to synthesize a folate-coupled PLGA-PEG derivative [133]. The amine group of an antibody (e.g., Herceptin®) can be linked to the carboxylic acid groups on the outer surface of PLGA derivative-based NPs via *N*-(3-dimethylaminopropyl)-*N′*-ethylcarbodiimide hydrochloride (EDC) and *N*-hydroxysuccinimide (NHS)-coupled reactions [129]. For peptide labeling, cyclic Arg-Gly-Asp (cRGD)-thiol (SH) was reacted with maleimide-functionalized PLGA-PEG NPs to prepare cRGD-linked PLGA-PEG NPs [128].

4.3. Verification of Tumor Targetability by In Vivo Imaging

Passive and active tumor-targeting approaches guiding drug delivery and cancer imaging can be assessed using several in vivo imaging techniques. In vivo and ex vivo imaging data can provide data on the pattern of biodistribution of fabricated NPs in the body. Interestingly, in vivo imaging can show the real-time distribution of fabricated NPs and the current status of cancer tissue without the need to sacrifice experimental animals. PLGA-based NPs guided by real-time imaging can increase the therapeutic efficacies of drug cargos. Recently, several studies have reported the in vivo tumor targeting capability of PLGA-based NPs by bioimaging techniques (Table 3).

Table 3. Verification of tumor-targeting capability by in vivo imaging.

Polymer	Drug	Targeting Material	Target Receptor (Cell Line)	Imaging Technique	Imaging Modality	Ref.
PLGA-mPEG	Platinum(II) prodrug	cRGD	Integrin (SKOV-3 cells)	US and NIRF	PFH and Cy7	[128]
PLGA-PEG-COOH	PTX	Herceptin	HER2 receptor (SKBR-3 cells)	PA and US	PFH and SPIO	[129]
PLGA-PEG-COOH	DOX	AS1411 aptamer	Nucleolin receptor (C26 cells)	MR	SPIO	[134]
PLGA-PEG	DOX	Biotin	Biotin receptor (4T1 cells)	FL	DOX	[135]
PLGA-PEG-COOH	DOX	FA	Folate receptor (Bel-7402 cells)	US and MR	PFH and Fe_3O_4	[133]
mPEG-PLGA-PLL	PTX	Anti-CA19-9 Ab	CA19-9 (capan-1 cells)	FL	DiR	[123]
Maleimide-PEG-PLGA	Curcumin	c(RGDf(N-me)V)	$\alpha_v\beta_3$, $\alpha_v\beta_5$, and $\alpha_5\beta_1$ integrins (C6 cells)	FL	DiR	[124]
PLGA	DTX	Angiopep-2	LRP-1 (U87-MG cells)	NIRF and X-ray	IR780 and gold nanoshell	[130]
PLGA-Glc	DTX	Glucose	Glucose transporter (Hep-2 cells)	NIRF	Cy5.5	[70]
PLGA	DTX	HA	CD44 receptor (MDA-MB-231 cells)	NIRF	Cy5.5	[65]
PLGA-PEG	Curcumin and PTX	T7 (HAIYPRH) peptide	Tf receptor (U87 cells)	FL, X-ray, and MR	DiR and MNP	[136]
PLGA	ZnPc	Anti-VEGFR-2 Ab	VEGFR-2 (MDA-MB-231 cells)	PA and US	ZnPc and PFH	[137]

Antibody (Ab); cyclic Arg-Gly-Asp (cRGD); 1,1′-dioctadecyl-3,3,3′,3′-tetramethylindotricarbocyanineiodide (DIR); docetaxel (DTX); doxorubicin (DOX); fluorescence (FL); folic acid (FA); hyaluronic acid (HA); low-density lipoprotein receptor-related protein-1 (LRP-1); magnetic nanoparticle (MNP); magnetic resonance (MR); methoxypolyethylene glycol (mPEG); near-infrared fluorescence (NIRF); paclitaxel (PTX); perfluorohexane (PFH); photoacoustic (PA); phthalocyanine zinc (ZnPc); poly((D,L)lactic-glycolic)acid–star glucose (PLGA-Glc); polyethylene glycol (PEG); poly-L-lysine (PLL); superparamagnetic iron oxide (SPIO); transferrin (Tf); ultrasound (US); vascular endothelial growth factor receptor (VEGFR).

Lipid-platinum prodrug (Pt(IV)) conjugate-loaded PLGA-PEG-cRGD NPs have been designed, and glutathione (GSH)-sensitive and US-triggered anticancer activities have been assessed [128]. cRGD-modified Pt(IV) NPs can target the tumor site via an EPR effect (passive tumor targeting) and cRGD-integrin receptor interactions (active tumor targeting). Under US exposure in the tumor region, the NP shell can be cracked, releasing the lipid-Pt(IV) prodrug. This can then adsorb onto the cellular membrane due to its amphiphilicity and move into the internal cellular space via passive diffusion. cRGD-modified Pt(IV) NPs were transported into the internal space of cancer cells via receptor-mediated endocytosis. Prodrug and NPs were released from the endosome in response to endogenous GSH. A combination of US and cRGD-modified Pt(IV) NPs enhanced the production of reactive oxygen species (ROS), resulting in mitochondrial-mediated apoptosis in cancer cells. The tumor-targeting efficiency of cRGD-modified Pt(IV) NPs was further verified with Cy7 incorporation by NIRF imaging in SKOV-3 tumor-bearing mouse models.

HER2-targeting PLGA NPs including PFH, paclitaxel (PTX), and superparamagnetic iron oxide (SPIO) were fabricated and their photothermal/chemo-therapeutic efficacies guided by photoacoustic (PA)/US imaging were evaluated [129]. Herceptin was conjugated to the outer surface of PLGA-based NPs to target the HER2 receptor. SPIO and PFH were included in the NPs for PA and US imaging, respectively. SPIO can convert external near-infrared (NIR) light to thermal energy and can thus be used for the photothermal ablation of tumors. It can then be combined with the chemotherapeutic effects of PTX for the treatment of breast cancers. Photothermal heating of SPIO can be transferred to PLGA polymer, which can make the structure of the polymer rubbery. Then, a drug with poor aqueous solubility (PTX) can be diffused from the NPs. The tumor-targeting efficiency of Herceptin-modified NPs was assessed by photoacoustic (PA)/US bimodal imaging in the SKBR-3 tumor-xenograft mouse model [129]. Under NIR laser irradiation, Herceptin-modified NPs containing PHF, PTX, and SPIO exerted superior tumor growth inhibition based on the synergism of photothermal- and chemo-therapeutic efficacy.

Angiopep-2-linked PLGA@Au NPs including docetaxel (DTX) were prepared and then NIR laser-triggered drug release and chemo-photothermal therapeutic efficacies were evaluated [130]. Organic-inorganic hybrid NPs based on a core-shell structure were designed with an outer Au shell that can be used for photothermal therapy (PTT) by converting the NIR laser to heat energy and as an X-ray imaging agent. Angiopep-2 carried by NPs can be efficiently internalized in U87MG cells via receptor-mediated endocytosis and have presented improved anticancer activity. X-ray and NIR thermal imaging analyses were performed to demonstrate the tumor-targeting efficiency and therapeutic potentials. Angiopep-2-conjugated Au nanoshell/PLGA/DTX NPs exhibited the anti-glioma activity in U87MG tumor-bearing mouse models [130].

PLGA NPs coated with amphiphilic HA derivative (HA-ceramide [HACE]) were developed to target the CD44 receptor for drug delivery [65]. HACE was composed of a hydrophilic backbone (HA) and a hydrophobic segment (CE); thus, PLGA NPs can be entrapped in the internal hydrophobic cavity of self-assembled HACE nanostructures. DTX was encapsulated in PLGA-based NPs as a poorly water-soluble chemotherapeutic agent. Higher levels of HACE-coated PLGA NPs were internalized by cancer cells expressing the CD44 receptor- (MDA-MB-231 cells) compared with cancer cells negative for the CD44 receptor (NIH3T3 cells). In mice bearing MDA-MB-231 tumors, HACE-PLGA NPs accumulated at higher levels in tumor tissue compared with PLGA NPs.

5. In Vivo Anticancer Activities of PLGA-based NPs

5.1. *Parameters for Assessing In Vivo Antitumor Activity*

Various PLGA NPs developed as anticancer therapies have been applied to animals to demonstrate superiority versus conventional interventions. Currently, standard techniques used to assess in vivo antitumor activity include tumor size measurement and survival analysis. Specifically, cancer cell-lines are xenografted in animals, who are often immunocompromised, and the tumor volume or survival rate is monitored over time in response to treatment. Tumor volume is determined using the modified ellipsoid formula: (tumor length $\times$ tumor width^2)/2 [138,139]. However, in some models where direct tumor measurements are not available (e.g., tumor inside the skull, lung, or liver), the tumor in the scanned image or the weight of the dissected tumor can be used to substitute for volume data [140,141]. The survival rate is defined as the percentage of survivors in a group over a specific period after diagnosis. From the survival rate versus time function (i.e., Kaplan–Meier curve), the median survival value can be estimated and used to assess the effectiveness of the treatments [142,143].

5.2. *Key Factors for Improved Antitumor Efficacy*

Most PLGA NPs developed for anticancer therapy share therapeutic advantages, such as passive targeting via the EPR effect and controlled drug release (Figure 4). Moreover, further chemical or physical modifications with other compounds provide specific functions not provided by the unmodified NPs. These properties have been translated into significant improvements in antitumor activity, as shown in Table 4.

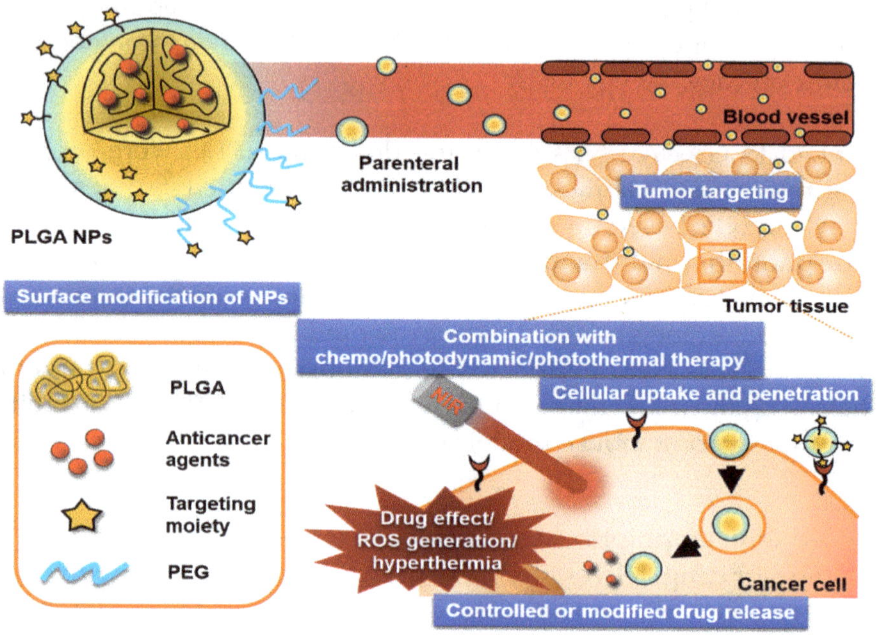

Figure 4. Crucial factors that affect the antitumor activities of PLGA NPs. Polyethylene glycol (PEG); reactive oxygen species (ROS).

5.2.1. Controlled Release and EPR Effect

The clinical value of anticancer agents is often highly compromised due to the dose-limiting severe side effects (e.g., renal and gastrointestinal toxicities). Many approaches using PLGA NPs have been developed to avoid the accumulation of drug in normal tissues (Table 4). Moreno et al. reported that cisplatin (CP)-loaded PLGA NPs exhibited comparable antitumor efficacy to free CP [144]. However, the PLGA NPs presented reduced systemic toxicity in terms of body weight and blood urea nitrogen (BUN). The authors suggested that the results were due to the controlled release of CP and the passive targeting of PLGA NPs, as well as the induction of apoptosis.

PEGylation is one of the most extensively studied strategies to enhance the antitumor efficacy of PLGA NPs, and increases the circulation time of NPs in the bloodstream. This pharmacokinetic advantage increases the chance of tumors being targeted by NPs. Interestingly, CP-loaded NPs prepared with the mPEG-PLGA copolymer resulted in an enhanced survival rate compared with free CP, which was not observed when using the unmodified PLGA NPs [144,145]. Similarly, mPEG-PLGA NPs co-loaded with gemcitabine (GEM) and betulinic acid (BA) resulted in a significant reduction in tumor volume compared with GEM + BA solution in mice with Ehrlich ascites carcinoma xenografts [146].

5.2.2. Targeted Delivery

The surface modification of PLGA NPs with tumor-targeting moieties (i.e., active-targeting strategy) can also enhance anticancer activity [147]. Typical examples can be found in studies using PTX-loaded PLGA NPs, in which the targeting moieties were tethered with the aid of PEG linkers. Liang et al. reported that the addition of FA, a small molecule ligand of folate receptor, to the surface of PTX-loaded PLGA NPs resulted in increased reduction in tumor volume compared with unmodified NPs in HEC-1A tumor-xenografted mice [148]. A comparable improvement was observed in studies exploiting peptides (iNGR; CRNGRGPDC) as a tumor-targeting moiety. The median survival of mice bearing intracranial U87-MG glioblastoma was 1.6-fold longer following treatment with PTX-loaded iNGR-PEG-PLGA NPs compared with unmodified NPs [149]. Aptamer (AS1411) conjugation also augmented the tumor inhibitory activity of PLGA NPs. The average tumor volume in C6 tumor-xenografted mice following treatment with PTX-loaded AS1411-PEG-PLGA NPs was reduced by 33% compared with those treated with the non-targeted NPs [140].

The targeting moieties can be attached indirectly. The most straightforward approach was based on the charge-charge interaction between the targeting moiety and the NP surface. This was demonstrated by Wu et al., who coated the surface of PLGA NPs modified with a positively charged surfactant, vitamin E-oligo(methyl diglycol L-glutamate) with the anionic polymer, HA [143]. In that study, the HA-coated PLGA (HPLGA) NPs loaded with DTX prolonged median survival 1.4-fold compared with free DTX in orthotopic A549-Luc lung xenograft model. Another approach has exploited the strong binding affinity between avidin and biotin. Biotin-conjugated RVG29 (fragment of the rabies virus coat protein) was successfully attached to avidin-palmitate anchored on the surface of camptothecin (CPT)-loaded PLGA NPs; however, no significant difference was found in median survival compared with the biotin-attached CPT-loaded PLGA NPs (control) in mice bearing intracranial glioblastoma [142]. However, doxorubicin (DOX)-loaded lecithin hybridized PLGA NPs resulted in a reduced mean tumor area (9.6 ± 10.7 mm^2) compared with free DOX (21.7 ± 13.4 mm^2) in orthotopic glioblastoma rat models [141]. This was attributed to the adsorption of apolipoprotein A-1, an endogenous targeting moiety in the bloodstream, to the lecithin-rich surface of NP after systemic administration.

5.2.3. Cellular Uptake and Penetration

Factors regarding cellular uptake and penetration are also closely related to the antitumor activity of PLGA NPs. One interesting approach was reported by Zhang et al. [150], who co-loaded methenamine mandelate (MM), a urinary antibacterial agent, with $NaHCO_3$ in PLGA NPs. Following the entry of NPs cancer cells via the endo-lysosomal pathway, $NaHCO_3$ generates CO_2 bubbles due to the acidic nature of endo-lysosomes. The bubbles broke down the structural integrity of the NPs and the subsequent release of MM resulted in formaldehyde production in the cancer cells. This pH-responsive drug release resulted in greater inhibition of tumor growth in MCF-7 tumor xenografted mice compared with NPs without $NaHCO_3$. Another approach reported by Wang et al. utilized CPP to decorate the surface of PLGA NPs [90]. In that study, tumor penetration and intranuclear delivery of DOX were achieved by the alkyl-chained LMWP anchored in PLGA NPs, resulting in near complete arrest of tumor growth in MCF-7/ADR tumor-xenografted mice.

5.2.4. Combination with Photodynamic Therapy (PDT) and/or PTT

PDT and PTT have gained much attention based on their effectiveness in cancer treatment [7, 43,151,152]. Combination treatment with chemotherapy, PDT, and PTT using multifunctional PLGA NPs has been investigated. A photosensitizer (e.g., 5-aminolevulinic acid, hypocrellin A, meso-tetra hydroxyphenylchlorine [mTHPC], pheophorbide a [Pba], and PpIX) and/or photothermal agents (e.g., ICG) can be introduced into PLGA NPs by encapsulation or adsorption [153–158]. FA-modified PLGA NPs including Pba have been fabricated, and enhanced anticancer activities based on PDT against gastric cancer (MKN28 tumor) after intravenous injection have been demonstrated [155]. Peng et al. reported the use of polydopamine (PDA) and D-α-tocopheryl polyethylene glycol 1000 succinate (TPGS)-coated DTX-loaded PLGA NPs [159]. When co-treated with NIR laser irradiation, this nanoplatform resulted in an approximately 10-fold reduction in tumor size and weight compared with Taxotere®, a commercial formulation of DTX, in MCF-7/ADR tumor-xenografted mice. This result was explained by the augmented photothermal conservation property by PDA and the reduced multi-drug resistance by TPGS. Similarly, gold- or polyaniline-modified PLGA NPs also resulted in effective tumor suppression in the presence of NIR irradiation [130,160]. These therapeutic advancements were ascribed to the synergistic effects of chemo/photodynamic/photothermal therapy.

Table 4. Summary of successful in vivo cancer therapy using various types of PLGA NPs.

Drug@Formulation	Target (Cell Line)	Functions	Therapeutic Benefits	Ref.
As_2O_3@PLGA-PEG/LA NPs	Liver cancer (HepG2 cells)	EPR effect; controlled release of As_2O_3	1.49- and 1.09-fold reduction in tumor volume compared with saline and free As_2O_3, respectively, in HepG2 tumor-bearing mice	[147]
CBP/ICG@FA-PEG-PLGA NPs	Breast cancer (MCF-7 cells)	EPR effect; targeted delivery via the folate receptor; combination of chemo, photodynamic, and photothermal therapy	The strongest tumor growth suppression potentials in NPs with NIR laser irradiation group rather than the other group	[157]
CPT@RVG-PLGA NPs	Glioblastoma (GL261-Luc2 cells)	Brain-specific delivery of CPT	Prolonged tumor doubling time and increased median survival (3.15/23 days) compared with either saline (2.46/16.5 days) or blank RVG-PLGA (2.50/19 days) in mice bearing intracranial GL261-Luc2 gliomas	[142]
CP@PLGA NPs	Colon cancer (DHD/K12PROb cells)	Higher activation of caspase-3-mediated apoptosis	Comparable reduction in tumor volume with free CP in DHD/K12PROb tumor-xenografted mice	[144]
CP@mPEG-PLGA NPs	Colorectal cancer (HT 29 cells)	EPR effect; prolonged CP residence in the systemic circulation	Increased survival rate of HT 29 tumor-bearing mice compared with saline, free CP, or blank NPs	[145]
DOX@lecithin-PLGA NPs	Glioblastoma (GB 101/8 cells)	Adsorption of apolipoprotein A-1 on the surface of the NPs and subsequent improvement of endocytosis into vascular endothelial cells via lipoprotein receptors	Reduced mean tumor area (9.6 ± 10.7 mm^2) compared with vehicle (32.1 ± 3.8 mm^2) and free DOX (21.7 ± 13.4 mm^2) in rats with orthotopic glioblastoma	[141]
DOX@LMWP/PLGA NPs	Breast cancer (MCF-7/ADR cells)	Targeted nuclear delivery of DOX; tumor penetration by breaking down the diffusion barriers caused by interstitial fluid pressure	Near-complete tumor growth arrest in MCF-7/ADR tumor-bearing mice compared with vehicle, free DOX, or DOX-loaded PLGA NPs	[90]
DTX@HPLGA NPs	Lung cancer (A549-Luc cells)	Enhanced colloidal stability; superior tumor selectivity *in vivo*	Improved median survival (46 days) compared with vehicle (20 days), free DTX (34 days), and blank HPLGA NPs (24 days) in orthotopic A549-Luc lung xenografts	[143]
DTX@PLGA-PDA-TPGS NPs + NIR	Drug-resistant breast cancer (MCF-7/ADR cells)	Improved photothermal conservation by PDA; inhibition of P-glycoprotein by TPGS	Approximate 10-fold reduction in tumor size and weight compared with Taxotere®	[159]
DTX@ANG/GS/PLGA NPs + NIR	Glioblastoma (U87-MG cells)	DTX accumulation in the tumor; heat-induced tumor cell damage	The greatest tumor inhibition rate among all groups comprising saline, 808 nm irradiation, free DTX, GS/PLGA/DTX NPs, and ANG/GS/PLGA/DTX NPs.	[130]
GEM/BA@mPEG-PLGA NPs	Ehrlich ascites carcinoma (EAC cells)	Combination drug delivery; improved pharmacokinetic properties	Reduced mean tumor volume (195.5 mm^3) compared with saline (1236.5 mm^3), GEM solution (553.1 mm^3), GEM NPs (367.8 mm^3), or GEM + BA solution (213.5 mm^3) in mice bearing Ehrlich tumors	[146]
MM@$NaHCO_3$/PLGA NPs	Breast cancer (MCF-7 cells)	EPR effect; pH-responsive degradation of NPs due to CO_2 bubbles generated from $NaHCO_3$ and subsequent rapid release of MM in lysosomes	Highest tumor growth inhibition compared with vehicle, blank NPs, or MM–loaded NPs in MCF-7 tumor-xenografted mice	[150]
MTX@PANI-LT-PLGA NPs + NIR	Breast cancer (MDA-MB-231 cells)	Targeting somatostatin receptors by LT modification; hyperthermia effect	Higher tumor suppression compared with saline, free MTX, PANI PLGA NPs, MTX/PANI PLGA NPs, or MTX/PANI LT-PLGA NPs in mice	[160]
PTX@FA-PEG-PLGA NPs	Endometrial carcinoma (HEC-1A cells)	EPR effect; targeted delivery via the folate receptor	Higher anti-tumor efficacy than free PTX and non-targeted NPs in mice	[148]

Table 4. *Cont.*

Drug@Formulation	Target (Cell Line)	Functions	Therapeutic Benefits	Ref.
PTX@AS1411-PEG-PLGA NPs	Glioma (C6 cells)	Targeted delivery to the tumor and angiogenic blood vessels by AS1411 aptamer	The highest average tumor inhibition based on tumor volume and weight (81.68 and 79.93%), compared with non-targeted NPs (66.95 and 68.69%) and Taxol® (68.69 and 46.75%)	[140]
PTX@iNGR-PEG-PLGA NPs	Glioblastoma (U87-MG cells)	Targeted delivery to angiogenic blood vessels and tumor penetration by iNGR	Prolonged median survival (42.5 days) compared with saline (17.5 days), PTX-loaded PEG-PLGA NPs (27 days), Taxol® (21.5 days), and PTX-loaded cNGR-PEG-PLGA NPs (34 days) in mice bearing intracranial U87-MG glioblastoma	[149]

Adriamycin (ADR); angiopep-2 (ANG); betulinic acid (BA); camptothecin (CPT); carboplatin (CBP); cisplatin (CP); CNGRC peptide (cNGR); CRNGRGPDC peptide (iNGR); D-α-tocopheryl polyethylene glycol 1000 succinate (TPGS); docetaxel (DTX); doxorubicin (DOX); enhanced permeability and retention (EPR); folic acid (FA); fragment of rabies virus coat protein (RVG); gemcitabine (GEM); gold nanoshell (GS); hyaluronic acid-coated PLGA (HPLGA); indocyanine green (ICG); lactose acid (LA); lanreotide (LT); low molecular weight protamine (LMWP); luciferase (Luc); methenamine mandelate (MM); methotrexate (MTX); methoxypolyethylene glycol (mPEG); near-infrared (NIR); paclitaxel (PTX); polyaniline (PANI); polydopamine (PDA); polyethylene glycol (PEG).

6. In Vivo Pharmacokinetics of PLGA-Based NPs

The pharmacokinetics of DTX-loaded PEGylated PLGA NPs (DTX-PEG-PLGA NPs) was assessed in Balb/C mice bearing C26 tumors [161]. The PEGylated NPs exhibited a markedly delayed plasma clearance (CL) as shown in Table 5. Following the administration of DTX-PEG-PLGA NPs, the plasma DTX levels remained much higher after 24 h compared with those of free DTX solution and DTX-loaded PLGA NPs. In contrast, the DTX solution and DTX-loaded PLGA NPs were quickly eliminated from the systemic circulation and their plasma concentrations 2 h after dosing were low. These data suggest that the NPs with a steric PEG barrier would prevent their rapid uptake by a mononuclear phagocyte system and improve their circulatory half-life. Shah et al. reported the pharmacokinetics of PTX-loaded PLGA NPs surface-modified with Tf and Pluronic® P85 in male Sprague-Dawley (SD) rats bearing C6 glioma [89]. PTX in solution administered intravenously was rapidly cleared from blood whereas PTX loaded in different NP formulations was retained in blood for longer, indicating the long circulation properties of drug-loaded NPs (Table 5). This increase in residence time may be attributed to decreased opsonization from blood due to the smaller size (less than 200 nm) and hydrophilicity (imparting stealthiness) of the NPs [162].

Milane et al. reported the biodistribution and pharmacokinetics of polymer-blend (PLGA-PEG-EGFR-targeting peptide) NPs loaded with lonidamine in an orthotopic animal model of multidrug-resistant breast cancer [163]. As shown in Table 5, the NPs containing EGFR-targeting peptide (targeted NPs) increase the plasma AUC, MRT, and $t_{1/2}$ of lonidamine relative to lonidamine administered as a solution. Furthermore, the targeted NPs decrease the tumor λ_z, increase the tumor MRT, and increase the AUC relative to drug solution. Collectively, although exact mechanisms remain unclear, the NP formulations improve the tumor pharmacokinetics relative to drug solution, with the targeted NPs providing a slight advantage in terms of the pharmacokinetic parameters of lonidamine relative to the non-targeted NPs.

The comparative pharmacokinetics of platinum (Pt)-loaded PLGA-PEG NPs and Pt prodrug was evaluated in male SD rats following intravenous administration of the maximal tolerated doses of the compounds (40 and 20 mg/kg, respectively) [164]. Pt remaining in the systemic circulation 1 h after administration was 77% following administration of Pt-PLGA-b-PEG-NPs and 15.6% following administrated of the Pt prodrug, whereas this value for CP has been reported as 1.5% in the literature [165]. The mean AUC for total Pt in the blood was about 26% of that observed in plasma (Table 5), suggesting that Pt is not extensively distributed in red blood cells. After a single intravenous dose of the Pt-loaded NPs, both the liver and spleen showed the highest Pt concentration at 24 h. In the kidney, which is the primary target organ of cisplatin toxicity, the Pt-loaded NPs resulted in lower Pt levels than the Pt prodrug. The lower Pt level in the kidney indicated that the NP system would exhibit reduced nephrotoxicity compared with that of CP. Notably, the 24-h cumulative Pt excretion after Pt-loaded PLGA-PEG NPs was about 17 times less than after cisplatin treatment. This difference is probably due to the characteristics of Pt compounds, which can bind to protein or other tissue compositions firmly through covalent bonds.

Table 5. Summary of in vivo pharmacokinetic parameters altered by PLGA-based NPs.

Drug@Formulation	Animal Model	Pharmacokinetic Alterations	Ref.
DTX@PEG-PLGA NPs	Balb/C mice bearing C26 tumors	▪ Plasma CL (mL/h/kg): 407.1 in solution; 148.4 in DTX-PEG-PLGA NPs	[161]
PTX@P85/Tf-PLGA NPs	SD rats bearing C6 glioma	▪ Plasma AUC (μg·h/mL): 108.23 in solution; 362.52 in PLGA-NPs; 391.54 in P85-PLGA-NPs; 551.83 in Tf-PLGA-NPs ▪ Plasma $t_{1/2}$ (h): 2.1 in solution; 3.96 in PLGA-NPs; 4.33 in P85-PLGA-NPs; 5.43 in Tf-PLGA-NPs	[162]
Lonidamine@PLGA-PEG-EGFR peptide NPs	Female nude mice xenografted with MDA-MB-231 tumors	● Plasma ▪ AUC (μg·h/mL): 768.8 in solution; 992.44 in PLGA-PEG NPs; 1316.01 in PLGA-PEG-EGFR NPs ▪ MRT (h): 2.36 in solution; 3.77 in PLGA-PEG NPs; 4.38 in PLGA-PEG-EGFR NPs ▪ $t_{1/2}$ (h): 1.67 in solution; 3.92 in PLGA-PEG NPs; 4.16 in PLGA-PEG-EGFR NPs ● Tumor ▪ AUC (μg·h/mL): 4.58 in solution; 32.09 in PLGA-PEG NPs; 49.96 in PLGA-PEG-EGFR NPs ▪ MRT (h): 1.94 in solution; 4.46 in PLGA-PEG NPs; 7.25 in PLGA-PEG-EGFR NPs ▪ λ_z (h): 0.63 in solution; 0.26 in PLGA-PEG NPs; 0.13 in PLGA-PEG-EGFR NPs	[163]
Pt@PLGA-PEG NPs	SD rats	● Plasma ▪ $AUC_{0–24\,h}$ (μg·h/mL): 14.7 in Pt prodrug; 48.9 in PLGA-PEG NPs ▪ V_d (mL/kg): 210.9 in Pt prodrug; 43.2 in PLGA-PEG NPs ● Blood ▪ $AUC_{0–24\,h}$ (μg·h/mL): 3.8 in Pt prodrug; 12.7 in PLGA-PEG NPs ▪ V_d (mL/kg): 678.7 in Pt prodrug; 81.9 in PLGA-PEG NPs	[164]
ICG@PEG/FA-PLGA NPs	Female NCr mice xenografted with MDA-MB-231 tumors	▪ $AUC_{0–12\,h}$ ratio (PEG/FA-PLGA NPs: PLGA NPs): 3.45 in plasma;2.94 in tumor; 0.87 in liver	[166]
Bufalin@PEG-PLGA-PLL-RGD NPs	Mice bearing colon cancer	▪ $t_{1/2}$ (h): 3.35 in solution; 7.17 in PEG-PLGA-PLL-RGD NPs ▪ MRT (h): 3.45 in solution; 7.63 in PEG-PLGA-PLL-RGD NPs ▪ V_d (L/kg): 63.37 in solution; 187.83 in PEG-PLGA-PLL-RGD NPs	[167]
DTX@PLGA/HA NPs	SD rats	▪ AUC (μg·h/L): 6110 in solution; 9394 in PLGA NPs; 23,175 in PLGA/HA NPs ▪ V_d (L/kg): 6.94 in solution; 7.52 in PLGA NPs; 3.16 in PLGA/HA NPs	[168]
DTX@PLGA-PEG-Apt NPs	SD rats	▪ AUC (ng·h/mL): 1393.6 in solution; 3996.9 in PLGA-PEG NPS; 3807.4 in PLGA-PEG-Apt NPs ▪ CL (L/h): 3.588 in solution; 1.251 in PLGA-PEG NPS; 1.313 in PLGA-PEG-Apt NPs ▪ V_d (L): 0.501 in solution; 0.165 in PLGA-PEG NPS; 0.166 in PLGA-PEG-Apt NPs	[169]

Aptamer (Apt); Arg-Gly-Asp (RGD); docetaxel (DTX); epidermal growth factor receptor (EGFR); folic acid (FA); hyaluronic acid (HA); indocyanine green (ICG); platinum (Pt); Pluronic® P85 (P85); polyethylene glycol (PEG); poly-L-lysine (PLL); Sprague-Dawley (SD); transferrin (Tf).

Ma et al. reported the tissue distribution of ICG-loaded PLGA NPs modified with PEG and FA in mice xenografted with MDA-MB-231 tumors, which present high expression of folate receptor [166]. As shown in Table 5, the plasma $AUC_{0–12\,h}$ in the dual-modified PLGA NPs was higher than the corresponding $AUC_{0–12\,h}$ in the non-modified PLGA NPs, except for the $AUC_{0–12\,h}$ in liver, which was lower. Such an increase and decrease confirmed the function of PEG, which enabled the NPs to circulate longer in blood and partially escape elimination by the liver. The tumor $AUC_{0–12\,h}$ of the dual-modified PLGA NPs was three-fold higher than that of the non-modified PLGA NPs, strongly demonstrating the tumor-targeting ability of the dual-modified PLGA NPs. Since both PEG and FA were present on the dual-modified NPs, it is difficult for this study to reveal which factor contributed more for tumor targeting. However, it is speculated that longer systemic circulation is a prerequisite for tumor targeting via an EPR effect, and simultaneously FA enhances the affinity of the NPs with folate receptor-expressing tumor cells, resulting in the accumulation and intracellular uptake.

A pharmacokinetic study investigating bufalin-loaded NPs comprised of mPEG, PLGA, PLL, and cRGD was performed in mice with SW620 colon cancer [167]. In plasma, bufalin was detectable even 24 h after injection in mice treated with bufalin-loaded mPEG-PLGA-PLL-cRGD NPs (BNPs), while bufalin was not detected in the plasma of mice treated with free bufalin. The MRT and elimination half-life of BNPs were significantly greater than those of free bufalin (Table 5). Huang et al. reported the pharmacokinetics of biodegradable DTX-loaded self-assembled NPs made of PLGA/HA block copolymers (PLGA/HA NPs) in SD rats [168]; both DTX-loaded PLGA and the PLGA/HA NPs resulted in some increase in the plasma levels of DTX compared with free DTX. The V_d for the PLGA/HA NPs was only half of that reported for PLGA NPs or free DTX, indicating greater retention of active DTX in plasma circulation when loaded into PLGA/HA NPs. As shown in Table 5, the AUC for the PLGA/HA NPs was 2.5- and 3.8-fold higher than that of the PLGA NPs and free DTX, probably due to HA shell. Collectively, the PLGA/HA NPs could prolong the circulation of DTX in the plasma.

Chen et al. reported the pharmacokinetics of DTX-loaded PLGA-PEG NPs modified with anti-prostate-specific membrane antigen (PSMA) aptamer in LNCaP tumor-xenografted BALB/c mice for targeted delivery of DTX to prostate tumors [169]. The CL and V_d of DTX decreased when DTX was applied in encapsulated formulations, suggesting favorable conditions for enhanced systemic exposure, which is reflected by the increases in AUC (Table 5). The DTX solution presented higher distribution to the heart and lower distribution to other organs, including the liver, spleen, lung, and kidney, compared with PLGA-PEG-apt NPs. Generally, NPs administered intravenously are readily entrapped in the RES, a unique microstructure abundant in the spleen, liver, and lung [170].

In a previous study [171], curcumin, a clinically promising anticancer phytochemical, exhibited a very short half-life of ~8 min following intravenous dosing as a free form in female BALB/c nude mice. However, PLGA-PEG NPs conjugated with EGFR-targeting GE11 peptide for breast cancer therapy prolonged the half-life to ~6 h. This provided further evidence that the sustained release of curcumin from the NP formulation and/or protection from elimination in the systemic circulation could prolong the period of tumor exposure to curcumin. Recently, it was reported that anti-EGFR protein-anchored PLGA-PEG NPs (immunonanoparticle, INP) for breast cancer therapy significantly enhanced tumor PTX concentrations by approximately 93-fold, compared to PLGA-PEG NPs and free PTX in athymic mice [94]. Paolini et al. developed galactosamine-modified PLGA NPs with a hydrodynamic diameter of 63 nm for the liver-specific delivery of bergamottin, a natural CYP3A4-inhibiting compound [172]. The bergamottin-loaded PLGA-galactosamine NPs efficiently inhibited CYP3A4 in vitro, and the highest accumulation was observed in hepatocytes. Compared with DTX treatment alone in nude mice bearing MDA-MB-231 tumors, co-treatment with NPs significantly improved the delay in tumor growth and demonstrated a major improvement in overall survival (survival rate of 67% versus 0% at day 55). Ahmad et al. assessed in situ intestinal transport and in vivo pharmacokinetics of DTX-loaded CS-coated PLGA NPs (DTX-CS-PLGA NPs), which were developed for target therapy of intestinal cancer [173]. DTX-CS-PLGA and DTX-PLGA NPs, along with GF120918, presented a 5- and 2.2-fold enhancement, respectively, in apparent intestinal permeability in a rat ileum permeation study. Similarly, significantly higher C_{max}, T_{max}, and AUC were observed following administration of DTX-CS-PLGA and DTX-PLGA NPs compared with free DTX suspension in rats. The higher T_{max} is consistent with the sustained in vitro release profile, whereas the higher C_{max} and AUC for the nanoformulations may be attributed to the enhanced intestinal absorption of DTX. The possible mechanisms of the enhanced DTX absorption include encapsulation of DTX, protecting it from GI shielding, avoiding CYP and P-glycoprotein recognition, and endocytosis into enterocytes (direct uptake of NPs) [173].

7. Current Status and Challenges of PLGA-Based Formulations for Clinical Applications

There have been many developments in PLGA-based formulations for the diagnosis and therapy of diseases in research status [59–62]. Several pharmaceutical products based on PLGA have been prescribed as follows: Arestin® (minocycline HCl, microsphere, periodontal; OraPharma), Bydureon® (exenatide, microsphere, subcutaneous; AstraZeneca PLC), Eligard® (leuprolide acetate, in situ forming gel, subcutaneous; Tolmar Pharmaceuticals, Inc.), Lupron depot® (leuprolide acetate, microsphere, intramuscular; AbbVie Inc.), Ozurdex® (dexamethasone, implant, intravitreal; Allergan), Signifor LAR® (pasireotide pamoate, microsphere, intramuscular; Norvatis Pharmaceuticals Corp.), Vivitrol® (Naltrexone, microsphere, intramuscular; Alkermes, Inc.), and Zoladex® (goserelin acetate, implant, subcutaneous; AstraZeneca PLC). Micellar structure based on mPEG-poly(D,L-lactide) including PTX has been also developed and used in clinics as Genexol® PM (Samyang Biopharm). Unfortunately, there was little progress in the commercialization of PLGA-based NPs for cancer imaging and therapy. For the clinical translation of developed PLGA NPs, following drawbacks should be overcome; poor drug loading capacity (in spite of high drug encapsulation efficiency), high initial burst release rate of drug, generation of acidic products after its biodegradation, difficulty in scale-up process, and nanotoxicology [174]. In view of the toxicological issue, the influences of degraded products (LA and GA) of PLGA to the major organs and tissues were investigated [175]. In that literature [175], the oral administration of PLGA NPs in rats exhibited minimal toxicities on liver and intestine and no toxicity in brain, kidney, and lung. Recent endeavors in the areas of regulation and mass production may accelerate the launch of PLGA-based nanoformulations for cancer therapy in the market.

8. Conclusions

A variety of nanosystems based on PLGA or PLGA derivatives have been developed for cancer imaging and treatment. Because of the biocompatibility and biodegradability of PLGA, its potential for clinical application may be high compared with that of other materials. As naive PLGA-based NPs can only target tumors passively through the EPR effect, several functional groups (i.e., targeting ligands) have been introduced as active tumor-targeting strategies. Chemical or physical modulation of PLGA NPs can control drug cargo release, endocytosis in cancer cells, in vivo tumor targeting efficiency, in vivo anticancer activities, and in vivo pharmacokinetics following their intravenous administration. However, for clinical application, mass production process of those PLGA-based NPs should be established and the safety of surface-engineered PLGA NPs has to be thoroughly identified. The introduction of biosafe or commercially available functional materials into PLGA-based NPs may augment their anticancer efficacy and attenuate unwanted adverse effects.

Author Contributions: Conceptualization, I.-S.Y., H.-J.C.; investigation, K.-T.K., J.-Y.L., I.-S.Y., H.-J.C.; writing—original draft preparation, K.-T.K., J.-Y.L., I.-S.Y., H.-J.C.; writing—review and editing, I.-S.Y., D.-D.K., H.-J.C.; visualization, K.-T.K., J.-Y.L., I.-S.Y., H.-J.C.; funding acquisition, H.-J.C.

References

1. Choi, Y.H.; Han, H.K. Nanomedicines: Current status and future perspectives in aspect of drug delivery and pharmacokinetics. *J. Pharm. Investig.* **2018**, *48*, 43–60. [CrossRef] [PubMed]
2. Elzoghby, A.O.; Hemasa, A.L.; Freag, M.S. Hybrid protein-inorganic nanoparticles: From tumor-targeted drug delivery to cancer imaging. *J. Control. Release* **2016**, *243*, 303–322. [CrossRef] [PubMed]
3. Fan, W.; Yung, B.C.; Chen, X. Stimuli-responsive NO release for on-demand gas-sensitized synergistic cancer therapy. *Angew. Chem. Int. Ed.* **2018**, *57*, 8383–8394. [CrossRef] [PubMed]
4. Fang, R.H.; Jiang, Y.; Fang, J.C.; Zhang, L. Cell membrane-derived nanomaterials for biomedical applications. *Biomaterials* **2017**, *128*, 69–83. [CrossRef] [PubMed]

5. Gao, M.; Yu, F.; Lv, C.; Choo, J.; Chen, L. Fluorescent chemical probes for accurate tumor diagnosis and targeting therapy. *Chem. Soc. Rev.* **2017**, *46*, 2237–2271. [CrossRef] [PubMed]
6. Gu, Z.; Zhu, S.; Yan, L.; Zhao, F.; Zhao, Y. Graphene-based smart platforms for combined cancer therapy. *Adv. Mater.* **2019**, *31*, 1800662. [CrossRef] [PubMed]
7. Guo, X.; You, J. Near infrared light-controlled therapeutic molecules release of nanocarriers in cancer therapy. *J. Pharm. Investig.* **2017**, *47*, 297–316. [CrossRef]
8. Hu, Y.; Mignani, S.; Majoral, J.P.; Shen, M.; Shi, X. Construction of iron oxide nanoparticle-based hybrid platforms for tumor imaging and therapy. *Chem. Soc. Rev.* **2018**, *47*, 1874–1900. [CrossRef]
9. Guan, Q.; Li, Y.A.; Li, W.Y.; Dong, Y.B. Photodynamic therapy based on nanoscale metal-organic frameworks: From material design to cancer nanotherapeutics. *Chem. Asian J.* **2018**, *13*, 3122–3149. [CrossRef]
10. Jeon, G.; Ko, Y.T. Enhanced photodyamic therapy via photosensitizer-loaded nanoparticles for cancer treatment. *J. Pharm. Investig.* **2019**, *49*, 1–8. [CrossRef]
11. Le, Q.V.; Choi, J.; Oh, Y.K. Nano delivery systems and cancer immunotherapy. *J. Pharm. Investig.* **2018**, *48*, 527–539. [CrossRef]
12. Lee, M.K. Clinical usefulness of liposomal formulations in cancer therapy: Lessons from the experiences of doxorubicin. *J. Pharm. Investig.* **2019**, *49*, 203–214. [CrossRef]
13. Liu, Y.; Bhattarai, P.; Dai, Z.; Chen, X. Photothermal therapy and photoacoustic imaging via nanotheranostics in fighting cancer. *Chem. Soc. Rev.* **2019**, *48*, 2053–2108. [CrossRef] [PubMed]
14. Raichur, V.; Devi, V.K. Formulation and evaluation of osteotropic drug delivery system of methotrexate with a potential for passive bone targeting. *J. Pharm. Investig.* **2017**, *47*, 335–347. [CrossRef]
15. Sobh, R.A.; Nasr, H.E.; Moustafa, A.B.; Mohamed, W.S. Tailoring of anticancer drugs loaded in MWCNT/Poly(MMA-*co*-HEMA) nanosphere composite by using in situ microemulsion polymerization. *J. Pharm. Investig.* **2019**, *49*, 45–55. [CrossRef]
16. Sun, Q.; Barz, M.; De Geest, B.G.; Diken, M.; Hennink, W.E.; Kiessling, F.; Lammers, T.; Shi, Y. Nanomedicine and macroscale materials in immuno-oncology. *Chem. Soc. Rev.* **2019**, *48*, 351–381. [CrossRef] [PubMed]
17. Tang, H.; Zheng, Y.; Chen, Y. Materials chemistry of nanoultrasonic biomedicine. *Adv. Mater.* **2017**, *29*, 1604105. [CrossRef] [PubMed]
18. Tang, W.L.; Tang, W.H.; Li, S.D. Cancer theranostic applications of lipid-based nanoparticles. *Drug Discov. Today* **2018**, *23*, 1159–1166. [CrossRef] [PubMed]
19. Wang, H.; Li, X.; Tse, B.W.; Yang, H.; Thorling, C.A.; Liu, Y.; Touraud, M.; Chouane, J.B.; Liu, X.; Roberts, M.S.; et al. Indocyanine green-incorporating nanoparticles for cancer theranostics. *Theranostics* **2018**, *8*, 1227–1242. [CrossRef]
20. Youn, Y.S.; Kwag, D.S.; Lee, E.S. Multifunctional nano-sized fullerenes for advanced tumor therapy. *J. Pharm. Investig.* **2017**, *47*, 1–10. [CrossRef]
21. Golombek, S.K.; May, J.N.; Theek, B.; Appold, L.; Drude, N.; Kiessling, F.; Lammers, T. Tumor targeting via EPR: Strategies to enhance patient responses. *Adv. Drug Deliv. Rev.* **2018**, *130*, 17–38. [CrossRef] [PubMed]
22. Maeda, H. Macromolecular therapeutics in cancer treatment: The EPR effect and beyond. *J. Control. Release* **2012**, *164*, 138–144. [CrossRef] [PubMed]
23. Maeda, H.; Wu, J.; Sawa, T.; Matsumura, Y.; Hori, K. Tumor vascular permeability and the EPR effect in macromolecular therapeutics: A review. *J. Control. Release* **2000**, *65*, 271–284. [CrossRef]
24. Nichols, J.W.; Bae, Y.H. EPR: Evidence and fallacy. *J. Control. Release* **2014**, *190*, 451–464. [CrossRef] [PubMed]
25. Maeda, H.; Nakamura, H.; Fang, J. The EPR effect for macromolecular drug delivery to solid tumors: Improvement of tumor uptake, lowering of systemic toxicity, and distinct tumor imaging in vivo. *Adv. Drug Deliv. Rev.* **2013**, *65*, 71–79. [CrossRef] [PubMed]
26. Fang, J.; Nakamura, H.; Maeda, H. The EPR effect: Unique features of tumor blood vessels for drug delivery, factors involved, and limitations and augmentation of the effect. *Adv. Drug Deliv. Rev.* **2011**, *63*, 136–151. [CrossRef] [PubMed]
27. Danhier, F.; Feron, O.; Préat, V. To exploit the tumor microenvironment: Passive and active tumor targeting of nanocarriers for anti-cancer drug delivery. *J. Control. Release* **2010**, *148*, 135–146. [CrossRef]
28. Jeong, J.Y.; Hong, E.H.; Lee, S.Y.; Lee, J.Y.; Song, J.H.; Ko, S.H.; Shim, J.S.; Choe, S.; Kim, D.D.; Ko, H.J.; et al. Boronic acid-tethered amphiphilic hyaluronic acid derivative-based nanoassemblies for tumor targeting and penetration. *Acta Biomater.* **2017**, *53*, 414–426. [CrossRef]

29. Lee, J.Y.; Chung, S.J.; Cho, H.J.; Kim, D.D. Phenylboronic acid-decorated chondroitin sulfate A-based theranostic nanoparticles for enhanced tumor targeting and penetration. *Adv. Funct. Mater.* **2015**, *25*, 3705–3717. [CrossRef]
30. Lee, S.Y.; Cho, H.J. Amine-functionalized poly(lactic-*co*-glycolic acid) nanoparticles for improved cellular uptake and tumor penetration. *Colloids Surf. B Biointerfaces* **2016**, *148*, 85–94. [CrossRef]
31. Lee, S.Y.; Cho, H.J. Mitochondria targeting and destabilizing hyaluronic acid derivative-based nanoparticles for the delivery of lapatinib to triple-negative breast cancer. *Biomacromolecules* **2019**, *20*, 835–845. [CrossRef] [PubMed]
32. Lee, S.Y.; Ko, S.H.; Shim, J.S.; Kim, D.D.; Cho, H.J. Tumor targeting and lipid rafts disrupting hyaluronic acid-cyclodextrin-based nanoassembled structure for cancer therapy. *ACS Appl. Mater. Interfaces* **2018**, *10*, 36628–36640. [CrossRef] [PubMed]
33. Lee, S.Y.; Koo, J.S.; Yang, M.; Cho, H.J. Application of temporary agglomeration of chitosan-coated nanoparticles for the treatment of lung metastasis of melanoma. *J. Colloid Interface Sci.* **2019**, *544*, 266–275. [CrossRef] [PubMed]
34. Lee, S.Y.; Park, J.H.; Ko, S.H.; Shim, J.S.; Kim, D.D.; Cho, H.J. Mussel-inspired hyaluronic acid derivative nanostructures for improved tumor targeting and penetration. *ACS Appl. Mater. Interfaces* **2017**, *9*, 22308–22320. [CrossRef] [PubMed]
35. Li, C.; Zhang, Y.; Chen, G.; Hu, F.; Zhao, K.; Wang, Q. Engineered multifunctional nanomedicine for simultaneous stereotactic chemotherapy and inhibited osteolysis in an orthotopic model of bone metastasis. *Adv. Mater.* **2017**, *29*, 1605754. [CrossRef] [PubMed]
36. Sun, Q.; Ojha, T.; Kiessling, F.; Lammers, T.; Shi, Y. Enhancing tumor penetration of nanomedicines. *Biomacromolecules* **2017**, *18*, 1449–1459. [CrossRef] [PubMed]
37. Tian, B.; Li, J.; Pang, R.; Dai, S.; Li, T.; Weng, Y.; Jin, Y.; Hua, Y. Gold nanoparticles biosynthesized and functionalized using a hydroxylated tetraterpenoid trigger gene expression changes and apoptosis in cancer cells. *ACS Appl. Mater. Interfaces* **2018**, *10*, 37353–37363. [CrossRef] [PubMed]
38. Yang, J.; Li, L.; Kopeček, J. Biorecognition: A key to drug-free macromolecular therapeutics. *Biomaterials* **2019**, *190–191*, 11–23. [CrossRef] [PubMed]
39. Bhushan, B.; Khanadeev, V.; Khlebtsov, B.; Khlebtsov, N.; Gopinath, P. Impact of albumin based approaches in nanomedicine: Imaging, targeting and drug delivery. *Adv. Colloid Interface Sci.* **2017**, *246*, 13–39. [CrossRef]
40. De Matteis, V.; Cascione, M.; Toma, C.C.; Leporatti, S. Silver nanoparticles: Synthetic routes, in vitro toxicity and theranostic applications for cancer disease. *Nanomaterials* **2018**, *8*, 319. [CrossRef]
41. Dykman, L.A.; Khlebtsov, N.G. Multifunctional gold-based nanocomposites for theranostics. *Biomaterials* **2016**, *108*, 13–34. [CrossRef] [PubMed]
42. Hong, S.H.; Choi, Y. Mesoporous silica-based nanoplatforms for the delivery of photodynamic therapy agents. *J. Pharm. Investig.* **2018**, *48*, 3–17. [CrossRef] [PubMed]
43. Kim, H.S.; Lee, D.Y. Photothermal therapy with gold nanoparticles as an anticancer medication. *J. Pharm. Investig.* **2017**, *47*, 19–26. [CrossRef]
44. Kim, S.; Lee, S.Y.; Cho, H.J. Berberine and zinc oxide-based nanoparticles for the chemo-photothermal therapy of lung adenocarcinoma. *Biochem. Biophys. Res. Commun.* **2018**, *501*, 765–770. [CrossRef] [PubMed]
45. Koo, J.S.; Lee, S.Y.; Azad, M.O.K.; Kim, M.; Hwang, S.J.; Nam, S.; Kim, S.; Chae, B.J.; Kang, W.S.; Cho, H.J. Development of iron(II) sulfate nanoparticles produced by hot-melt extrusion and their therapeutic potentials for colon cancer. *Int. J. Pharm.* **2019**, *558*, 388–395. [CrossRef] [PubMed]
46. Lee, J.J.; Lee, S.Y.; Park, J.H.; Kim, D.D.; Cho, H.J. Cholesterol-modified poly(lactide-*co*-glycolide) nanoparticles for tumor-targeted drug delivery. *Int. J. Pharm.* **2016**, *509*, 483–491. [CrossRef] [PubMed]
47. Lee, J.S.; Youn, Y.H.; Kwon, I.K.; Ko, N.R. Recent advances in quantum dots for biomedical applications. *J. Pharm. Investig.* **2018**, *48*, 209–214. [CrossRef]
48. Lee, J.Y.; Chung, S.J.; Cho, H.J.; Kim, D.D. Iodinated hyaluronic acid oligomer-based nanoassemblies for tumor-targeted drug delivery and cancer imaging. *Biomaterials* **2016**, *85*, 218–231. [CrossRef]
49. Lee, J.Y.; Park, J.H.; Lee, J.J.; Lee, S.Y.; Chung, S.J.; Cho, H.J.; Kim, D.D. Polyethylene glycol-conjugated chondroitin sulfate A derivative nanoparticles for tumor-targeted delivery of anticancer drugs. *Carbohydr. Polym.* **2016**, *151*, 68–77. [CrossRef]

50. Lee, J.Y.; Termsarasab, U.; Lee, M.Y.; Kim, D.H.; Lee, S.Y.; Kim, J.S.; Cho, H.J.; Kim, D.D. Chemosensitizing indomethacin-conjugated chitosan oligosaccharide nanoparticles for tumor-targeted drug delivery. *Acta Biomater.* **2017**, *57*, 262–273. [CrossRef]
51. Lee, J.Y.; Termsarasab, U.; Park, J.H.; Lee, S.Y.; Ko, S.H.; Shim, J.S.; Chung, S.J.; Cho, H.J.; Kim, D.D. Dual CD44 and folate receptor-targeted nanoparticles for cancer diagnosis and anticancer drug delivery. *J. Control. Release* **2016**, *236*, 38–46. [CrossRef] [PubMed]
52. Lee, S.Y.; Cho, H.J. An α-tocopheryl succinate enzyme-based nanoassembly for cancer imaging and therapy. *Drug Deliv.* **2018**, *25*, 738–749. [CrossRef] [PubMed]
53. Oberli, M.A.; Reichmuth, A.M.; Dorkin, J.R.; Mitchell, M.J.; Fenton, O.S.; Jaklenec, A.; Anderson, D.G.; Langer, R.; Blankschtein, D. Lipid nanoparticle assisted mRNA delivery for potent cancer immunotherapy. *Nano Lett.* **2017**, *17*, 1326–1335. [CrossRef] [PubMed]
54. Park, J.H.; Cho, H.J.; Yoon, H.Y.; Yoon, I.S.; Ko, S.H.; Shim, J.S.; Cho, J.H.; Park, J.H.; Kim, K.; Kwon, I.C.; et al. Hyaluronic acid derivative-coated nanohybrid liposomes for cancer imaging and drug delivery. *J. Control. Release* **2014**, *174*, 98–108. [CrossRef] [PubMed]
55. Sarisozen, C.; Pan, J.; Dutta, I.; Torchilin, V.P. Polymers in the co-delivery of siRNA and anticancer drugs to treat multidrug-resistant tumors. *J. Pharm. Investig.* **2017**, *47*, 37–49. [CrossRef]
56. Sim, T.; Lim, C.; Hoang, N.H.; Oh, K.T. Recent advance of pH-sensitive nanocarriers targeting solid tumors. *J. Pharm. Investig.* **2017**, *47*, 383–394. [CrossRef]
57. Tasciotti, E. Smart cancer therapy with DNA orgami. *Nat. Biotechnol.* **2018**, *36*, 234–235. [CrossRef]
58. Zhu, B.; Wang, L.; Li, J.; Fan, C. Precisely tailored DNA nanostructures and their theranostic applications. *Chem. Rec.* **2017**, *17*, 1213–1230. [CrossRef]
59. Martins, C.; Sousa, F.; Araújo, F.; Sarmento, B. Functionalizing PLGA and PLGA derivatives for drug delivery and tissue regeneration applications. *Adv. Healthc. Mater.* **2018**, *7*, 1701035. [CrossRef]
60. Swider, E.; Koshkina, O.; Tel, J.; Cruz, L.J.; de Vries, I.J.M.; Srinivas, M. Customizing poly(lactic-*co*-glycolic acid) particles for biomedical applications. *Acta Biomater.* **2018**, *73*, 38–51. [CrossRef]
61. Danhier, F.; Ansorena, E.; Silva, J.M.; Coco, R.; Le Breton, A.; Préat, V. PLGA-based nanoparticles: An overview of biomedical applications. *J. Control. Release* **2012**, *161*, 505–522. [CrossRef] [PubMed]
62. Mir, M.; Ahmed, N.; Rehman, A.U. Recent applications of PLGA based nanostructures in drug delivery. *Colloids Surf. B Biointerfaces* **2017**, *159*, 217–231. [CrossRef] [PubMed]
63. Chen, H.; Li, F.; Yao, Y.; Wang, Z.; Zhang, Z.; Tan, N. Redox dual-responsive and O_2-evolving theranostic nanosystem for highly selective chemotherapy against hypoxic tumors. *Theranostics* **2019**, *9*, 90–103. [CrossRef] [PubMed]
64. Gao, M.; Liang, C.; Song, X.; Chen, Q.; Jin, Q.; Wang, C.; Liu, Z. Erythrocyte-membrane-enveloped perfluorocarbon as nanoscale artificial red blood cells to relieve tumor hypoxia and enhance cancer radiotherapy. *Adv. Mater.* **2017**, *29*, 1701429. [CrossRef] [PubMed]
65. Park, J.H.; Lee, J.Y.; Termsarasab, U.; Yoon, I.S.; Ko, S.H.; Shim, J.S.; Cho, H.J.; Kim, D.D. Development of poly(lactic-*co*-glycolic) acid nanoparticles-embedded hyaluronic acid–ceramide-based nanostructure for tumor-targeted drug delivery. *Int. J. Pharm.* **2014**, *473*, 426–433. [CrossRef] [PubMed]
66. Saneja, A.; Arora, D.; Kumar, R.; Dubey, R.D.; Panda, A.K.; Gupta, P.N. CD44 targeted PLGA nanomedicines for cancer chemotherapy. *Eur. J. Pharm. Sci.* **2018**, *121*, 47–58. [CrossRef] [PubMed]
67. Acharya, S.; Sahoo, S.K. PLGA nanoparticles containing various anticancer agents and tumour delivery by EPR effect. *Adv. Drug Deliv. Rev.* **2011**, *63*, 170–183. [CrossRef]
68. Ding, D.; Zhu, Q. Recent advances of PLGA micro/nanoparticles for the delivery of biomacromolecular therapeutics. *Mater. Sci. Eng. C Mater. Biol. Appl.* **2018**, *92*, 1041–1060. [CrossRef]
69. Lee, S.Y.; Cho, H.J. Dopamine-conjugated poly(lactic-*co*-glycolic acid) nanoparticles for protein delivery to macrophages. *J. Colloid Interface Sci.* **2017**, *490*, 391–400. [CrossRef]
70. Park, J.H.; Cho, H.J.; Kim, D.D. Poly((D,L)lactic-glycolic)acid–star glucose nanoparticles for glucose transporter and hypoglycemia-mediated tumor targeting. *Int. J. Nanomed.* **2017**, *12*, 7453–7467. [CrossRef]
71. Allahyari, M.; Mohit, E. Peptide/protein vaccine delivery system based on PLGA particles. *Hum. Vaccin. Immunother.* **2016**, *12*, 806–828. [CrossRef] [PubMed]
72. Rezvantalab, S.; Drude, N.I.; Moraveji, M.K.; Guvener, N.; Koons, E.K.; Shi, Y.; Lammers, T.; Kiessling, F. PLGA-based nanoparticles in cancer treatment. *Front. Pharmacol.* **2018**, *9*, 1260. [CrossRef] [PubMed]

73. Dinarvand, R.; Sepehri, N.; Manoochehri, S.; Rouhani, H.; Atyabi, F. Polylactide-*co*-glycolide nanoparticles for controlled delivery of anticancer agents. *Int. J. Nanomed.* **2011**, *6*, 877–895. [CrossRef] [PubMed]
74. Booysen, L.L.; Kalombo, L.; Brooks, E.; Hansen, R.; Gilliland, J.; Gruppo, V.; Lungenhofer, P.; Semete-Makokotlela, B.; Swai, H.S.; Kotze, A.F.; et al. In vivo/in vitro pharmacokinetic and pharmacodynamic study of spray-dried poly-(DL-lactic-*co*-glycolic) acid nanoparticles encapsulating rifampicin and isoniazid. *Int. J. Pharm.* **2013**, *444*, 10–17. [CrossRef] [PubMed]
75. Kapoor, D.N.; Bhatia, A.; Kaur, R.; Sharma, R.; Kaur, G.; Dhawan, S. PLGA: A unique polymer for drug delivery. *Ther. Deliv.* **2015**, *6*, 41–58. [CrossRef] [PubMed]
76. Lee, J.Y.; Kim, J.S.; Cho, H.J.; Kim, D.D. Poly(styrene)-*b*-poly(DL-lactide) copolymer-based nanoparticles for anticancer drug delivery. *Int. J. Nanomed.* **2014**, *9*, 2803–2813.
77. Rafiei, P.; Haddadi, A. Docetaxel-loaded PLGA and PLGA-PEG nanoparticles for intravenous application: Pharmacokinetics and biodistribution profile. *Int. J. Nanomed.* **2017**, *12*, 935–947. [CrossRef] [PubMed]
78. Sanna, V.; Roggio, A.M.; Posadino, A.M.; Cossu, A.; Marceddu, S.; Mariani, A.; Alzari, V.; Uzzau, S.; Pintus, G.; Sechi, M. Novel docetaxel-loaded nanoparticles based on poly(lactide-*co*-caprolactone) and poly(lactide-*co*-glycolide-*co*-caprolactone) for prostate cancer treatment: Formulation, characterization, and cytotoxicity studies. *Nanoscale Res. Lett.* **2011**, *6*, 260. [CrossRef]
79. Ashjari, M.; Khoee, S.; Mahdavian, A.R.; Rahmatolahzadeh, R. Self-assembled nanomicelles using PLGA-PEG amphiphilic block copolymer for insulin delivery: A physicochemical investigation and determination of CMC values. *J. Mater. Sci. Mater. Med.* **2012**, *23*, 943–953. [CrossRef]
80. Chen, X.; Chen, J.; Li, B.; Yang, X.; Zeng, R.; Liu, Y.; Li, T.; Ho, R.J.Y.; Shao, J. PLGA-PEG-PLGA triblock copolymeric micelles as oral drug delivery system: In vitro drug release and in vivo pharmacokinetics assessment. *J. Colloid Interface Sci.* **2017**, *490*, 542–552. [CrossRef]
81. Cai, Q.; Wang, L.; Deng, G.; Liu, J.; Chen, Q.; Chen, Z. Systemic delivery to central nervous system by engineered PLGA nanoparticles. *Am. J. Transl. Res.* **2016**, *8*, 749–764. [PubMed]
82. Chung, Y.I.; Kim, J.C.; Kim, Y.H.; Tae, G.; Lee, S.Y.; Kim, K.; Kwon, I.C. The effect of surface functionalization of PLGA nanoparticles by heparin- or chitosan-conjugated Pluronic on tumor targeting. *J. Control. Release* **2010**, *143*, 374–382. [CrossRef] [PubMed]
83. Hwang, H.S.; Shin, H.; Na, K. Combination of photodynamic therapy (PDT) and anti-tumor immunity in cancer therapy. *J. Pharm. Investig.* **2018**, *48*, 143–151. [CrossRef] [PubMed]
84. Kydd, J.; Jadia, R.; Velpurisiva, P.; Gad, A.; Paliwal, S.; Rai, P. Targeting strategies for the combination treatment of cancer using drug delivery systems. *Pharmaceutics* **2017**, *9*, 46. [CrossRef] [PubMed]
85. Li, K.; Ding, D.; Huo, D.; Pu, K.Y.; Thao, N.N.P.; Hu, Y.; Li, Z.; Liu, B. Conjugated polymer based nanoparticles as dual-modal probes for targeted in vivo fluorescence and magnetic resonance imaging. *Adv. Funct. Mater.* **2012**, *22*, 3107–3115. [CrossRef]
86. Chen, J.; Wu, Q.; Luo, L.; Wang, Y.; Zhong, Y.; Dai, H.B.; Sun, D.; Luo, M.L.; Wu, W.; Wang, G.X. Dual tumor-targeted poly(lactic-*co*-glycolic acid)-polyethylene glycol-folic acid nanoparticles: A novel biodegradable nanocarrier for secure and efficient antitumor drug delivery. *Int. J. Nanomed.* **2017**, *12*, 5745–5760. [CrossRef] [PubMed]
87. Liu, X.J.; Li, L.; Liu, X.J.; Li, Y.; Zhao, C.Y.; Wang, R.Q.; Zhen, Y.S. Mithramycin-loaded mPEG-PLGA nanoparticles exert potent antitumor efficacy against pancreatic carcinoma. *Int. J. Nanomed.* **2017**, *12*, 5255–5269. [CrossRef] [PubMed]
88. Lu, B.; Lv, X.; Le, Y. Chitosan-modified PLGA nanoparticles for control-released drug delivery. *Polymers* **2019**, *11*, 304. [CrossRef] [PubMed]
89. Shah, N.; Chaudhari, K.; Dantuluri, P.; Murthy, R.S.; Das, S. Paclitaxel-loaded PLGA nanoparticles surface modified with transferrin and Pluronic® P85, an in vitro cell line and in vivo biodistribution studies on rat model. *J. Drug Target.* **2009**, *17*, 533–542. [CrossRef] [PubMed]
90. Wang, H.; Zhao, Y.; Wang, H.; Gong, J.; He, H.; Shin, M.C.; Yang, V.C.; Huang, Y. Low-molecular-weight protamine-modified PLGA nanoparticles for overcoming drug-resistant breast cancer. *J. Control. Release* **2014**, *192*, 47–56. [CrossRef]
91. Lin, W.J.; Lee, W.C. Polysaccharide-modified nanoparticles with intelligent CD44 receptor targeting ability for gene delivery. *Int. J. Nanomed.* **2018**, *13*, 3989–4002. [CrossRef] [PubMed]

92. Mehdizadeh, M.; Rouhani, H.; Sepehri, N.; Varshochian, R.; Ghahremani, M.H.; Amini, M.; Gharghabi, M.; Ostad, S.N.; Atyabi, F.; Baharian, A.; et al. Biotin decorated PLGA nanoparticles containing SN-38 designed for cancer therapy. *Artif. Cells Nanomed. Biotechnol.* **2017**, *45*, 495–504. [CrossRef] [PubMed]
93. Bao, W.; Liu, R.; Wang, Y.; Wang, F.; Xia, G.; Zhang, H.; Li, X.; Yin, H.; Chen, B. PLGA-PLL-PEG-Tf-based targeted nanoparticles drug delivery system enhance antitumor efficacy via intrinsic apoptosis pathway. *Int. J. Nanomed.* **2015**, *10*, 557–566.
94. Venugopal, V.; Krishnan, S.; Palanimuthu, V.R.; Sankarankutty, S.; Kalaimani, J.K.; Karupiah, S.; Kit, N.S.; Hock, T.T. Anti-EGFR anchored paclitaxel loaded PLGA nanoparticles for the treatment of triple negative breast cancer. In-vitro and in-vivo anticancer activities. *PLoS ONE* **2018**, *13*, e0206109. [CrossRef] [PubMed]
95. Babu, A.; Amreddy, N.; Muralidharan, R.; Pathuri, G.; Gali, H.; Chen, A.; Zhao, Y.D.; Munshi, A.; Ramesh, R. Chemodrug delivery using integrin-targeted PLGA-chitosan nanoparticle for lung cancer therapy. *Sci. Rep.* **2017**, *7*, 14674. [CrossRef] [PubMed]
96. Ni, M.; Xiong, M.; Zhang, X.; Cai, G.; Chen, H.; Zeng, Q.; Yu, Z. Poly(lactic-*co*-glycolic acid) nanoparticles conjugated with CD133 aptamers for targeted salinomycin delivery to CD133+ osteosarcoma cancer stem cells. *Int. J. Nanomed.* **2015**, *10*, 2537–2554.
97. Foroozandeh, P.; Aziz, A.A. Insight into cellular uptake and intracellular trafficking of nanoparticles. *Nanoscale Res. Lett.* **2018**, *13*, 339. [CrossRef] [PubMed]
98. Kou, L.; Sun, J.; Zhai, Y.; He, Z. The endocytosis and intracellular fate of nanomedicines: Implication for rational design. *Asian J. Pharm. Sci.* **2013**, *8*, 1–10. [CrossRef]
99. Malinovskaya, Y.; Melnikov, P.; Baklaushev, V.; Gabashvili, A.; Osipova, N.; Mantrov, S.; Ermolenko, Y.; Maksimenko, O.; Gorshkova, M.; Balabanyan, V.; et al. Delivery of doxorubicin-loaded PLGA nanoparticles into U87 human glioblastoma cells. *Int. J. Pharm.* **2017**, *524*, 77–90. [CrossRef]
100. Sahay, G.; Alakhova, D.Y.; Kabanov, A.V. Endocytosis of nanomedicines. *J. Control. Release* **2010**, *145*, 182–195. [CrossRef]
101. Trindade, I.C.; Pound-Lana, G.; Pereira, D.G.S.; de Oliveira, L.A.M.; Andrade, M.S.; Vilela, J.M.C.; Postacchini, B.B.; Mosqueira, V.C.F. Mechanisms of interaction of biodegradable polyester nanocapsules with non-phagocytic cells. *Eur. J. Pharm. Sci.* **2018**, *124*, 89–104. [CrossRef]
102. Alshaer, W.; Hillaireau, H.; Fattal, E. Aptamer-guided nanomedicines for anticancer drug delivery. *Adv. Drug Deliv. Rev.* **2018**, *134*, 122–137. [CrossRef] [PubMed]
103. Salatin, S.; Yari Khosroushahi, A. Overviews on the cellular uptake mechanism of polysaccharide colloidal nanoparticles. *J. Cell. Mol. Med.* **2017**, *21*, 1668–1686. [CrossRef] [PubMed]
104. Kim, C.H.; Lee, S.G.; Kang, M.J.; Lee, S.; Choi, Y.W. Surface modification of lipid-based nanocarriers for cancer cell-specific drug targeting. *J. Pharm. Investig.* **2017**, *47*, 203–227. [CrossRef]
105. Ghosh, D.; Peng, X.; Leal, J.; Mohanty, R.P. Peptides as drug delivery vehicles across biological barriers. *J. Pharm. Investig.* **2018**, *48*, 89–111. [CrossRef] [PubMed]
106. Kreuter, J. Drug delivery to the central nervous system by polymeric nanoparticles: What do we know? *Adv. Drug Deliv. Rev.* **2014**, *71*, 2–14. [CrossRef]
107. Zhang, Z.; Wang, X.; Li, B.; Hou, Y.; Yang, J.; Yi, L. Development of a novel morphological paclitaxel-loaded PLGA microspheres for effective cancer therapy: In vitro and in vivo evaluations. *Drug Deliv.* **2018**, *25*, 166–177. [CrossRef] [PubMed]
108. Wang, M.; Zhang, Y.; Feng, J.; Gu, T.; Dong, Q.; Yang, X.; Sun, Y.; Wu, Y.; Chen, Y.; Kong, W. Preparation, characterization, and in vitro and in vivo investigation of chitosan-coated poly (D,L-lactide-*co*-glycolide) nanoparticles for intestinal delivery of exendin-4. *Int. J. Nanomed.* **2013**, *8*, 1141–1154.
109. Alibolandi, M.; Ramezani, M.; Abnous, K.; Hadizadeh, F. AS1411 aptamer-decorated biodegradable polyethylene glycol-poly(lactic-*co*-glycolic acid) nanopolymersomes for the targeted delivery of gemcitabine to non-small cell lung cancer in vitro. *J. Pharm. Sci.* **2016**, *105*, 1741–1750. [CrossRef]
110. Wei, J.; Sun, J.; Liu, Y. Enhanced targeting of prostate cancer-initiation cells by salinomycin-encapsulated lipid-PLGA nanoparticles linked with CD44 antibodies. *Oncol. Lett.* **2019**, *17*, 4024–4033.
111. Kou, L.; Yao, Q.; Sivaprakasam, S.; Luo, Q.; Sun, Y.; Fu, Q.; He, Z.; Sun, J.; Ganapathy, V. Dual targeting of l-carnitine-conjugated nanoparticles to OCTN2 and $ATB^{0,+}$ to deliver chemotherapeutic agents for colon cancer therapy. *Drug Deliv.* **2017**, *24*, 1338–1349. [CrossRef] [PubMed]

112. Li, L.; Di, X.; Wu, M.; Sun, Z.; Zhong, L.; Wang, Y.; Fu, Q.; Kan, Q.; Sun, J.; He, Z. Targeting tumor highly-expressed LAT1 transporter with amino acid-modified nanoparticles: Toward a novel active targeting strategy in breast cancer therapy. *Nanomedicine* **2017**, *13*, 987–998. [CrossRef]
113. Cespedes, A.; Perez, M.J.; Gomara, M.J.; Wandosell, F.; Haro, I. Atorvastatin in PLGA-PEG nanoparticles derivatized with the HIV-TAT peptide protects neuronal cultures in an oxygen-glucose deprivation (OGD) model. *Am. J. Nanotechnol. Nanomed.* **2018**, *1*, 55–63.
114. Choi, D.H.; Park, Y.S. Arginine-rich peptide coated PLGA nanoparticles enhance polymeric delivery of antisense $HIF_{1\alpha}$-oligonucleotide to fully differentiated stiff adipocytes. *Toxicol. Environ. Health Sci.* **2019**, *11*, 1–10. [CrossRef]
115. Nottelet, B.; Darcos, V.; Coudane, J. Aliphatic polyesters for medical imaging and theranostic applications. *Eur. J. Pharm. Biopharm.* **2015**, *97*, 350–370. [CrossRef]
116. Reul, R.; Tsapis, N.; Hillaireau, H.; Sancey, L.; Mura, S.; Recher, M.; Nicolas, J.; Coll, J.L.; Fattal, E. Near infrared labeling of PLGA for in vivo imaging of nanoparticles. *Polym. Chem.* **2012**, *3*, 694–702. [CrossRef]
117. Ratzinger, G.; Agrawal, P.; Körner, W.; Lonkai, J.; Sanders, H.M.; Terreno, E.; Wirth, M.; Strijkers, G.J.; Nicolay, K.; Gabor, F. Surface modification of PLGA nanospheres with Gd-DTPA and Gd-DOTA for high-relaxivity MRI contrast agents. *Biomaterials* **2010**, *31*, 8716–8723. [CrossRef] [PubMed]
118. Subramanian, S.; Pandey, U.; Gugulothu, D.; Patravale, V.; Samuel, G. Modification of PLGA nanoparticles for improved properties as a 99mTc-labeled agent in sentinel lymph node detection. *Cancer Biother. Radiopharm.* **2013**, *28*, 598–606. [CrossRef]
119. Nomikou, N.; Curtis, K.; McEwan, C.; O'Hagan, B.M.G.; Callan, B.; Callan, J.F.; McHale, A.P. A versatile, stimulus-responsive nanoparticle-based platform for use in both sonodynamic and photodynamic cancer therapy. *Acta Biomater.* **2017**, *49*, 414–421. [CrossRef]
120. Sivakumar, B.; Aswathy, R.G.; Romero-Aburto, R.; Mitcham, T.; Mitchel, K.A.; Nagaoka, Y.; Bouchard, R.R.; Ajayan, P.M.; Maekawa, T.; Sakthikumar, D.N. Highly versatile SPION encapsulated PLGA nanoparticles as photothermal ablators of cancer cells and as multimodal imaging agents. *Biomater. Sci.* **2017**, *5*, 432–443. [CrossRef]
121. Li, Q.; Li, C.; Tong, W. Nile red loaded PLGA nanoparticles surface modified with Gd-DTPA for potential dual-modal imaging. *J. Nanosci. Nanotechnol.* **2016**, *16*, 5569–5576. [CrossRef] [PubMed]
122. Yang, C.; Vu-Quang, H.; Husum, D.M.U.; Tingskov, S.J.; Vinding, M.S.; Nielsen, T.; Song, P.; Nielsen, N.C.; Nørregaard, R.; Kjems, J. Theranostic poly(lactic-*co*-glycolic acid) nanoparticle for magnetic resonance/infrared fluorescence bimodal imaging and efficient siRNA delivery to macrophages and its evaluation in a kidney injury model. *Nanomedicine* **2017**, *13*, 2451–2462. [CrossRef] [PubMed]
123. Xing, L.; Shi, Q.; Zheng, K.; Shen, M.; Ma, J.; Li, F.; Liu, Y.; Lin, L.; Tu, W.; Duan, Y.; et al. Ultrasound-mediated microbubble destruction (UMMD) facilitates the delivery of CA19-9 targeted and paclitaxel loaded mPEG-PLGA-PLL nanoparticles in pancreatic cancer. *Theranostics* **2016**, *6*, 1573–1587. [CrossRef] [PubMed]
124. Zhang, X.; Li, X.; Hua, H.; Wang, A.; Liu, W.; Li, Y.; Fu, F.; Shi, Y.; Sun, K. Cyclic hexapeptide-conjugated nanoparticles enhance curcumin delivery to glioma tumor cells and tissue. *Int. J. Nanomed.* **2017**, *12*, 5717–5732. [CrossRef] [PubMed]
125. Vats, M.; Mishra, S.K.; Baghini, M.S.; Chauhan, D.S.; Srivastava, R.; De, A. Near infrared fluorescence imaging in nano-therapeutics and photo-thermal evaluation. *Int. J. Mol. Sci.* **2017**, *18*, 924. [CrossRef] [PubMed]
126. da Silva, C.L.; Del Ciampo, J.O.; Rossetti, F.C.; Bentley, M.V.; Pierre, M.B. Improved in vitro and in vivo cutaneous delivery of protoporphyrin IX from PLGA-based nanoparticles. *Photochem. Photobiol.* **2013**, *89*, 1176–1184. [CrossRef] [PubMed]
127. Shen, X.; Li, T.; Chen, Z.; Xie, X.; Zhang, H.; Feng, Y.; Li, S.; Qin, X.; Yang, H.; Wu, C.; et al. NIR-light-triggered anticancer strategy for dual-modality imaging-guided combination therapy via a bioinspired hybrid PLGA nanoplatform. *Mol. Pharm.* **2019**, *16*, 1367–1384. [CrossRef] [PubMed]
128. Huang, H.; Dong, Y.; Zhang, Y.; Ru, D.; Wu, Z.; Zhang, J.; Shen, M.; Duan, Y.; Sun, Y. GSH-sensitive Pt(IV) prodrug-loaded phase-transitional nanoparticles with a hybrid lipid-polymer shell for precise theranostics against ovarian cancer. *Theranostics* **2019**, *9*, 1047–1065. [CrossRef]
129. Guo, Y.; Wang, X.Y.; Chen, Y.L.; Liu, F.Q.; Tan, M.X.; Ao, M.; Yu, J.H.; Ran, H.T.; Wang, Z.X. A light-controllable specific drug delivery nanoplatform for targeted bimodal imaging-guided photothermal/chemo synergistic cancer therapy. *Acta Biomater.* **2018**, *80*, 308–326. [CrossRef]

130. Hao, Y.; Zhang, B.; Zheng, C.; Ji, R.; Ren, X.; Guo, F.; Sun, S.; Shi, J.; Zhang, H.; Zhang, Z.; et al. The tumor-targeting core-shell structured DTX-loaded PLGA@Au nanoparticles for chemo-photothermal therapy and X-ray imaging. *J. Control. Release* **2015**, *220*, 545–555. [CrossRef]
131. Hahn, M.A.; Singh, A.K.; Sharma, P.; Brown, S.C.; Moudgil, B.M. Nanoparticles as contrast agents for in-vivo bioimaging: Current status and future perspectives. *Anal. Bioanal. Chem.* **2011**, *399*, 3–27. [CrossRef] [PubMed]
132. Sah, H.; Thoma, L.A.; Desu, H.R.; Sah, E.; Wood, G.C. Concepts and practices used to develop functional PLGA-based nanoparticulate systems. *Int. J. Nanomed.* **2013**, *8*, 747–765. [CrossRef] [PubMed]
133. Tang, H.; Guo, Y.; Peng, L.; Fang, H.; Wang, Z.; Zheng, Y.; Ran, H.; Chen, Y. In vivo targeted, responsive, and synergistic cancer nanotheranostics by magnetic resonance imaging-guided synergistic high-intensity focused ultrasound ablation and chemotherapy. *ACS Appl. Mater. Interfaces* **2018**, *10*, 15428–15441. [CrossRef] [PubMed]
134. Mosafer, J.; Abnous, K.; Tafaghodi, M.; Mokhtarzadeh, A.; Ramezani, M. In vitro and in vivo evaluation of anti-nucleolin-targeted magnetic PLGA nanoparticles loaded with doxorubicin as a theranostic agent for enhanced targeted cancer imaging and therapy. *Eur. J. Pharm. Biopharm.* **2017**, *113*, 60–74. [CrossRef] [PubMed]
135. Singh, Y.; Durga Rao Viswanadham, K.K.; Kumar Jajoriya, A.; Meher, J.G.; Raval, K.; Jaiswal, S.; Dewangan, J.; Bora, H.K.; Rath, S.K.; Lal, J.; et al. Click biotinylation of PLGA template for biotin receptor oriented delivery of doxorubicin hydrochloride in 4T1 cell-induced breast cancer. *Mol. Pharm.* **2017**, *14*, 2749–2765. [CrossRef] [PubMed]
136. Cui, Y.; Zhang, M.; Zeng, F.; Jin, H.; Xu, Q.; Huang, Y. Dual-targeting magnetic PLGA nanoparticles for codelivery of paclitaxel and curcumin for brain tumor therapy. *ACS Appl. Mater. Interfaces* **2016**, *8*, 32159–32169. [CrossRef] [PubMed]
137. Chen, Y.L.; Liu, F.Q.; Guo, Y.; Cheng, J.; Yang, L.; Lu, M.; Li, P.; Xu, J.; Yu, T.; Wang, Z.G.; et al. PA/US dual-modality imaging to guide VEGFR-2 targeted photothermal therapy using ZnPc-/PFH-loaded polymeric nanoparticles. *Biomater. Sci.* **2018**, *6*, 2130–2143. [CrossRef] [PubMed]
138. Euhus, D.M.; Hudd, C.; Laregina, M.C.; Johnson, F.E. Tumor measurement in the nude mouse. *J. Surg. Oncol.* **1986**, *31*, 229–234. [CrossRef] [PubMed]
139. Tomayko, M.M.; Reynolds, C.P. Determination of subcutaneous tumor size in athymic (nude) mice. *Cancer Chemother. Pharmacol.* **1989**, *24*, 148–154. [CrossRef]
140. Guo, J.; Gao, X.; Su, L.; Xia, H.; Gu, G.; Pang, Z.; Jiang, X.; Yao, L.; Chen, J.; Chen, H. Aptamer-functionalized PEG–PLGA nanoparticles for enhanced anti-glioma drug delivery. *Biomaterials* **2011**, *32*, 8010–8020. [CrossRef] [PubMed]
141. Wohlfart, S.; Khalansky, A.S.; Gelperina, S.; Maksimenko, O.; Bernreuther, C.; Glatzel, M.; Kreuter, J. Efficient chemotherapy of rat glioblastoma using doxorubicin-loaded PLGA nanoparticles with different stabilizers. *PLoS ONE* **2011**, *6*, e19121. [CrossRef] [PubMed]
142. Cook, R.L.; Householder, K.T.; Chung, E.P.; Prakapenka, A.V.; DiPerna, D.M.; Sirianni, R.W. A critical evaluation of drug delivery from ligand modified nanoparticles: Confounding small molecule distribution and efficacy in the central nervous system. *J. Control. Release* **2015**, *220*, 89–97. [CrossRef] [PubMed]
143. Wu, J.; Deng, C.; Meng, F.; Zhang, J.; Sun, H.; Zhong, Z. Hyaluronic acid coated PLGA nanoparticulate docetaxel effectively targets and suppresses orthotopic human lung cancer. *J. Control. Release* **2017**, *259*, 76–82. [CrossRef] [PubMed]
144. Moreno, D.; Zalba, S.; Navarro, Í.; De Ilarduya, C.T.; Garrido, M.J. Pharmacodynamics of cisplatin-loaded PLGA nanoparticles administered to tumor-bearing mice. *Eur. J. Pharm. Biopharm.* **2010**, *74*, 265–274. [CrossRef] [PubMed]
145. Mattheolabakis, G.; Taoufik, E.; Haralambous, S.; Roberts, M.L.; Avgoustakis, K. In vivo investigation of tolerance and antitumor activity of cisplatin-loaded PLGA-mPEG nanoparticles. *Eur. J. Pharm. Biopharm.* **2009**, *71*, 190–195. [CrossRef] [PubMed]
146. Saneja, A.; Kumar, R.; Mintoo, M.J.; Dubey, R.D.; Sangwan, P.L.; Mondhe, D.M.; Panda, A.K.; Gupta, P.N. Gemcitabine and betulinic acid co-encapsulated PLGA–PEG polymer nanoparticles for improved efficacy of cancer chemotherapy. *Mater. Sci. Eng. C* **2019**, *98*, 764–771. [CrossRef] [PubMed]

147. Song, X.; You, J.; Shao, H.; Yan, C. Effects of surface modification of As_2O_3-loaded PLGA nanoparticles on its anti-liver cancer ability: An in vitro and in vivo study. *Colloids Surf. B Biointerfaces* **2018**, *169*, 289–297. [CrossRef] [PubMed]
148. Liang, C.; Yang, Y.; Ling, Y.; Huang, Y.; Li, T.; Li, X. Improved therapeutic effect of folate-decorated PLGA–PEG nanoparticles for endometrial carcinoma. *Bioorg. Med. Chem.* **2011**, *19*, 4057–4066. [CrossRef] [PubMed]
149. Kang, T.; Gao, X.; Hu, Q.; Jiang, D.; Feng, X.; Zhang, X.; Song, Q.; Yao, L.; Huang, M.; Jiang, X.; et al. iNGR-modified PEG-PLGA nanoparticles that recognize tumor vasculature and penetrate gliomas. *Biomaterials* **2014**, *35*, 4319–4332. [CrossRef] [PubMed]
150. Zhang, L.; Hao, W.; Xu, L.; Gao, Y.; Wang, X.; Zhu, D.; Chen, Z.; Zhang, X.; Chen, H.; Mei, L. A pH-sensitive methenamine mandelate-loaded nanoparticle induces DNA damage and apoptosis of cancer cells. *Acta Biomater.* **2017**, *62*, 246–256. [CrossRef]
151. Deng, K.; Li, C.; Huang, S.; Xing, B.; Jin, D.; Zeng, Q.; Hou, Z.; Lin, J. Recent progress in near infrared light triggered photodynamic therapy. *Small* **2017**, *13*, 1702299. [CrossRef]
152. Li, T.; Yan, L. Functional polymer nanocarriers for photodynamic therapy. *Pharmaceuticals* **2018**, *11*, 133. [CrossRef] [PubMed]
153. Bœuf-Muraille, G.; Rigaux, G.; Callewaert, M.; Zambrano, N.; Van Gulick, L.; Roullin, V.G.; Terryn, C.; Andry, M.C.; Chuburu, F.; Dukic, S.; et al. Evaluation of mTHPC-loaded PLGA nanoparticles for in vitro photodynamic therapy on C6 glioma cell line. *Photodiagn. Photodyn. Ther.* **2019**, *25*, 448–455. [CrossRef] [PubMed]
154. Lin, X.; Yan, S.Z.; Qi, S.S.; Xu, Q.; Han, S.S.; Guo, L.Y.; Zhao, N.; Chen, S.L.; Yu, S.Q. Transferrin-modified nanoparticles for photodynamic therapy enhance the antitumor efficacy of hypocrellin A. *Front. Pharmacol.* **2017**, *8*, 815. [CrossRef] [PubMed]
155. Son, J.; Yang, S.M.; Yi, G.; Roh, Y.J.; Park, H.; Park, J.M.; Choi, M.G.; Koo, H. Folate-modified PLGA nanoparticles for tumor-targeted delivery of pheophorbide a in vivo. *Biochem. Biophys. Res. Commun.* **2018**, *498*, 523–528. [CrossRef] [PubMed]
156. Xin, Y.; Liu, T.; Yang, C. Development of PLGA-lipid nanoparticles with covalently conjugated indocyanine green as a versatile nanoplatform for tumor-targeted imaging and drug delivery. *Int. J. Nanomed.* **2016**, *11*, 5807–5821. [CrossRef]
157. Vivek, R.; Varukattu, N.; Chandrababu, R.; Alok, S.; Thondhi, P.; Alagarsamy, V.; Kannan, S. Multifunctional nanoparticles for trimodal photodynamic therapy-mediated photothermal and chemotherapeutic effects. *Photodiagn. Photodyn. Ther.* **2018**, *23*, 244–253. [CrossRef] [PubMed]
158. Wang, X.; Shi, L.; Tu, Q.; Wang, H.; Zhang, H.; Wang, P.; Zhang, L.; Huang, Z.; Zhao, F.; Luan, H.; et al. Treating cutaneous squamous cell carcinoma using 5-aminolevulinic acid polylactic-*co*-glycolic acid nanoparticle-mediated photodynamic therapy in a mouse model. *Int. J. Nanomed.* **2015**, *10*, 347–355.
159. Peng, Y.; Nie, J.; Cheng, W.; Liu, G.; Zhu, D.; Zhang, L.; Liang, C.; Mei, L.; Huang, L.; Zeng, X. A multifunctional nanoplatform for cancer chemo-photothermal synergistic therapy and overcoming multidrug resistance. *Biomater. Sci.* **2018**, *6*, 1084–1098. [CrossRef] [PubMed]
160. Nguyen, H.T.; Dai Phung, C.; Thapa, R.K.; Pham, T.T.; Tran, T.H.; Jeong, J.-H.; Ku, S.K.; Choi, H.-G.; Yong, C.S.; Kim, J.O. Multifunctional nanoparticles as somatostatin receptor-targeting delivery system of polyaniline and methotrexate for combined chemo–photothermal therapy. *Acta Biomater.* **2018**, *68*, 154–167. [CrossRef] [PubMed]
161. Senthilkumar, M.; Mishra, P.; Jain, N.K. Long circulating PEGylated poly(D,L-lactide-*co*-glycolide) nanoparticulate delivery of Docetaxel to solid tumors. *J. Drug Target.* **2008**, *16*, 424–435. [CrossRef] [PubMed]
162. Moghimi, S.M.; Muir, I.S.; Illum, L.; Davis, S.S.; Kolb-Bachofen, V. Coating particles with a block co-polymer (poloxamine-908) suppresses opsonization but permits the activity of dysopsonins in the serum. *Biochim. Biophys. Acta* **1993**, *1179*, 157–165. [CrossRef]
163. Milane, L.; Duan, Z.F.; Amiji, M. Pharmacokinetics and biodistribution of lonidamine/paclitaxel loaded, EGFR-targeted nanoparticles in an orthotopic animal model of multi-drug resistant breast cancer. *Nanomedicine* **2011**, *7*, 435–444. [CrossRef]
164. Dhar, S.; Kolishetti, N.; Lippard, S.J.; Farokhzad, O.C. Targeted delivery of a cisplatin prodrug for safer and more effective prostate cancer therapy in vivo. *Proc. Natl. Acad. Sci. USA* **2011**, *108*, 1850–1855. [CrossRef]

165. Avgoustakis, K.; Beletsi, A.; Panagi, Z.; Klepetsanis, P.; Karydas, A.G.; Ithakissios, D.S. PLGA-mPEG nanoparticles of cisplatin: In vitro nanoparticle degradation, in vitro drug release and in vivo drug residence in blood properties. *J. Control. Release* **2002**, *79*, 123–135. [CrossRef]

166. Ma, Y.; Sadoqi, M.; Shao, J. Biodistribution of indocyanine green-loaded nanoparticles with surface modifications of PEG and folic acid. *Int. J. Pharm.* **2012**, *436*, 25–31. [CrossRef]

167. Yin, P.; Wang, Y.; Qiu, Y.; Hou, L.; Liu, X.; Qin, J.; Duan, Y.; Liu, P.; Qiu, M.; Li, Q. Bufalin-loaded mPEG-PLGA-PLL-cRGD nanoparticles: Preparation, cellular uptake, tissue distribution, and anticancer activity. *Int. J. Nanomed.* **2012**, *7*, 3961–3969. [CrossRef]

168. Huang, J.; Zhang, H.; Yu, Y.; Chen, Y.; Wang, D.; Zhang, G.; Zhou, G.; Liu, J.; Sun, Z.; Sun, D.; et al. Biodegradable self-assembled nanoparticles of poly(D,L-lactide-*co*-glycolide)/hyaluronic acid block copolymers for target delivery of docetaxel to breast cancer. *Biomaterials* **2014**, *35*, 550–566. [CrossRef]

169. Chen, Z.; Tai, Z.; Gu, F.; Hu, C.; Zhu, Q.; Gao, S. Aptamer-mediated delivery of docetaxel to prostate cancer through polymeric nanoparticles for enhancement of antitumor efficacy. *Eur. J. Pharm. Biopharm.* **2016**, *107*, 130–141. [CrossRef]

170. Choi, S.J.; Choy, J.H. Layered double hydroxide nanoparticles as target-specific delivery carriers: Uptake mechanism and toxicity. *Nanomedicine* **2011**, *6*, 803–814. [CrossRef]

171. Jin, H.; Pi, J.; Zhao, Y.; Jiang, J.; Li, T.; Zeng, X.; Yang, P.; Evans, C.E.; Cai, J. EGFR-targeting PLGA-PEG nanoparticles as a curcumin delivery system for breast cancer therapy. *Nanoscale* **2017**, *9*, 16365–16374. [CrossRef] [PubMed]

172. Paolini, M.; Poul, L.; Berjaud, C.; Germain, M.; Darmon, A.; Bergere, M.; Pottier, A.; Levy, L.; Vibert, E. Nano-sized cytochrome P450 3A4 inhibitors to block hepatic metabolism of docetaxel. *Int. J. Nanomed.* **2017**, *12*, 5537–5556. [CrossRef] [PubMed]

173. Ahmad, N.; Alam, M.A.; Ahmad, R.; Naqvi, A.A.; Ahmad, F.J. Preparation and characterization of surface-modified PLGA-polymeric nanoparticles used to target treatment of intestinal cancer. *Artif. Cells Nanomed. Biotechnol.* **2018**, *46*, 432–446. [CrossRef] [PubMed]

174. Sharma, S.; Parmar, A.; Kori, S.; Sandhir, R. PLGA-based nanoparticles: A new paradigm in biomedical applications. *Trends Anal. Chem.* **2016**, *80*, 30–40. [CrossRef]

175. Navarro, S.M.; Morgan, T.W.; Astete, C.E.; Stout, R.W.; Coulon, D.; Mottram, P.; Sabliov, C.M. Biodistribution and toxicity of orally administered poly(lactic-*co*-glycolic) acid nanoparticles to F344 rats for 21 days. *Nanomedicine* **2016**, *11*, 1653–1669. [CrossRef] [PubMed]

4

Factorial Design as a Tool for the Optimization of PLGA Nanoparticles for the Co-Delivery of Temozolomide and O6-Benzylguanine

Maria João Ramalho, Joana A. Loureiro, Manuel A. N. Coelho and Maria Carmo Pereira *

LEPABE—Laboratory for Process Engineering, Environment, Biotechnology and Energy, Faculty of Engineering, University of Porto, Rua Dr. Roberto Frias, 4200-465 Porto, Portugal
* Correspondence: mcsp@fe.up.pt

Abstract: Poly(D,L-lactic-*co*-glycolic) (PLGA) nanoparticles (NPs) have been widely studied for several applications due to their advantageous properties, such as biocompatibility and biodegradability. Therefore, these nanocarriers could be a suitable approach for glioblastoma multiforme (GBM) therapy. The treatment of this type of tumours remains a challenge due to intrinsic resistance mechanisms. Thus, new approaches must be envisaged to target GBM tumour cells potentially providing an efficient treatment. Co-delivery of temozolomide (TMZ) and O6-benzylguanine (O6BG), an inhibitor of DNA repair, could provide good therapeutic outcomes. In this work, a fractional factorial design (FFD) was employed to produce an optimal PLGA-based nanoformulation for the co-loading of both molecules, using a reduced number of observations. The developed NPs exhibited optimal physicochemical properties for brain delivery (dimensions below 200 nm and negative zeta potential), high encapsulation efficiencies (EE) for both drugs, and showed a sustained drug release for several days. Therefore, the use of an FFD allowed for the development of a nanoformulation with optimal properties for the co-delivery of TMZ and O6BG to the brain.

Keywords: drug delivery; experimental design; fractional factorial design; O6-methylguanine DNA methyltransferase (MGMT) protein; glioblastoma multiforme

---

1. Introduction

Nanomedicine has been arousing increasing interest, since it allows the early diagnosis and monitoring of several diseases and also can increase the efficacy of conventional pharmacological treatments by enabling their controlled delivery [1–4]. Several materials have been widely studied for nanoparticles (NPs) development. Among polymeric materials, poly(D,L-lactic-*co*-glycolic) (PLGA) is perhaps the most used, due to being FDA-approved, biocompatible, biodegradable, and having tunable physicochemical properties [5]. Since these polymeric NPs allow the release of drugs in a controlled and sustained manner for long periods, the required drug doses and administration frequency can be minimized, decreasing the toxicity of the encapsulated drug [6]. Additionally, PLGA NPs are up-taken by endocytic mechanism, circumventing the p-glycoprotein-mediated cellular efflux, enabling drug accumulation in the target cells. Also, since this polymer can be easily functionalized with different materials, the design of NPs with diverse targeting moieties can be achieved [7].

Therefore, several efforts have been conducted in seeking the development of PLGA NPs for novel therapies with several therapeutic drugs without reducing their bioavailability or activity. The entrapment of therapeutic drugs in PLGA NPs also allow a reduction in their toxicity, and therefore these NPs have been extensively studied for cancer treatment. Most particularly, several attempts to encapsulate temozolomide (TMZ) in PLGA NPs for brain delivery have been conducted [8]. TMZ, the gold standard treatment for glioblastoma multiforme (GBM), presents several limitations, as it has low bioavailability and high toxicity, reducing its pharmacological activity [9]. Therefore, TMZ encapsulation in a nanocarrier emerges as a suitable approach to increase its chemotherapeutic efficacy, since it will avoid drug elimination after administration and increase its accumulation in the target tissues. GBM is the brain cancer with a high mortality rate, since its classical therapy fails to effectively cure the disease [10]. Thus, it is urgent to find new approaches for its treatment.

In fact, different PLGA delivery nanosystems were developed for TMZ in the last decade. Jain et al., 2014 developed PLGA NPs for TMZ entrapment. Although exhibiting promising results, modifying the NPs' surface with a targeting moiety to improve the specificity of the nanocarriers could be a suitable strategy to enhance its efficiency [11]. Later, Ananta et al., 2016 prepared PLGA NPs that were not able to maintain a favorable sustained release of TMZ [12]. Also, some authors used active targeting strategies to increase the NPs specificity to GBM cells. In fact, Jain et al., 2011 modified the surface of PLGA NPs with transferrin molecules to promote transport across the blood–brain barrier (BBB). The developed nanocarriers enhanced the accumulation and cytotoxic effect of TMZ in mice's brains [13]. Lee et al., 2016 also functionalized PLGA NPs with folate molecules to increase the NPs accumulation in target cells, but the prepared nanosystems did not exhibit good encapsulation efficiency (EE) values [14]. Our group (2018) also developed anti-transferrin receptor monoclonal antibody modified PLGA NPs for the delivery of TMZ. The obtained results showed that PLGA NPs are a promising approach for GBM treatment with TMZ [15].

However, GBM patients usually exhibit low sensitivity to therapy due to intrinsic resistance mechanisms. The O6-methylguanine DNA methyltransferase (MGMT) protein is highlighted as one of the main causes of therapeutic failure of TMZ [16]. Therefore, new strategies to decrease resistance to therapy are necessary. A promising approach is the use of molecules that are able to revert or inhibit these intrinsic resistance mechanisms. Most recently, co-treatment with O6-benzylguanine (O6BG) has been explored to decrease the resistance to TMZ's therapy by binding to the MGMT protein, leading to its inhibition, and consequently hindering the repair of the damaged DNA [17,18]. Nanoencapsulation of O6BG may reduce its toxicity in healthy tissues by targeted delivery. Accumulation of O6BG in healthy tissues is undesirable to avoid inactivation of the MGMT protein in these tissues, and consequently exacerbates the toxicity of alkylating agents, such as TMZ [19].

Also, systemic administration of two free drugs usually leads to infective pharmacological activity and, consequently, treatment failure, due to differences in the biodistribution profile of each drug [20]. Therefore, the entrapment of both drugs in NPs should address this problem. In fact, to increase therapeutic efficiency, the co-loading of TMZ with other molecules in PLGA NPs has also already been studied for glioblastoma therapy. Xu et al., 2016 proposed the co-delivery of TMZ with paclitaxel using PLGA NPs [21]. Until this moment, to the best of our knowledge, the co-encapsulation of TMZ and O6BG in a nanosystem was not reported. Thus, the aim of this work was to prepare a nanocarrier for the co-loading of both drugs.

However, the use of PLGA NPs faces a few limitations because of their poor loading capacity and the typical initial burst release. Additionally, the production of PLGA NPs requires different stages that can present high costs and be difficult to scale-up, such as centrifugation and dialysis. Also, it can be challenging to entrap hydrophilic drugs, since those exhibit a high partition into the aqueous phase during NPs preparation [6]. Therefore, is necessary to optimize the preparation methods. As well, usually the entrapment of two distinct molecules, with different physicochemical properties such as hydrophilicity and molecular weight, can be a challenging task. Though, high encapsulation of both drugs is desirable to increase the nanosystem efficiency and to reduce the amount of administered polymer. Also, it is essential to control the physicochemical properties of the developed NPs, such as size and surface charge, since these parameters control their biological fate, biodistribution, and toxicity, therefore affecting their therapeutic potential [22,23].

Therefore, experimental design could be a suitable approach to optimize the nanoformulation. In fact, in the last years, experimental design has been used for the optimization of drug-loaded NPs [24,25]. This is because a nanoformulation design requires full knowledge of the correlation between the experimental factors and the obtained NPs properties. To obtain an optimized nanoformulation using a conventional screening method (evaluating the effect of one experimental variable at a time) is expensive and time-consuming. Experimental design is therefore a validated and useful tool for the development and optimization of experimental procedures with a lower number of observations while still providing the desired information on the correlation between the experimental and the response variables. The obtained model can then be used for predicting future observations within the original design range [26]. Different types of experimental designs can be used, and in this work, a fractional factorial design (FFD) is proposed. When several experimental variables are being studied, FFD is a rapid and reliable tool, allowing the exploration of a maximum number of variables, while requiring less experimental observations, and still obtaining the desired information. However, since it uses only a partial combination of factors, some information about possible interactions can be lost [27].

Thus, the effect of five experimental variables on the physicochemical properties of the developed PLGA NPs and encapsulation efficiency (EE) of both drugs was studied in this work. The studied experimental factors were the amounts of TMZ, O6BG, surfactant, organic solvent, and polymer.

2. Materials and Methods

2.1. Materials

TMZ (MW 194.15, purity ≥99%) was purchased from Selleck Chemicals (Munich, Germany). O6BG (MW 241.25, purity ≥98%) was obtained from Abcam (Cambridge, UK). PLGA Resomer® RG503H (50:50; MW 24,000–38,000), poly(vinyl alcohol) (PVA) Mowiol® 4-88 (MW 31,000), phosphate buffer saline (PBS) and dichloromethane were acquired from Sigma–Aldrich (St. Louis, MO, USA). Uranyl acetate was provided by electron microscopy sciences (Hatfield, UK).

2.2. Preparation of TMZ+O6BG-Loaded PLGA NPs

For the synthesis of PLGA NPs loading, both TMZ and O6BG, a variation of the single emulsion–solvent evaporation method, were used [28]. Known amounts of PLGA, TMZ, and O6BG were dissolved in a dichloromethane solution. A 2% (*w*/*v*) PVA solution was added drop-by-drop to the prepared organic solution. Then, the solution was vortexed (Genius 3, ika®vortex, Germany) and placed in an ultrasonic bath at an ultrasonic frequency of 45 kHz (Ultrasonic cleaner, VWR™, Kuala Lumpur, Malaysia) to yield an oil-in-water (o-in-w) emulsion.

The emulsion was then poured into a 0.2% (*w*/*v*) PVA solution and maintained in unremitting agitation in a magnetic stirrer (800 rpm, Colorsquid, ika®, Staufen, Germany) until complete organic solvent evaporation (6 h). The suspension was then filtered using a membrane with a pore size of 200 nm, (polyethersulfone membrane syringe filter, VWR, Radnor, PA, USA) and stored at 4 °C overnight to increase the NPs' stability, avoiding their aggregation. After, the samples were centrifuged for 30 min at 14100× *g* (MiniSpin®plus, Eppendorf, Hamburg, Germany), to separate NPs from the non-encapsulated drug. The supernatant containing the non-encapsulated drug was saved for analysis.

2.3. Experimental Design and Data Analysis

High and comparable EE values for each drug are a prerequisite for the co-loading in the same NPs. In preliminary studies, it was verified that the co-encapsulation of TMZ and O6BG reduced the encapsulation of each drug alone. Thus, it was necessary to optimize the entrapment of both drugs. Also, it was important to control the physicochemical properties of the developed NPs, since these parameters influence the therapeutic efficacy and toxicity of the NPs. To obtain an optimized formulation, it is useful to study how the several experimental parameters influence the entire production process.

Therefore, a 2^{5-2} FFD was implemented using the Minitab Statistical Software (Minitab Inc., State college, PA, USA) to determine the effect of different experimental factors on the PLGA NPs features. The studied independent variables were the amount of both used drugs, the quantity of surfactant and organic solvent, and the amount of polymer. A variation of a full factorial design, in which only a subset of the total runs was performed, took place. The chosen factors of interest were varied on two levels (determined in preliminary studies) according to the experimental plan presented in Table 1. Two replicates were conducted for each combination and for center levels, and the order of the experiments was randomly sorted to avoid any bias.

Table 1. Process and formulation parameters of the used FFD.

Parameter	Component	Units	Applied Level		
			Low Level (−1)	Centre Level (0)	High Level (+1)
X_1	m_{TMZ}	mg	0.250	0.625	1
X_2	m_{O6BG}	mg	0.250	0.625	1
X_3	$\%_{PVA}$	% (w/v)	2	3	4
X_4	V_{DCM}	mL	0.50	0.75	1
X_5	m_{PLGA}	mg	10	15	20

Note: m_{TMZ}—Mass of TMZ; m_{O6BG}—Mass of O6BG; $\%_{PVA}$—percent weight per volume of PVA; V_{DCM}—Volume of dichloromethane; m_{PLGA}—mass of PLGA.

The observed response dependent variables were the NPs size, PdI, zeta potential values, and EE of both TMZ and O6BG. For the experimental design, 18 formulations were prepared, and an outline of the experimental plan and its results is shown in Table 2.

Table 2. Outline of the experimental design and results. The experimental levels (low, centre, and high) are represented by the coded values of −1, 0, and +1, respectively.

Run Order	Coded Independent Variables					Measured Dependent Variables				
	X_1	X_2	X_3	X_4	X_5	Mean Size (nm)	PdI	Zeta Potential (mV)	EE (%)	
									TMZ	O6BG
1	+1	+1	−1	+1	−1	183	0.148	−26.2	55.1	78.5
2	−1	+1	+1	−1	−1	202	0.110	−26.7	38.7	74.1
3	0	0	0	0	0	173	0.115	−23.4	45.1	71.6
4	+1	+1	−1	+1	−1	179	0.165	−24.1	56.7	80.8
5	−1	−1	−1	+1	+1	178	0.132	−24.4	53.5	94.0
6	−1	+1	−1	−1	+1	193	0.158	−22.4	52.3	91.6
7	+1	−1	−1	−1	−1	162	0.158	−27.5	31.8	99.0
8	0	0	0	0	0	178	0.127	− 22.1	44.7	77.3
9	−1	−1	+1	+1	−1	192	0.190	−27.0	42.6	79.7
10	+1	+1	+1	+1	+1	171	0.142	−20.3	27.2	78.5
11	+1	−1	+1	−1	+1	200	0.137	−22.7	40.3	99.8
12	+1	−1	+1	−1	+1	205	0.109	−22.5	46.3	99.6
13	+1	+1	+1	+1	+1	180	0.118	−22.3	28.9	82.6
14	+1	−1	−1	−1	−1	176	0.125	−28.0	36.6	99.5
15	−1	+1	−1	−1	+1	189	0.130	−21.7	50.9	95.5
16	−1	−1	−1	+1	+1	172	0.158	−23.4	54.5	98.0
17	−1	−1	+1	+1	−1	184	0.146	−26.2	46.7	78.1
18	−1	+1	+1	−1	−1	205	0.141	−27.5	36.5	76.9

The applied experimental design accounts for main terms and two-factor interactions terms. The latter refers to two different variables that interact with each other, creating a combined effect on the response that independently would not occur. Therefore, the main effects and the two-factor interactions are accounted for in the used regression model. Thus, regression equations were obtained for each studied dependent variable to quantify the relationship between these and all the experimental independent variables. The experimental data was then fitted to the following polynomial regression Equation (1) [29]:

$$Y = \beta_0 + \sum_{i=1}^{5} \beta_i X_i + \sum \beta_{ij} X_i X_j \quad (1)$$

in which Y is the predicted response; β_0 is the intercept term and the remaining term; $X_{i,j}$ is the studied levels of the independent variables; and $\beta_{j,i}$ is the fitted coefficients for $X_{i,j}$.

The statistical regression models for the different dependent variables were fitted independently. Additionally, the polynomial equations were statistically validated using ANOVA (Analysis of Variance) by statistical significance of coefficients, R^2 values, and normal distribution of the residues. Minitab Statistical Software was also used for the statistical analysis of the data.

2.4. *TMZ+O6BG-Loaded PLGA NPs Physicochemical Characterization*

2.4.1. Dynamic Light Scattering for Size Determination

The mean diameter and size distribution of the prepared NPs were evaluated by dynamic light scattering (DLS). The measurements were performed in a ZetaSizer Nano ZS (Malvern Instruments, Worcestershire, UK). The attained data is given in intensity distribution. The intensity-weighted mean diameter (Z-average) is given. For the optimized formulation, at least three independent measurements were performed, and obtained results are expressed as the mean and standard deviation (SD). Statistical analysis was performed using the *t*-student test, and p-values ≤ 0.05 were considered significant.

2.4.2. Laser Doppler Velocimetry Method for Zeta Potential Determination

The zeta potential values of the prepared NPs were determined by laser doppler velocimetry method. The measurements were also performed in a ZetaSizer Nano ZS (Malvern Instruments, Worcestershire, UK). The analysis was performed using the dielectric constant of water. For the optimized formulation, at least three independent measurements were performed, and obtained results are expressed as the mean and SD. Statistical analysis was performed using the *t*-student test.

2.4.3. Transmission Electron Microscopy for Morphological Analysis

The morphological analysis of the NPs was obtained by transmission electron microscopy (TEM). The NPs were prepared on copper grids (Formvar/Carbon-400 mesh Copper, Agar Scientific, Essex, UK) and negatively stained. For that, 10 µL of samples were stained with 2% (*v*/*v*) uranyl acetate for 45 s, and air-dried. This is a heavy metal salt able to scatter electrons, enhancing the contrast to better visualize the samples [30]. Then, the NPs were visualized using a JEM 1400 electron microscope (Jeol, Tokyo, Japan) at an accelerating voltage of 80 kV.

2.5. *TMZ+O6BG-Loaded PLGA NPs Stability Studies*

The stability of the prepared PLGA NPs was analysed through size and zeta potential variations. PLGA NPs' dispersions in ultrapure water were stored at 4 °C and DLS measurements were performed at different timepoints to evaluate variations in PLGA NPs size and zeta potential values. These measurements were performed weekly, for 6 weeks. For optimized nanoformulation, three independent samples were used.

2.6. *Drug Encapsulation Efficiency of TMZ+O6BG-PLGA NPs*

The TMZ and O6BG EE values of the prepared PLGA NPs were assessed by UV–Vis spectrophotometry, using the following Equation (2):

$$EE = \frac{total\ amount\ of\ drug - \ amount\ of\ free\ drug}{total\ amount\ of\ drug} \times 100 \tag{2}$$

Non-encapsulated TMZ and O6BG molecules were separated from the NPs colloidal suspension by centrifugation (30 min, 14100× *g*, MiniSpin®plus, Eppendorf, Germany) and quantified (UV-1700 PharmaSpec UV-Vis spectrophotometer, Shimadzu, Kyoto, Japan) at 240 nm and 329 nm for O6BG and TMZ, respectively. The results were correlated to control samples corresponding to total amount of drug. For the optimized formulation, three independent experiments were conducted, and obtained results are expressed as the mean and SD. Statistical analysis was performed using the *t*-student test.

2.7. In Vitro Release of TMZ and O6BG from PLGA NPs

To assess the drug release profile of the developed NPs, in vitro dialysis studies were performed for 20 days at 37 °C. For that, a cellulose dialysis membrane (Float-A-Lyzer G2, CE, 10KDa, SpectrumLabs, Los Angles, CA, USA) was rinsed in ultrapure water for 24 h before the beginning of the experiments and equilibrated with release medium 1 h before the dialysis.

A known amount of TMZ+O6BG-PLGA NPs diluted in 2 mL of release medium was placed into the inner space of the dialysis membrane. The outside space was filled with a known volume of release medium to ensure sink conditions. PBS (pH 7.4, 0.01 M) was used as the release buffer to mimic the physiological salt concentrations and pH of blood plasma. The dialysis membrane was kept in continuous stirring at 200 rpm at 37 °C, simulating the physiological temperature. The amount of drug release at predetermined timepoints (0, 6, and 24 h; and day 3, 6, 8, 9, 11, 13, 16, and 20) was quantified by UV-Vis spectrophotometry (UV-1700 PharmaSpec UV-Vis spectrophotometer, Shimadzu, Kyoto, Japan). A solution of TMZ and O6BG in PBS was used as control. For the optimized formulation, three independent experiments were conducted, and obtained results are expressed as the mean and SD. Statistical analysis was performed using the *t*-student test.

The TMZ and O6BG release curves, representing the percentage of drug released in function of time, were then plotted by the following Equation (3):

$$\%\ drug\ released = \frac{amount\ of\ drug\ released\ at\ time\ t}{amount\ of\ encapsulated\ drug} \times 100 \tag{3}$$

3. Results and Discussion

3.1. Statistical Analysis of Experimental Data

The applied experimental design allowed the identification of the experimental factors influencing the physicochemical properties of the NPs, astheir size and the encapsulation efficiency of both drugs on the polymeric matrix. Since zeta potential (≤ -20 mV) and PdI values (<0.2) were always inside the desired range, they were not considered for this model.

Previous nanoformulation studies were conducted to identify the five major experimental variables that affect the PLGA NPs properties, such as size and EE of both drugs. The amount of TMZ, O6BG, surfactant, organic solvent, and polymer were chosen and varied in two levels. The levels choice was based on the knowledge acquired in the preliminary experiments. All other parameters, such as type of surfactant and organic solvent, aqueous to organic phase ratio, time of sonication, ultrasonic frequency of sonication, process temperature, and emulsification and evaporation processes, were maintained constantly.

The mathematical model (Equation (1)) was fitted to the data and statistical analysis was performed using ANOVA (Table 3). As Table 3 shows, the model is statistically significant ($p < 0.05$) with insignificant lack of fit ($p > 0.05$) for all the chosen responses. Hence, the linear model was acceptable for response prediction within the range of experimental variables.

Table 3. Results of analysis of variance (ANOVA) for the regression models. Non-significant factors are marked as blue.

Source	Size, Y_1 (nm)				EE of TMZ, Y_2 (%)				EE of O6BG, Y_3 (%)			
	SS	df	*F*-Value	*p*-Value	SS	Df	*F*-Value	*p*-Value	SS	df	*F*-Value	*p*-Value
Model	4192.98	7	17.06	0.0001	1381.55	7	41.63	<0.0001	4311.36	7	35.96	<0.0001
X_1	12.20	1	8.92	0.0199	55.29	1	11.66	0.0244	170.83	1	9.97	0.0586
X_2	117.63	1	14.74	0.0200	41.70	1	8.80	0.0510	190.31	1	11.11	0.0520
X_3	3452.85	1	30.67	<0.0001	194.24	1	40.97	0.0001	1788.94	1	104.45	<0.0001
X_4	49.99	1	1.42	0.1263	46.25	1	9.76	0.0208	134.43	1	7.85	0.0745
X_5	100.42	1	11.41	0.0224	260.82	1	55.02	<0.0001	1843.34	1	107.63	<0.0001
X_2X_3	313.15	1	23.14	0.0057	350.60	1	74.20	<0.0001	173.67	1	10.14	0.0577
X_2X_5	146.75	1	18.42	0.0176	432.64	1	91.26	<0.0001	9.83	1	0.57	0.8480
Residual	351.06	10			47.40	10			171.27	10		
Lack of Fit	46.42	1	1.37	0.2716	2.77	1	0.56	0.4742	29.41	1	1.87	0.2051
Pure Error	304.64	9			44.64	9			141.86	9		
Cor Total	4544.04	17			1428.95	17			4482.63	17		
R^2		0,9227				0,9668				0,9618		

Figure 1 also shows a satisfactory agreement between experimental observations and predicted response, proving that the applied regression model is suitable for the determination of the optimal experimental settings for the preparation of NPs.

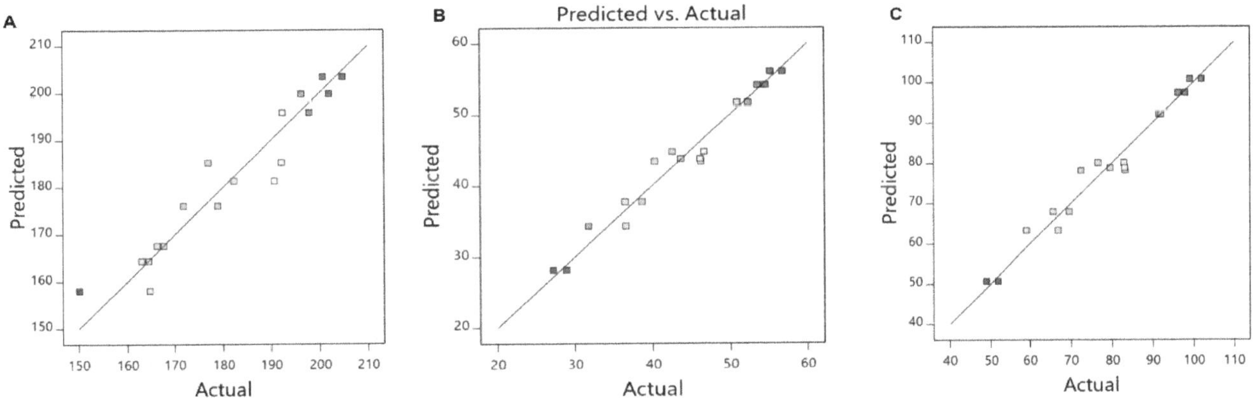

Figure 1. Graphical plots of the experimental values versus the model predicted values for (**A**) mean size, (**B**) EE for TMZ, and (**C**) EE for O6BG. Red dots indicate high values and blue dots low values, respectively.

The statistical analysis of the obtained results also allowed the determination of the regression coefficient (RC) values that describes the direction of the relationship between an experimental variable and the variable response. A negative sign before a factor indicates that the response decreases, whereas a positive sign shows that the response increases with the experimental factor. With the RC values, it was possible to obtain the polynomial regression equation for each studied response, quantifying the relationship between each of the studied experimental variables and the response. The non-significant factors ($p > 0.05$) were excluded from the mathematical model, allowing the reduction in complexity of the attained equations.

Response surface analysis and contour graphs were plotted based on the determined model polynomial function in a three and a two-dimensional model, respectively, illustrating the effect of the chosen significant independent factors on each observed response. The effect of all the independent variables on each dependent variable was studied and the effects of the most significant variables are discussed in detail below.

3.1.1. Effect on NPs' Size

The size of the NPs is a critical property, influencing its half-life, biodistribution, and cellular internalization. The size of the NPs ranged from 162 nm (sample 7) to 205 nm (sample 12). Almost all the studied variables significantly affected the size of the NPs ($p < 0.05$), as shown in Table 3.

The polynomial Equation (4) describes the relationship between the significant studied experimental variables ($p < 0.05$) and the size of the NPs:

$$\begin{aligned} Size = \ & 134.9 - 9.67\, amount\ TMZ\ (mg) + 83.9\, amount\ O6BG\ (mg) \\ & + 15.05\, amount\ PVA\ (\%) + 1.644\, amount\ PLGA\ (mg) \\ & - 13.41\, amount\ O6BG\ (mg) \times amount\ PVA\ (\%) \\ & - 2.541\, amount\ O6BG\ (mg) \times amount\ PLGA\ (mg) \end{aligned} \quad (4)$$

The experimental factor that most significantly affected NPs size was the amount of surfactant, which exhibited a positive effect on the size of the NPs. Thus, an increase in PVA concentration led to an increase in NP size. Although using a high quantity of surfactant can induce the creation and stabilization of smaller NPs due to a reduction of the interfacial tension between the polymer and the external aqueous phase [31], the opposite effect was verified. This may be explained by the increased viscosity of the aqueous phase when increasing the PVA concentration. A higher viscosity decreases the shear stress, originating emulsion droplets with larger sizes. Also, higher amounts of surfactant can promote the coalescence of the NPs, yielding NPs with larger diameters [32]. Also, some studies report that residual PVA remains at the surface, contributing to the size increase [33].

Additionally, the amount of PLGA also exhibited a significantly positive effect on the size of the NPs ($p < 0.05$). Increasing the polymer amount increases the viscosity of the organic phase, decreasing the shear stress, as mentioned above. Also, the augmented viscosity hampers the diffusion of the organic solvent into the aqueous phase, leading to the formation of larger emulsion droplets, originating larger NPs after solvent evaporation [34].

Higher initial loading of O6BG positively affected the NPs size ($p < 0.05$), since it will result in higher drug loading, as will be discussed later. The contrary was observed for TMZ amount ($p < 0.05$), since higher amounts of TMZ will decrease its entrapment, as will also be discussed later.

Response surface analysis and contour graphs were plotted (Figure 2) based on this model polynomial function. Contour and surface response plots allowed visual identification of the optimal levels of each factor, to choose the most suitable values for the development of an optimal formulation. Both response surface and contour plots (Figure 2A,B) showed that the lower the amount of PVA and PLGA, the lower the NPs size, as already predicted by the calculated positive RC values (Equation (4)). Thus, optimal nanoformulation with small dimensions would fall into the low and central levels of both factors.

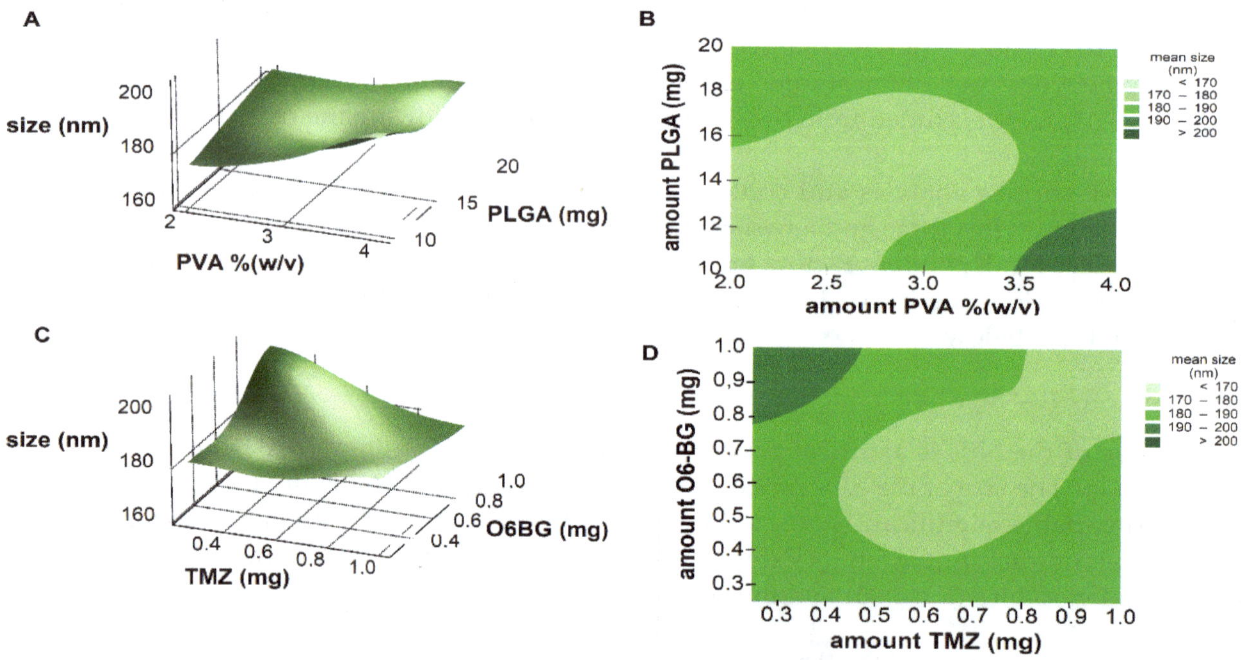

Figure 2. (**A**) Response surface plot and (**B**) contour plot showing the effect of two factors (amount of PVA and PLGA) on the resulting NPs size. (**C**) Response surface plot and (**D**) contour plot showing the effect of two factors (amount of TMZ and O6BG) on the resulting NPs size.

In addition to all the five factors significantly affecting the NPs size, some significant two-factor interactions were observed (Table 3). Interaction plots on Figure 3 show high interaction between two factors. Each point in the interaction plot shows the mean size values at different combinations of factor levels. As the lines are not parallel, with different slopes, the plot indicates that there is an interaction between the two factors [35]. The same is verified in all the attained interaction plots.

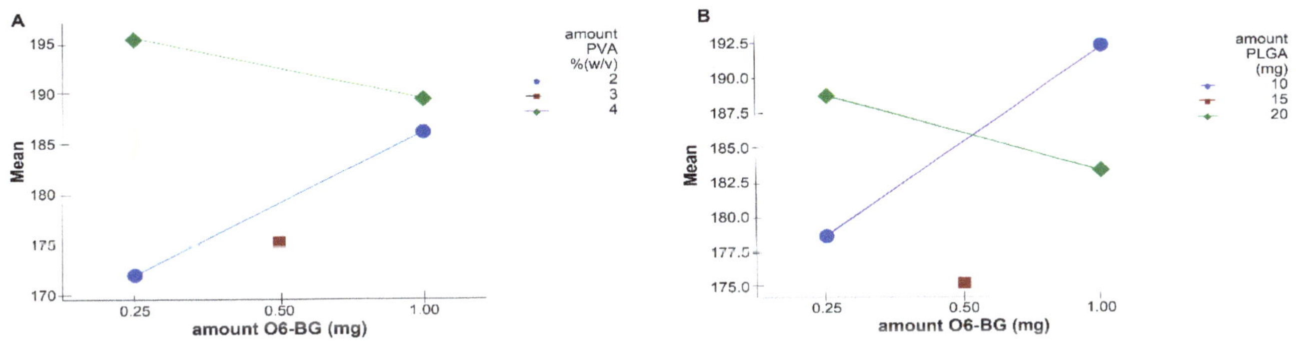

Figure 3. Interaction plots for size data means showing significant two-way interaction terms for the independent variables. Solid blue lines display factor at low level, whereas dashed green lines are the high level of the factors. (**A**) interaction term X_2X_3: amount of O6BG/amount of surfactant, (**B**) X_2X_5: amount of O6BG/amount of PLGA.

The main effects can be confused with the two-factor interactions, which explains the results obtained in Figure 2. Although Equation (4) predicts that the lower the amount of TMZ and the higher the amount of O6BG, the higher the NPs size, optimal values fall into high levels of both TMZ and O6BG. As shown in Figure 3A,B, at low levels of both PLGA and PVA amounts, O6BG positively affects the size of the NPs. On the other hand, at high levels of PLGA and PVA, increasing the O6BG amount decreases the size of the NPs.

3.1.2. Effect on the Encapsulation Efficiency of TMZ

High encapsulation of the drug is desirable to increase the nanosystem efficiency and to reduce the amount of administered polymer. The EE values for TMZ in the prepared NPs ranged from 27.2 (sample 10) to 56.7% (sample 4).

The polynomial Equation (5) describes the relationship between the significant studied experimental variables ($p < 0.05$) and the EE of TMZ:

$$\begin{aligned} EE\%\ TMZ = \ & 11.84 - 8.80\ amount\ TMZ\ (mg) - 3.40\ amount\ PVA\ (\%) \\ & + 7.95\ amount\ DCM\ (mL) + 1.461\ amount\ PLGA\ (mg) \\ & -13.87\ amount\ O6BG(mg) \times amount\ PVA\ (\%) \\ & - 2.153\ amount\ O6BG\ (mg) \times amount\ PLGA\ (mg) \end{aligned} \quad (5)$$

EE values were significantly influenced by almost all the studied independent variables, as shown by the calculated p-values on Table 3. All the experimental variables show a positive effect on the EE of TMZ, except PVA concentration and TMZ amount. PLGA had a positive effect on the EE of TMZ. As already mentioned, a higher amount of PLGA polymer results in larger NPs and, consequently, higher encapsulation of the drug. Also, the increased viscosity caused by higher PLGA concentration mentioned above could complicate the diffusion of TMZ molecules into the aqueous phase, enhancing the drug's entrapment into the NPs' polymeric matrix [36]. On the other hand, increased volumes of organic solvent increased drug solubility, therefore increasing drug entrapment.

Also, the encapsulation of TMZ decreased with PVA concentration due to a higher partition of TMZ molecules into the aqueous phase during emulsification, decreasing the EE values. It is reported that drug molecules can diffuse out from the oil nanodroplets and solubilize in PVA micelles at the aqueous phase [37]. Increasing the TMZ amount may cause saturation of the organic phase, leading to the partition of the drug molecules to the aqueous phase, lowering its entrapment in the polymeric matrix.

Response surface analysis and contour graphs (Figure 4) show that the optimal formulation would be prepared with low amounts of PVA and TMZ, and high amounts of PLGA and organic solvent.

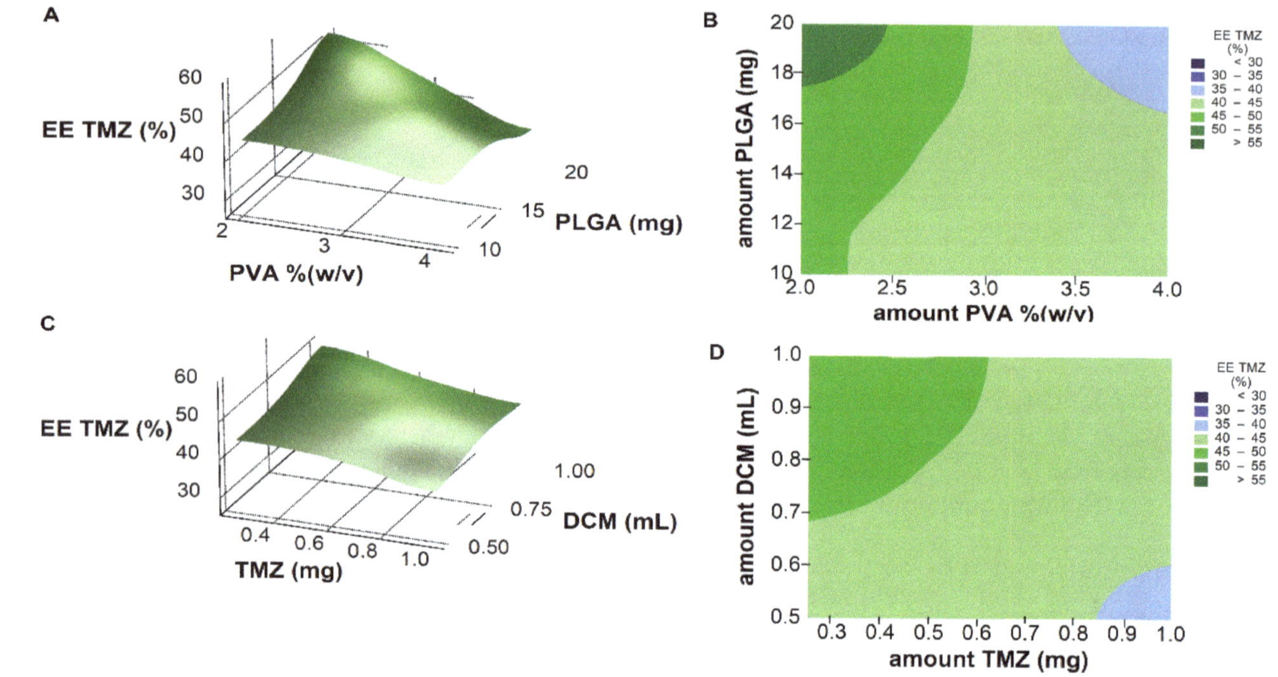

Figure 4. (**A**) Response surface plot and (**B**) contour plot showing the effect of two factors (amount of PVA and PLGA, respectively) on the resulting EE TMZ values. (**C**) Response surface plot and (**D**) contour plot showing the effect of two factors (amount of TMZ and DCM, respectively) on the resulting EE TMZ values.

All five studied variables were part of an extensive interaction system. A significant two-factor interaction of O6BG amount with both PLGA and PVA amounts (Table 3) was verified ($p < 0.05$), as shown in Figure 5.

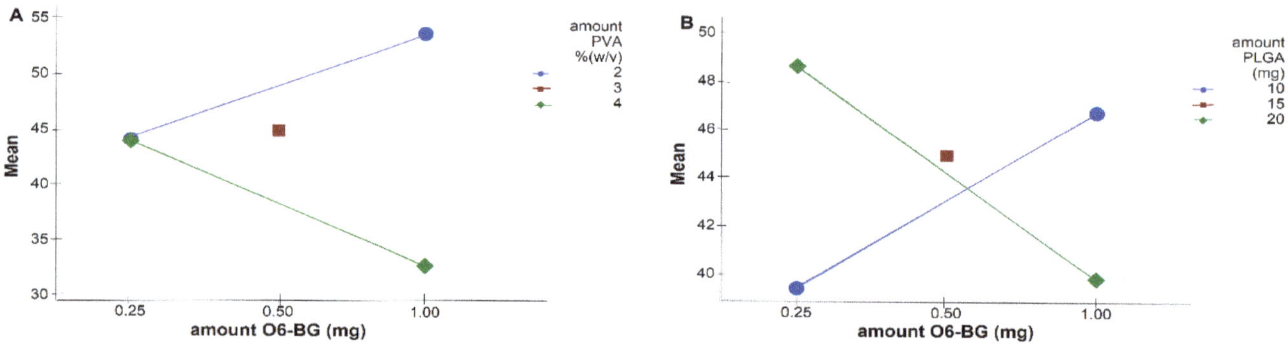

Figure 5. Interaction plots for EE of TMZ data means showing significant two-way interaction terms for the dependent variables. Solid blue lines display factors at a low level, whereas green dashed lines are the high level of the factors. (**A**) interaction term X_2X_3: amount of O6BG/amount of surfactant, (**B**) X_2X_5: amount of O6BG/amount of PLGA.

The described two-factor interaction between the PVA and O6BG amounts shows a significant PVA concentration effect and interaction term (Figure 5A). There is a difference among the means of the two PVA levels, but not a difference in the means among O6BG amount. This proves that although the amount of O6BG did not show a significant direct effect on the EE values, the interaction term exists. The amount of O6BG affected the nanoformulation at both low and high PVA amounts. At low PVA levels, the O6BG amount showed a positive effect in the TMZ encapsulation. The opposite was observed at high PVA amounts.

The same is verified in the two-factor interaction between the PLGA and O6BG amounts (Figure 5B).

3.1.3. Effect on the Encapsulation Efficiency of O6BG

The EE values of O6BG in the prepared NPs ranged from 70.9 (sample 3) to 99.8% (sample 11).

The polynomial Equation (6) describes the relationship between the significant studied experimental variables ($p < 0.05$) and the EE of O6BG:

$$E\%\ O6BG = 104.4 - 4.12\, amount\ PVA\ (\%) + 0.854\, amount\ PLGA\ (mg) \quad (6)$$

PVA and PLGA amounts were the only studied independent variables that significantly influenced the EE values, as shown by the calculated *p*-values on Table 3. While PLGA concentration showed a positive effect on the EE of O6BG, PVA concentration exhibited a negative influence. In fact, increasing PVA concentration hampered the encapsulation of the drug, since it enhanced the partition of O6BG molecules into the aqueous phase during emulsification, decreasing the encapsulation efficiencies values [37]. Also, as already mentioned, higher amounts of PLGA polymer resulted in larger NPs and, consequently, higher encapsulation of the drug. Also, the increased viscosity caused by higher PLGA concentration mentioned above could complicate the diffusion of O6BG molecules into the aqueous phase, enhancing the drug's entrapment into the NPs' polymeric matrix [36].

Response surface analysis and contour graphs (Figure 6) show that predicted optimal nanoformulation with high O6BG molecules entrapment would fall into the high levels of PLGA and low levels of surfactant concentration. No significant two-factor interactions were observed.

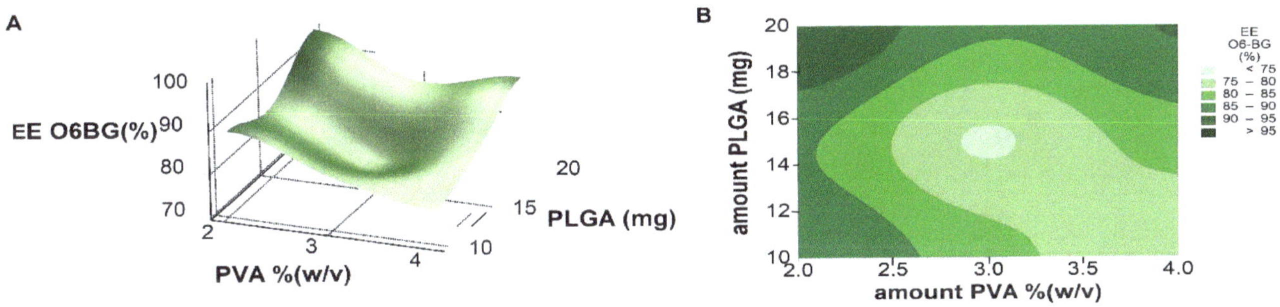

Figure 6. (**A**) Response surface plot and (**B**) contour plot showing the effect of two factors (amount of PLGA and PVA, respectively) on the resulting EE values.

3.2. *Nanoformulation Optimization and Physicochemical Characterization*

The optimization process was performed by determining the optimal experimental values, which were obtained by solving the three determined polynomial regression equations and grid searching in the response surface graphs or contour plots applying the following criteria: to minimize the particle size (Y_1), and to maximize the EE values for both drugs (Y_2 and Y_3). The optimum levels of the formulation factors are presented in Table 4.

Table 4. Optimal formulation parameters for the PLGA NPs determined by the experimental design.

Parameter	Component	Units	Optimal Value
X_1	m_{TMZ}	mg	1
X_2	m_{O6BG}	mg	1
X_3	$\%_{PVA}$	% (*w*/*v*)	0.5
X_4	V_{DCM}	mL	1
X_5	m_{PLGA}	mg	15

A formulation checkpoint was prepared according to the predicted model to validate the reliability and the precision of the factorial design, using these optimal experimental conditions. The checkpoint formulation was prepared in triplicates and the properties of the attained NPs were within the range of the predicted values, as shown in Table 5.

Table 5. Validation of the model by comparing the predicted values with the observed experimental values. The experimental data is given as the mean ± SD ($n = 3$).

	Size (Y_1) (nm)	EE TMZ (Y_2) (%)	EE O6BG (Y_3) (%)
Predicted values	173 (164–180)	68 (63–73)	89 (83–95)
Experimental values	177 ± 4	63 ± 4	90 ± 4
Experimental error	2%	7%	1%

Higher encapsulation verified for O6BG can be explained by its greater affinity for the organic phase, compared with TMZ. While TMZ exhibits a log P value of 0.36, for O6BG, log P is 1.66 (values obtained from Marvin Sketch Calculator software. Chemaxon™,Version 16.4.25, Budapest, Hungary).

The developed NPs exhibit mean dimensions suitable for brain delivery. Although PdI and zeta potential values were not considered for the model, they were also determined for the checkpoint formulations. The developed NPs exhibited zeta potential values of −22 ± 1 mV and PdI values of 0.19 ± 0.01. The high negative zeta potential values are associated with low toxicity [38] and suggest that the NPs are stable [39]. In fact, all the nanoformulations prepared in the 18 runs of the FFD (data not shown) and the checkpoint formulations proved to be stable in storage conditions for at least six weeks, as shown in Figure 7.

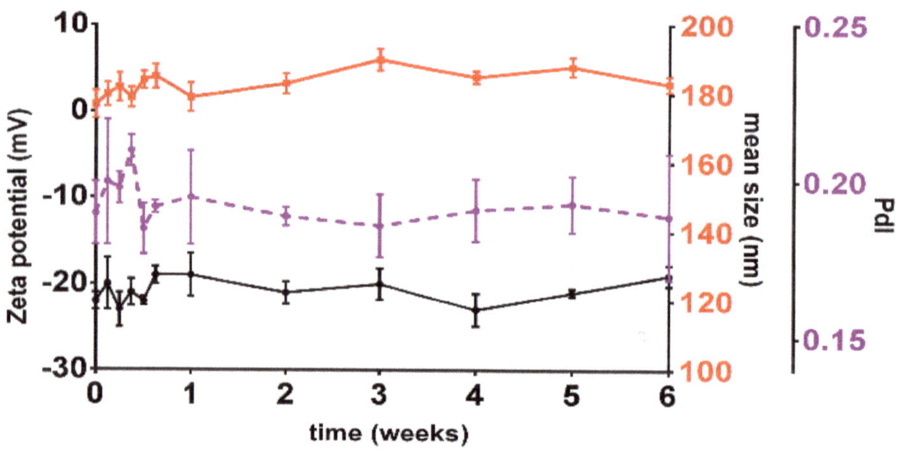

Figure 7. Stability of the prepared checkpoint nanoformulations. Black line: Graphical representation of variations in zeta potential values over 6 weeks (data plotted on the left Y-axis); Red line: Graphical representation of variations in mean sizes over 6 weeks (data plotted on the first right Y-axis); Purple line: Graphical representation of variations in PdI values over 6 weeks (data plotted on the second right Y-axis). Results are given as mean ± SD ($n = 3$).

The stability of the prepared colloidal suspension NPs is granted by a PVA layer on the NP's surface. During the NPs preparation, the PVA molecules adsorb on the surface of the resultant nanodroplets acting as a mechanic barrier that prevent coalescence and avoid NPs' aggregation [40]. TEM image (Figure 8) shows this stabilizer layer around the NPs' surface. Also, the attained PdI values suggest that the colloidal suspension is monodisperse. Therefore, it can be concluded that the method followed for the preparation of PLGA NPs produced well-stabilized monodisperse O6BG+TMZ-loaded PLGA NPs.

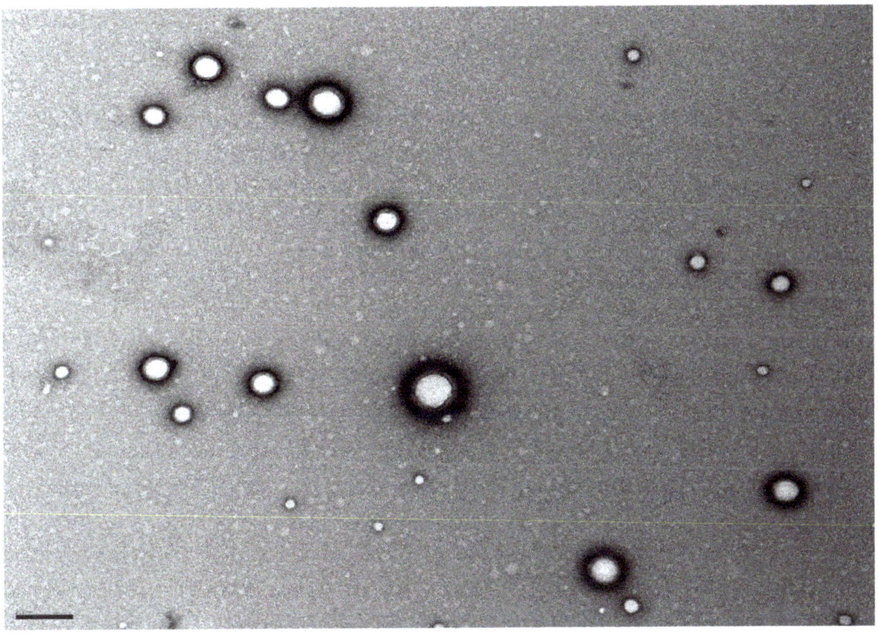

Figure 8. TEM photograph showing the morphology of the developed PLGA NPs. Scale bar is 200 nm.

3.3. Drug Release from the PLGA NPs

For the evaluation of the in vitro release profile of the developed NPs, the dialysis method was used. To simulate the physiological conditions (temperature, salt concentration, and pH), the release studies were conducted at 37 °C in PBS (10 mM, pH 7.4). The release curves were plotted and are shown in Figure 9.

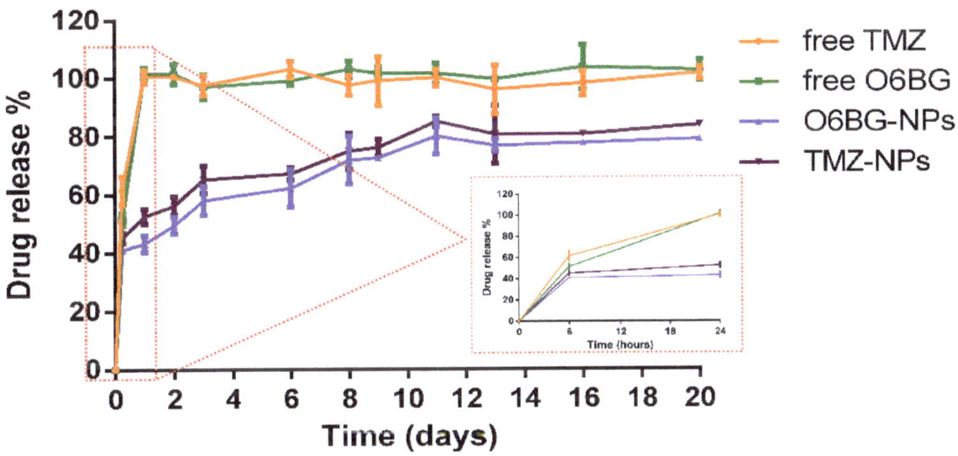

Figure 9. In vitro release of TMZ and O6BG from PLGA NPs in PBS (10 mM, pH 7.4) at 37 °C. Free TMZ and O6BG were used as control. Results are given as mean ± SD ($n = 3$). An enlargement of the first time points—6 and 24 h—is presented to highlight the burst effect.

PLGA NPs showed an initial burst release for both drugs, due to the presence of the drug molecules adsorbed at the NPs' surface. As Figure 9 depicts, at the first 24 h, 48 ± 3% of the total TMZ and 43 ± 3% of the total O6BG were released. Then, both drugs located at the polymeric matrix of the NPs were released in a slower and controlled manner that was prolonged for 20 days.

A faster release for TMZ was verified in comparison to O6BG. The PLGA NPs exhibited a release of TMZ of 81 ± 1% after 20 days, while for O6BG, only about 79 ± 1% of the entrapped drug was released at day 20 (Figure 9). This may occur due to the higher affinity of TMZ to the aqueous buffer (lower log P values). However, the release profile is similar for the two drugs, due to the erosion of the polymer matrix that allows the release of both molecules.

The obtained release profile proved that the developed PLGA NPs are able to maintain the sustained and controlled release of both TMZ and O6BG, and therefore could be used for the co-delivery of entrapped molecules. Further optimization of the release profile to reduce the initial burst release may improve the efficiency of the nanovehicle.

4. Conclusions

PLGA NPs as drug delivery systems have gained increasing interest in the last years, due to their unique physicochemical properties, such as stability, biocompatibility, and biodegradability. Encapsulating drugs in PLGA NPs allows them to maximize their therapeutic effects and to minimize their side effects. Since the biological fate and toxicity of the NPs depend on their physicochemical properties, the developed nanosystems must meet several criteria to be appropriate for brain delivery.

PLGA NPs for the entrapment of both TMZ and O6BG for further GBM treatment were developed in this work. TMZ is the used drug for GBM chemotherapy, and despite its therapeutics effects being well-known, the drug is not able to effectively cure GBM patients. Intrinsic resistance mechanisms are of one of the major obstacles for GBM treatment, due to the DNA repair by the MGMT protein. To overcome this issue, co-therapy with TMZ and an inhibitor of the MGMT protein, O6BG, was proposed. O6BG is a guanine analogue able to inhibit the activity of the MGMT protein, hampering the DNA repair. Thus, O6BG could decrease the resistance to TMZ's therapy.

Hence, an optimized nanoformulation was developed in this work, and for that, FFD was used. FFD proved to be a suitable approach for the design of co-loaded NPs allowing to optimize the single emulsion solvent evaporation production process with a low replica number in a reliable and precise manner. The regression analysis of the results proved to adequate to identify the main experimental variables affecting the physicochemical properties of the developed NPs. The optimal experimental conditions were chosen, and the optimal nanoformulation was prepared using 1 mg of both drugs, 0.5% (*w*/*v*) of PVA, 1 mL of dichloromethane, and 15 mg of PLGA.

The developed NPs exhibited high encapsulation efficiencies for both drugs and showed a sustained drug release. Thus, it is expected that these nanocarriers will provide an effective brain delivery, allowing the drug to reach the brain at desirable doses, leading to a significant improvement on the GBM treatment.

PLGA NPs provide a novel and potentially efficient approach for the co-administration of TMZ and O6BG, presenting a potential solution for the intrinsic resistance mechanisms to TMZ due to MGMT high expression. Though these NPs could potentially overcome the limitations of the currently available therapies, future in vitro and in vivo tests are necessary to assess the nanosystem efficacy.

Author Contributions: All authors contributed to the conceptualization of the experiments. M.J.R. conducted the experiments, data analyses, and the writing of the manuscript. M.d.C.P contributed to the review and editing of the manuscript.

Acknowledgments: The authors are grateful to Simone Morais for her comments and suggestions during the preparation of this manuscript.

References

1. Hou, W.; Xia, F.; Alfranca, G.; Yan, H.; Zhi, X.; Liu, Y.; Peng, C.; Zhang, C.; de la Fuente, J.M.; Cui, D. Nanoparticles for multi-modality cancer diagnosis: Simple protocol for self-assembly of gold nanoclusters mediated by gadolinium ions. *Biomaterials* **2017**, *120*, 103–114. [CrossRef] [PubMed]

2. Darvishi Cheshmeh Soltani, R.; Jorfi, S.; Safari, M.; Rajaei, M.-S. Enhanced sonocatalysis of textile wastewater using bentonite-supported ZnO nanoparticles: Response surface methodological approach. *J. Environ. Manag.* **2016**, *179*, 47–57. [CrossRef] [PubMed]
3. Dalvand, A.; Nabizadeh, R.; Reza Ganjali, M.; Khoobi, M.; Nazmara, S.; Hossein Mahvi, A. Modeling of Reactive Blue 19 azo dye removal from colored textile wastewater using L-arginine-functionalized Fe3O4 nanoparticles: Optimization, reusability, kinetic and equilibrium studies. *J. Magn. Magn. Mater.* **2016**, *404*, 179–189. [CrossRef]
4. Andrade, S.; Ramalho, M.J.; Loureiro, J.A.; Pereira, M.C. Interaction of Natural Compounds with Biomembrane Models: A Biophysical Approach for the Alzheimer's Disease Therapy. *Colloids Surf. B Biointerfaces* **2019**, *180*, 83–92. [CrossRef] [PubMed]
5. Ramalho, M.J.; Pereira, M.C. Preparation and Characterization of Polymeric Nanoparticles: An Interdisciplinary Experiment. *J. Chem. Educ.* **2016**, *93*, 1446–1451. [CrossRef]
6. Makadia, H.K.; Siegel, S.J. Poly Lactic-co-Glycolic Acid (PLGA) as Biodegradable Controlled Drug Delivery Carrier. *Polymers* **2011**, *3*, 1377–1397. [CrossRef] [PubMed]
7. Danhier, F.; Ansorena, E.; Silva, J.M.; Coco, R.; Le Breton, A.; Preat, V. PLGA-based nanoparticles: An overview of biomedical applications. *J. Control Release* **2012**, *161*, 505–522. [CrossRef]
8. Mujokoro, B.; Adabi, M.; Sadroddiny, E.; Adabi, M.; Khosravani, M. Nano-structures mediated co-delivery of therapeutic agents for glioblastoma treatment: A review. *Mater. Sci. Eng C* **2016**, *69*, 1092–1102. [CrossRef]
9. Ramalho, M.J.; Andrade, S.; Coelho, M.Á.N.; Loureiro, J.A.; Pereira, M.C. Biophysical interaction of temozolomide and its active metabolite with biomembrane models: The relevance of drug-membrane interaction for Glioblastoma Multiforme therapy. *Eur. J. Pharm. Biopharm.* **2019**, *136*, 156–163. [CrossRef]
10. Shergalis, A.; Bankhead, A.; Luesakul, U.; Muangsin, N.; Neamati, N. Current Challenges and Opportunities in Treating Glioblastoma. *Pharmacol. Rev.* **2018**, *70*, 412. [CrossRef]
11. Jain, D.S.; Athawale, R.B.; Bajaj, A.N.; Shrikhande, S.S.; Goel, P.N.; Nikam, Y.; Gude, R.P. Unraveling the cytotoxic potential of Temozolomide loaded into PLGA nanoparticles. *DARU J. Pharm. Sci.* **2014**, *22*, 18. [CrossRef] [PubMed]
12. Ananta, J.S.; Paulmurugan, R.; Massoud, T.F. Temozolomide-loaded PLGA nanoparticles to treat glioblastoma cells: A biophysical and cell culture evaluation. *Neurol. Res.* **2016**, *38*, 51–59. [CrossRef] [PubMed]
13. Jain, A.; Chasoo, G.; Singh, S.K.; Saxena, A.K.; Jain, S.K. Transferrin-appended PEGylated nanoparticles for temozolomide delivery to brain: In vitro characterisation. *J. Microencapsul.* **2011**, *28*, 21–28. [CrossRef] [PubMed]
14. Lee, C.; Ooi, I. Preparation of temozolomide-loaded nanoparticles for glioblastoma multiforme targeting—Ideal versus reality. *Pharmaceuticals* **2016**, *9*, 54. [CrossRef] [PubMed]
15. Ramalho, M.J.; Sevin, E.; Gosselet, F.; Lima, J.; Coelho, M.A.N.; Loureiro, J.A.; Pereira, M.C. Receptor-mediated PLGA nanoparticles for glioblastoma multiforme treatment. *Int. J. Pharm.* **2018**, *545*, 84–92. [CrossRef] [PubMed]
16. Lee, S.Y. Temozolomide resistance in glioblastoma multiforme. *Genes Dis.* **2016**, *3*, 198–210. [CrossRef] [PubMed]
17. Warren, K.E.; Gururangan, S.; Geyer, J.R.; McLendon, R.E.; Poussaint, T.Y.; Wallace, D.; Balis, F.M.; Berg, S.L.; Packer, R.J.; Goldman, S.; et al. A phase II study of O6-benzylguanine and temozolomide in pediatric patients with recurrent or progressive high-grade gliomas and brainstem gliomas: A Pediatric Brain Tumor Consortium study. *J. Neuro Oncol.* **2012**, *106*, 643–649. [CrossRef]
18. Quinn, J.A.; Jiang, S.X.; Reardon, D.A.; Desjardins, A.; Vredenburgh, J.J.; Rich, J.N.; Gururangan, S.; Friedman, A.H.; Bigner, D.D.; Sampson, J.H.; et al. Phase II trial of temozolomide plus o6-benzylguanine in adults with recurrent, temozolomide-resistant malignant glioma. *J. Clin. Oncol.* **2009**, *27*, 1262–1267. [CrossRef]
19. Srivenugopal, S.K.; Rawat, A.; Niture, S.K.; Paranjpe, A.; Velu, C.; Venugopal, S.N.; Rao Madala, H.; Basak, D.; Punganuru, S.R. Posttranslational Regulation of O6-Methylguanine-DNA Methyltransferase (MGMT) and New Opportunities for Treatment of Brain Cancers. *Mini Rev. Med. Chem.* **2016**, *16*, 455–464. [CrossRef]
20. Miao, L.; Guo, S.; Zhang, J.; Kim, W.Y.; Huang, L. Nanoparticles with Precise Ratiometric Co-Loading and Co-Delivery of Gemcitabine Monophosphate and Cisplatin for Treatment of Bladder Cancer. *Adv. Funct. Mater.* **2014**, *24*, 6601–6611. [CrossRef]

21. Xu, Y.; Shen, M.; Li, Y.; Sun, Y.; Teng, Y.; Wang, Y.; Duan, Y. The synergic antitumor effects of paclitaxel and temozolomide co-loaded in mPEG-PLGA nanoparticles on glioblastoma cells. *Oncotarget* **2016**, *7*, 20890–20901. [CrossRef]
22. Hoshyar, N.; Gray, S.; Han, H.; Bao, G. The effect of nanoparticle size on in vivo pharmacokinetics and cellular interaction. *Nanomedicine* **2016**, *11*, 673–692. [CrossRef]
23. Blanco, E.; Shen, H.; Ferrari, M. Principles of nanoparticle design for overcoming biological barriers to drug delivery. *Nat. Biotechnol.* **2015**, *33*, 941. [CrossRef]
24. Wang, F.; Chen, L.; Jiang, S.; He, J.; Zhang, X.; Peng, J.; Xu, Q.; Li, R. Optimization of methazolamide-loaded solid lipid nanoparticles for ophthalmic delivery using Box–Behnken design. *J. Liposome Res.* **2014**, *24*, 171–181. [CrossRef]
25. Mazaheri, H.; Ghaedi, M.; Asfaram, A.; Hajati, S. Performance of CuS nanoparticle loaded on activated carbon in the adsorption of methylene blue and bromophenol blue dyes in binary aqueous solutions: Using ultrasound power and optimization by central composite design. *J. Mol. Liq.* **2016**, *219*, 667–676. [CrossRef]
26. Mäkelä, M. Experimental design and response surface methodology in energy applications: A tutorial review. *Energy Convers. Manag.* **2017**, *151*, 630–640. [CrossRef]
27. Papaneophytou, C.P.; Kontopidis, G. Statistical approaches to maximize recombinant protein expression in Escherichia coli: A general review. *Prot. Expr. Purif.* **2014**, *94*, 22–32. [CrossRef]
28. Ramalho, M.J.; Loureiro, J.A.; Gomes, B.; Frasco, M.F.; Coelho, M.A.; Pereira, M.C. PLGA nanoparticles as a platform for vitamin D-based cancer therapy. *Beilstein J. Nanotechnol.* **2015**, *6*, 1306–1318. [CrossRef]
29. Cun, D.; Jensen, D.K.; Maltesen, M.J.; Bunker, M.; Whiteside, P.; Scurr, D.; Foged, C.; Nielsen, H.M. High loading efficiency and sustained release of siRNA encapsulated in PLGA nanoparticles: Quality by design optimization and characterization. *Eur. J. Pharm. Biopharm.* **2011**, *77*, 26–35. [CrossRef]
30. Franken, L.E.; Boekema, E.J.; Stuart, M.C.A. Transmission Electron Microscopy as a Tool for the Characterization of Soft Materials: Application and Interpretation. *Adv. Sci.* **2017**, *4*, 1600476. [CrossRef]
31. Liu, Y.; Pan, J.; Feng, S.-S. Nanoparticles of lipid monolayer shell and biodegradable polymer core for controlled release of paclitaxel: Effects of surfactants on particles size, characteristics and in vitro performance. *Int. J. Pharm.* **2010**, *395*, 243–250. [CrossRef]
32. Tefas, L.R.; Tomu, Ţ.Ă.I.; Achim, M.; Vlase, L. Development and optimization of quercetin-loaded PLGA nanoparticles by experimental design. *Clujul Med.* **2015**, *88*, 214–223. [CrossRef]
33. Narayanan, K.; Subrahmanyam, V.M.; Venkata Rao, J. A Fractional Factorial Design to Study the Effect of Process Variables on the Preparation of Hyaluronidase Loaded PLGA Nanoparticles. *Enzyme Res.* **2014**, *2014*, 162962. [CrossRef]
34. Dos Santos, K.C.; da Silva, M.F.G.F.; Pereira-Filho, E.R.; Fernandes, J.B.; Polikarpov, I.; Forim, M.R. Polymeric nanoparticles loaded with the 3,5,3′-triiodothyroacetic acid (Triac), a thyroid hormone: Factorial design, characterization, and release kinetics. *Nanotechnol. Sci. Appl.* **2012**, *5*, 37–48. [CrossRef]
35. Calignano, F.; Manfredi, D.; Ambrosio, E.P.; Iuliano, L.; Fino, P. Influence of process parameters on surface roughness of aluminum parts produced by DMLS. *Int. J. Adv. Manuf. Technol.* **2013**, *67*, 2743–2751. [CrossRef]
36. Song, X.; Zhao, Y.; Hou, S.; Xu, F.; Zhao, R.; He, J.; Cai, Z.; Li, Y.; Chen, Q. Dual agents loaded PLGA nanoparticles: Systematic study of particle size and drug entrapment efficiency. *Eur. J. Pharm. Biopharm.* **2008**, *69*, 445–453. [CrossRef]
37. Sharma, N.; Madan, P.; Lin, S. Effect of process and formulation variables on the preparation of parenteral paclitaxel-loaded biodegradable polymeric nanoparticles: A co-surfactant study. *Asian J. Pharm. Sci.* **2016**, *11*, 404–416. [CrossRef]
38. Fröhlich, E. The role of surface charge in cellular uptake and cytotoxicity of medical nanoparticles. *Int. J. Nanomed.* **2012**, *7*, 5577. [CrossRef]
39. Ramalho, M.J.; Loureiro, J.A.; Gomes, B.; Frasco, M.F.; Coelho, M.A.N.; Pereira, M.C. PLGA nanoparticles for calcitriol delivery. In Proceedings of the 2015 IEEE 4th Portuguese Meeting on Bioengineering (ENBENG), Porto, Portugal, 26–28 February 2015; pp. 1–6. [CrossRef]
40. Sahoo, S.K.; Panyam, J.; Prabha, S.; Labhasetwar, V. Residual polyvinyl alcohol associated with poly (D, L-lactide-co-glycolide) nanoparticles affects their physical properties and cellular uptake. *J. Controll. Release* **2002**, *82*, 105–114. [CrossRef]

5

Monitoring the Fate of Orally Administered PLGA Nanoformulation for Local Delivery of Therapeutic Drugs

Lucia Morelli [1], Sara Gimondi [2], Marta Sevieri [2], Lucia Salvioni [1], Maria Guizzetti [1], Barbara Colzani [1], Luca Palugan [3], Anastasia Foppoli [3], Laura Talamini [2], Lavinia Morosi [2], Massimo Zucchetti [2], Martina Bruna Violatto [2], Luca Russo [2], Mario Salmona [2], Davide Prosperi [1,4], Miriam Colombo [1,*,†] and Paolo Bigini [2,*,†]

1 NanoBioLab, Dipartimento di Biotecnologie e Bioscienze, Università di Milano-Bicocca, Piazza della Scienza 2, 20126 Milano, Italy; luciaagnese.morelli@libero.it (L.M.); lucia.salvioni@unimib.it (L.S.); maria.guizzetti@gmail.com (M.G.); colzanib@gmail.com (B.C.); davide.prosperi@unimib.it (D.P.)

2 IRCCS Mario Negri Institute for Pharmacological Research; Via Mario Negri 2, 20157 Milano, Italy; sara.gimondi@gmail.com (S.G.); m.sevieri@campus.unimib.it (M.S.); laura.talamini@marionegri.it (L.T.); lavinia.morosi@marionegri.it (L.M.); massimo.zucchetti@marionegri.it (M.Z.); martina.violatto@marionegri.it (M.B.V.); luca.russo@marionegri.it (L.R.); mario.salmona@marionegri.it (M.S.)

3 Dipartimento di Scienze Farmaceutiche, Università di Milano, Via Giuseppe Colombo 71, 20133 Milano, Italy; luca.palugan@unimi.it (L.P.); anastasia.foppoli@unimi.it (A.F.)

4 Nanomedicine Laboratory, ICS Maugeri S.p.A. SB, Via S. Maugeri 10, 27100 Pavia, Italy

* Correspondence: miriam.colombo@unimib.it (M.C.); paolo.bigini@marionegri.it (P.B.)

† These authors contributed equally to this work.

Abstract: One of the goals of the pharmaceutical sciences is the amelioration of targeted drug delivery. In this context, nanocarrier-dependent transportation represents an ideal method for confronting a broad range of human disorders. In this study, we investigated the possibility of improving the selective release of the anti-cancer drug paclitaxel (PTX) in the gastro-intestinal tract by encapsulating it into the biodegradable nanoparticles made by FDA-approved poly(lactic-*co*-glycolic acid) (PLGA) and coated with polyethylene glycol to improve their stability (PLGA-PEG-NPs). Our study was performed by combining the synthesis and characterization of the nanodrug with in vivo studies of pharmacokinetics after oral administration in mice. Moreover, fluorescent PLGA-nanoparticles (NPs), were tested both in vitro and in vivo to observe their fate and biodistribution. Our study demonstrated that PLGA-NPs: (1) are stable in the gastric tract; (2) can easily penetrate inside carcinoma colon 2 ($CaCo_2$) cells; (3) reduce the PTX absorption from the gastrointestinal tract, further limiting systemic exposure; (4) enable PTX local targeting. At present, the oral administration of biodegradable nanocarriers is limited because of stomach degradation and the sink effect played by the duodenum. Our findings, however, exhibit promising evidence towards our overcoming these limitations for a more specific and safer strategy against gastrointestinal disorders.

Keywords: PLGA-NPs; nanomedicine; gastrointestinal tract; paclitaxel; in vivo imaging

---

1. Introduction

The generation of therapeutic methods that can improve the organ specificity of many different types of therapeutic agents is one of the major challenges of 21st-century pharmacology [1]. The availability of transport systems that can successfully improve the targeted release of administered substances would be, indeed, crucial in mitigating or even virtually eliminating the toxic side effects of already existing therapeutics. These improved transport systems can be used to limit the off-target spread and, consequently, reduce the potential side effects deriving from an unnecessary tropism [2]. Several strategies have been employed in the last years to improve the accuracy of drug targeting. Quite recently, our group and others have demonstrated that the systemic administration of anti-inflammatory and immunomodulatory agents, such as corticosteroids, can have a safer and more effective pharmacological profile when linked to a nanometric vector [3,4]. The potential prospects of nanocarriers for pharmacological purposes is extremely versatile complex. It is widely known that even the slightest modification of basic physicochemical strictures, such as the dimension, shape, and surface of the material itself, can indeed lead to a myriad of different results—causing a very vast range of reactions amongst the cells and organs of the host [5]. One of the primary and certainly most prominent, therapeutic strategies is the incorporation of the anti-neoplastic drug doxorubicin into liposomes for the treatment of tumors [6]. The first generation of nanoparticles (NPs) used for these purposes are mainly liposomes, polymeric micelles, and conjugates.

Since the turn of the century, the encapsulation of anti-neoplastic cytotoxic molecules inside NPs has been occurring with greater frequency. In 2004, an original formulation for the creation of nanocarriers to transport the anti-cancer drug paclitaxel (PTX) was developed [7,8]. In that case, different from other carriers, the biodegradable copolymer poly(lactic-*co*-glycolic acid) (PLGA) was utilized. In a more recent study, furthermore, it was shown that the systemic administration of PTX inside poly(lactic-*co*-glycolic acid)-polyethylene glycol-nanoparticles (PLGA-PEG-NPs), when functionalized with ANTI-EGFR, dramatically slows disease progression in triple-negative breast cancer-bearing mice, thus confirming the high efficacy, safety, and tenability of this material [9].

Nanoparticles utilizing FDA-approved PLGA, exhibit some important advantages. In particular, their biocompatibility causes low systemic toxicity in comparison to other polymers [10] and is highly versatile, allowing them to encapsulate various drugs, including small molecules and therapeutic biologics [11–13]. The importance of PLGA nanocarriers in biomedicine is further supported by evidence of its potential benefits in assisting drug transportation across biological barriers [14,15]. Most of their applications concern intravenous administration [16], but, in the last decade, many studies have been published regarding their potential efficacy in oral administration of drugs, even if the absorption efficiency needs to be more deeply investigated and optimized [17].

Although the majority of studies dealing with biodistribution, disease targeting, and therapeutic efficacy of NPs-based drug delivery systems has been conducted using systemic administration of nanoformulation, more recently the exploration of alternative routes, including topical [18,19], intranasal [20], intratracheal [21], and oral administration [22], are gaining increasing recognition.

Building on these advances, this work aimed to characterize the biodistribution of PTX alone or encapsulated in PEGylated PLGA-NPs after oral administration in healthy mice. This approach stems from the hope that, in so doing, the passage of the drug from the gastrointestinal (GI) tract to the bloodstream might be reduced, although not completely eliminating its release in the gut. While the active gastroduodenal absorption of PTX on oral ingestion is quite low, it is not possible to totally exclude systemic toxicity of both circulating cells and filter organs in the case of high doses or repeated cycles of chemotherapy. PLGA-NPs could, therefore, be useful to both protect the drug against gastric degradation and, at the same time, reduce the uptake by mucosae villi or Peyer's patches and the consequent release into the blood, while PEG grafting is expected to improve both the NPs stability and mucus-permeating properties in the GI tract [23,24]. In this study, PLGA-PEG-NPs were orally administered either loaded with PTX or labeled with a fluorophore (Rhodamine B), which allowed for the longitudinal tracking of NPs in both gastrointestinal and peripheral organs. This study could be of interest to understand the potentials of local delivery of anti-cancer agents in GI tumors by the oral administration of NPs, minimizing nonspecific absorption.

2. Materials and Methods

2.1. Nanoparticles Synthesis

2.1.1. Materials

PLGA (Resomer® RG 504 H, 50:50 lactide:glycolide, acid terminal, MW 38,000–54,000 g/mol), paclitaxel (PTX, MW 853.91 g/mol), rhodamine B (RhB, MW 479.01 g/mol); polyvinlyl alcohol (PVA, MW 9000–10,000 g/mol, 80% hydrolyzed); *N,N′*-dicyclohexylcarbodiimide (DCC, MW 206.33 g/mol, 99%); *N*-hydroxysuccinimide (NHS, MW 115.09 g/mol, 98%); dimethylamino pyridine (DMAP, MW 122.17 g/mol, 99%); ninhydrin (MW 178.14 g/mol); ethanolamine (MW 61.08 g/mol, ≥98%); dichloromethane (DCM, ≥99.8%); dimethyl sulfoxide (DMSO, ≥99.9%); acetonitrile anhydrous (ACN, 99.8%); methanol (MeOH, ≥99.9%) were purchased from Sigma–Aldrich Co (St Louis, MO, USA). Chloroform (≥99.8%) was purchased from Honeywell Riedel-de-Haën™ (Charlotte, NC, USA)). Poly (ethylene glycol) diamine (NH_2-PEG-NH_2, 6000 Da) was obtained from Rapp Polymer GmbH, (Tuebingen, Germany).

2.1.2. PLGA-PEG-RhB Synthesis

For activation of the carboxylic groups of PLGA, the polymer was dissolved in DCM (15 mL, 40 mg/mL) and the reaction was performed in a round flask for 4 h (250 rpm, RT, under inert gas) after the addition of DCC (30 mg) and NHS (15 mg). Then, the solution was diluted with diethyl ether, and the polymer was collected after precipitation (20 min, 6200× *g*, 4 °C) and evaporation of the residual organic phase. Next, the conjugation with NH_2-PEG-NH_2 (molar ratio PEG/PLGA = 2.7) was performed in 10 mL of $CHCl_3$ overnight (250 rpm, RT, under inert gas). To get rid of the unconjugated PEG, methanol (30 mL) was added, and the polymer was collected after precipitation twice [25]. The residual organic phase was then evaporated under reduced pressure, and the weight yield calculated (68.99 ± 14.94%). The degree of labeling was determined using the colorimetric ninhydrin assay (primary amine detection): Notably, 15 mg of the product (PLGA-PEG) was solubilized in DMSO (400 μL) then diluted with 100 μL of ninhydrin solution (3.5 mg/mL). Ethanolamine (18.75 mg/mL) and PLGA solutions were used as positive and negative controls, respectively. The samples were then incubated for 1 h at 65 °C (400 rpm), and the colored conjugate was detected by UV-Vis spectroscopy (Spectrophotometer Fluormax-Horiba Scientific, Rome, Italy) (λ = 600 nm), and the yield calculated using a calibration curve of ethanolamine standards. The obtained degree of labeling was 71.90 ± 12.70%.

Finally, RhB (molar ratio RhB/PLGA = 6.25) was added to the PLGA-PEG solution in $CHCl_3$ (15 mL) with an excess of DCC and DMAP. The reaction was carried out overnight (250 rpm, RT, under inert gas). At the end of the reaction, the solution was evaporated, and the product was solubilized with DCM (10 mL) and purified thrice by precipitation (20 min, 4 °C, 6200× *g*) after diethyl ether addition (20 mL). The reaction yield was 38.16 ± 13.50%. RhB linked was detected by fluorescence spectrometry ($\lambda_{exitation}$ 555 nm; $\lambda_{emission}$ 574 nm) and the degree of labeling calculated by the comparison with a calibration curve (1.43 ± 0.46 μg/mg).

2.1.3. Synthesis of PLGA-PEG-RhB-NPs and PTX-PLGA-PEG-RhB-NPs

NPs were synthesized according to the single emulsion method. PLGA-PEG-RhB solution (1 mL, 25 mg/mL in DCM) was emulsified with 8 mL of PVA 2% solution by sonicating twice (Sonifier Sound, Branson Ultrasonics, Shanghai, China; 30 s and 38% intensity) in an ice bath. The product was transferred immediately into a solution of PVA 2% (16 mL), allowing the organic solvent to evaporate (4 h, RT, 750 rpm). For PTX-PLGA-PEG-RhB-NPs synthesis, 5 mg of PTX was dissolved along with the polymer. After curing, NPs were collected by centrifugation at 19,500× *g*, 20 min, 4 °C (Heraeus Fresco 21; Thermo Fisher Scientific, Göteborg, Sweden), washed thrice with double distilled water and freeze-dried through an Alpha 1–2 LD freeze drier (Christ, Memmingen, Germany) at

0.500 mbar, −53 °C, 12 h, without the addition of any cryoprotectant. The process yield was calculated after the freeze-drying process, as the ratio between collected NPs and starting raw materials.

The amount of PTX loaded in the NPs was determined by HPLC analysis with UV detection (Waters Associates, Milford, MA, USA, model 2487 Variable Wavelength Detector, Wavelength: 230 nm). Briefly, 0.1 mL of the NPs solution was spiked with 5 μg of IS and extracted with 0.5 mL of CH_3CN. After vortex for 10 s, samples were centrifuged at 13,000 rpm for 10 min. The organic phase was separated and dried under nitrogen, and the residues were dissolved with 250 μL of the mobile phase. Fifty microliters of the reconstituted samples was injected into the HPLC system. The apparatus was equipped with a Symmetry C18 column (5 μm, 4.6 × 150 mm), the mobile phase was composed of 50% ammonium acetate buffer (0.01 M, pH 5), 40% acetonitrile, and 10% methanol with a flux rate of 1.3 mL/min and 30 min run time. NPs solution without drug was used to prepare the calibration curve by the addition of PTX in the range 10–100 μg/mL.

2.2. *Nanoparticles Characterization*

2.2.1. Dynamic Light Scattering (DLS) and Zeta Potential Measurements

All NPs were characterized in terms of size, size distribution, and Zeta potential through dynamic light scattering (DLS, Zetasizer Nano ZS; Malvern Instruments, Cambridge, UK) in ultrapure water at 1 mg/mL, at 25 °C. The scattered light from the NPs in suspension was used to calculate NPs' hydrodynamic diameter considering medium viscosity. NPs size distribution was described by the polydispersity index (PDI), where PDI $\leq$ 0.2 corresponds to the monodisperse NPs population.

2.2.2. Scanning Transmission Electron Microscopy (STEM) Analysis

PLGA-PEG-RhB-NPs were observed by a Zeiss SEM-FEG Gemini 500, operating at 30 kV in scanning transmission electron microscopy (STEM) mode (Zeiss, Germany). The NPs suspension was deposited onto a formvar-coated 200-mesh copper grid (Ted Pella, CA, USA), negatively stained with 1% uranyl acetate and allowed to dry before examination.

2.2.3. In Vitro Release Studies

PTX-PLGA-PEG-RhB-NPs equivalent to 8.75 μg of PTX were suspended in 1 mL of Tween/PBS and incubated at 37 °C with constant agitation. At predetermined time points (0.5, 1, 2, 4, 6, and 24 h), the suspension was centrifuged at 19,500× *g* for 15 min to separate NPs pellets and supernatants. PTX in the collected supernatants was analyzed with HPLC equipped with a UV detector (1260 Infinity II Series, Agilent Technologies, Palo Alto, CA, USA) and an Atlantis C18 column (25 cm × 4.6 mm, particle size 5 μm) (Supelco, St. Louis, MO, USA). The mobile phase was a mixture of acetonitrile and water (50:50) run in the isocratic mode at a flow rate of 1 mL/min. PTX was detected at 227 nm. PTX quantitation was performed using a calibration curve in a range of 1.25–40 μg/mL, and the results were expressed as a percentage of cumulative release (mean ± SD; $n = 4$).

2.2.4. Nanoparticles Stability in Different Buffers

The hydrodynamic dimension of the nanocarrier was analyzed in different conditions: Artificial saliva (pH 7.6; KH_2PO_4 1.9 mM, $NaHCO_3$ 17 mM, Na_2HPO_4 1.8 mM, NaCl 8.5 mM, KSCN 3.4 mM, Urea 2.2 mM, alpha-amylase 0.007 mM), intestinal fluid (pH 6; KH_2PO_4 49.96 mM, NaOH 0.0154 M, pancreatin 1 g/L), and gastric juice (pH 1.2; NaCl 300 mM, pepsin 0.9 mM, HCl 840 mM) that simulate the media in GI tract. The NPs (15 mg/mL) were incubated for 0, 1, 2, 4, 6, and 24 h and analyzed by DLS. Upon establishing the size stability, the samples were further analyzed with fluorescence spectroscopy ($\lambda_{exitation}$ 555 nm; $\lambda_{emission}$ 574 nm) to monitor the stability of RhB conjugation. The release of RhB after 24 h was then calculated after PLGA-PEG-RhB-NPs removal by centrifugation (mean ± SD; $n = 4$).

2.3. Cells

Carcinoma colon cells ($CaCo_2$) are a cell line derived from human colorectal adenocarcinoma and were purchased from ATCC® HTB-37™. $CaCo_2$ cells were grown as a single layer in adhesion in DMEM-High Glucose (Dulbecco's Modified Eagle Medium High Glucose-Biowest, Nuaillé, France) with the addition of 10% of fetal bovine serum (FBS) and 1% L-glutamine (200 mM), 100 U/mL penicillin, 0.1 mg per mL streptomycin. Cells were maintained at 37 °C and in a 5% CO_2 humidified atmosphere. The ability of PLGA-PEG-RhB-NPs and free RhB to be internalized by $CaCo_2$ cells was evaluated. For each condition, the experiment was conducted in triplicate. Cells were seeded at a density of 40,000 cells/well on 13 mm diameter slides in 24-well plates. Forty-eight hours after sowing, $CaCo_2$ cells were incubated with PLGA-PEG-RhB-NPs (100 μg/mL) and with RhB free (0.06 μg/mL) for 1, 4, and 24 h, while the wells destined for control did not receive any treatment. After incubation, the cells were washed with phosphate-buffer saline (PBS) three times and fixed with a 4% paraformaldehyde solution dissolved in PBS (0.1 M, pH 7.4) for 40 min and the vital nuclear dye Hoechst 33258 (2 μg/mL) was added to each well for 45 min. The slides thus obtained were assembled and analyzed with the Olympus BX51 epifluorescence microscope (Olympus, Tokyo, Japan). All acquisition parameters, including laser settings, were kept constant during all scans. To evaluate a possible cytotoxic effect of PLGA-PEG-RhB-NPs and free RhB, the metabolic activity of $CaCo_2$ cells was evaluated by RealTime-Glo™ MT Cell Viability Assay (Promega, Madison, WI, USA). Cells were seeded at 16,000 cells/well in 96 opaque-walled tissue culture plates and maintained at 37 °C. The RealTime-Glo reagents were added at the same time as the test compounds, according to the manufacturer's protocol. At selected time points (4 and 24 h), the cell viability was monitored by a plate-reading luminometer (GloMax® Discover Microplate Reader, Promega, Madison, WI, USA). For each condition, 6 replicates were prepared. The viability was expressed as a percentage compared to non-treated cells.

2.4. Animals

All procedures involving animals and their health were conducted so as to minimize the number of mice used and their collateral suffering, in accordance with institutional guidelines, national laws (DL n. 24, 4 March 2014; Authorization No. 19/2008 A) and international laws and agreements (EEC Council Directive 2010/63, 6 August 2013; NIH Guide to the Care and Use of Laboratory Animals, US National Research Council, 2008). The research project was first reviewed by the Internal Ethics Committee of the Mario Negri Institute and was subsequently approved by the ministry and designated with the before mentioned code (42/2016-PR).

All animals were housed in SPF (specific pathogen-free) conditions. The housing rooms had a temperature of 22 ± 1 °C, relative humidity values ± of 50 ± 10% and a 12 h light/dark cycle. Furthermore, the animals were kept in cages with free access to water and food.

2.5. Treatments

As regards pharmacokinetics, six weeks old CD1 mice were treated by oral gavage with 20 mg/kg of Cremophor PTX (n = 16) or PTX-PLGA-PEG-RhB-NPs (n = 16), three animals were treated with saline solution as control. Blood was collected in heparinized tubes, 30 min, 1, 4, and 24 h after treatment (4 animals for each group) and centrifuged to obtain plasma. After the mice were sacrificed, the stomach, duodenum, colon, and liver were collected and stored at −20 °C until analysis.

For the biodistribution studies, we recruited 5 animals for each experimental group. To reduce background fluorescence due to the food, mice were fed an AIN-76A diet without alfalfa (Mucedola s.r.l., Settimo Milanese, Italy) for two weeks before the analyzes. The dose of the different formulations was standardized on the quantity of RhB present and fixed at 0.6 mg/kg mouse based on previous experimental studies. Vehicle treated mice received the same volume of saline solution. Mice were sacrificed at 1, 4, or 24 h to follow the fate of RhB. The sacrifice was performed by cervical dislocation, and the stomach, intestine, liver, and blood were collected to perform ex vivo analyses. Plasma for fluorometric analysis was obtained from the blood collected. Finally, a piece of liver and GI tracts of three animals for each experimental group were frozen at −80 °C for cryostatic sections and histological analysis.

2.6. Molecular Imaging and Histology

The in vivo biodistribution of the different formulations was monitored over time using an optical fluorescence imaging system (IVIS Lumina XRMS, PerkinElmer, Waltham, MA, USA). Ex vivo scans of organs from mice sacrificed at 1, 4, and 24 h after the treatment were performed by the same instrument. The following acquisition parameters were used: Excitation filter: 580 nm, emission filter: 620 nm, exposure time: Auto, binning factor: Medium, f/Stop: 2, Field of View: D (for the gastro line—intestinal), C (for peripheral organs). Very importantly, the Living Image Software 4.3.1 (Perkin Elmer, Waltham, MA, USA) conjugated with the spectral unmixing system was used to separate the RhB signal from tissue autofluorescence, image processing, and fluorescence signal quantification analysis.

Longitudinal sections of 20 μm of thickness were prepared and then, after adhesion in glass slides, were incubated with a PBS solution of Hoechst 33258 (2 μg/mL, Sigma–Aldrich) for 45 min and, after three washes in PBS, observed at the Microscopy Virtual Slide (Olympus, Tokyo, Japan), to obtain rapid organ scans of the whole section with high anatomical resolution.

2.7. NPs Characterization from Homogenates and Biological Fluids

The fluorescence of PLGA-PEG-RhB-NPs was analyzed in tissues explanted from previously treated animals. The analyzed tissues were liver, stomach, intestine, and plasma. Each tissue sample was weighed, homogenized in PBS 1X according to a 1:4 weight ratio, and centrifuged at 1200 rpm for 10 min at 4 °C. For all samples, the analysis was performed using the Infinite® M200 multimode plate reader exciting at the wavelength of 500 nm and recording the signal at a range of emission wavelength from 550 to 560 nm. For the stability studies in solutions mimicking gastrointestinal fluids, the NPs were incubated in stock solutions as previously described [26].

2.8. Pharmacokinetics

The total concentration of PTX in the different biological matrices was determined by HPLC-UV, as previously described [27]. For the determination of PTX in organs, tissues were previously homogenized in 0.2 M CH_3COONH_4 pH 4.5. Each study sample (0.3 mL for plasma and 0.5 mL for homogenate tissues) was assayed together with five points of a standard calibration curve prepared in the corresponding control biological matrix obtained from untreated mice at concentrations ranging from 0.05 to 5 μg/sample. The limits of quantification (LOQ) were 0.16 μg/mL and 0.6 μg/g for plasma and organs, respectively.

2.9. Statistical Analysis

All data were expressed as mean ± SD, Student's t-test and p values were done using the GraphPad Prism version 6.00 for Windows (Graph-Pad Software, San Diego, CA, USA).

3. Results and Discussion

3.1. NPs Synthesis and Characterization

The protocol for the polymer modification was set up, and PLGA-PEG-RhB was employed to synthesize the NPs to be used as carriers for PTX. The covalently bound RhB chromophore allowed the tracking of the PLGA fate in vivo. The single emulsion method allowed us to obtain both unloaded and PTX-loaded NPs, having controlled size and homogenous size distributions (Table 1). As measured by DLS analysis, the encapsulation of PTX did not significantly change the dimensional features of NPs. Moreover, a negative Z-potential was observed as opposed to PLGA-PEG-NPs, where the free amines of PEG determined the surface properties. However, a small difference in net negative charge values between PLGA-PEG-RhB-NPs and PTX-PLGA-PEG-RhB-NPs was attributable to the intramolecular reorganization of portions of the polymer chains due to hydrophobic interaction with PTX. PTX loaded NPs were further characterized by STEM, which showed pseudospherical shaped nanoparticles with the size around 200 nm (Figure S1). PTX encapsulation efficiency detected by HPLC analysis was 10.87 ± 1.13%, while the calculated loading efficiency was 4.77 ± 0.15%, in line with previous studies [28]. The drug release performance was evaluated, and the test was conducted in PBS containing 0.2 *v*/*v* % Tween 80, considering both its poor solubility and the analysis detection limits [29]. As previously reported with similar experimental settings, a fast PTX dissolution was observed (80% within 4 h) (Figure S2) [30].

Table 1. NPs characterization and process yield. Data represent mean ± SD (n = 3).

Formulations	Size (nm ± SD)	PDI	Z-Potential (mV ± SD)	Process Yield (%, *w*/*w* ± SD)
PLGA-PEG-NPs	190.3 ± 12.7	0.078 ± 0.032	+17.9 ± 5.9	53.3 ± 7.7
PLGA-PEG-RhB-NPs	205.6 ± 18.6	0.168 ± 0.030	−18.2 ± 1.5	50.1 ± 13.4
PTX-PLGA-PEG-RhB-NPs	201.6 ± 26.2	0.205 ± 0.032	−13.3 ± 1.7	39.3 ± 7.3

Stability in Mimicking Biological Fluids

The first study was carried out to verify the potential role of PEG on the fate of PLGA-NPs in solutions mimicking saliva, gastric, and proximal intestinal fluid, respectively (Figure 1A,B). Longitudinal measurement of the NPs size by DLS was possible because, diversely from the serum, they are very poor in macromolecules, and the interference on the recording is almost zero. Figure 1A shows that the presence of the PEG confers to PLGA-NPs a long-lasting stability for at least 24 h after incubation. In contrast, the lack of PEG rapidly induced aggregation in NPs incubated in gastric fluid and, to a lesser extent in intestinal fluid. Since we aimed to conserve considerable stability up until the large intestine, we decided to carry on our studies using pegylated PLGA-NPs exclusively.

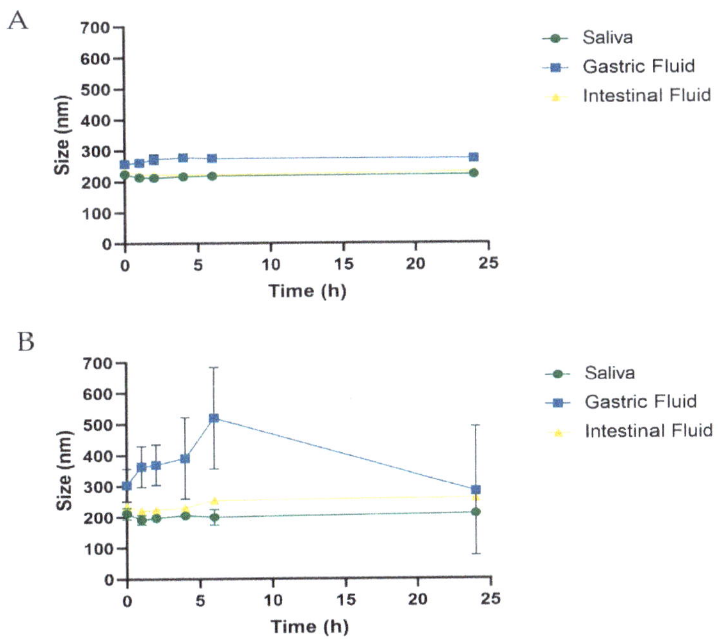

Figure 1. Graphics showing the diameter, measured by dynamic light scattering (DLS), after incubation of (**A**) pegylated or (**B**) not pegylated poly(lactic-*co*-glycolic acid)-nanoparticles (PLGA-NPs) in artificial fluids mimicking the saliva (green lines), the gastric juice (blue lines), or proximal intestinal fluid (yellow line). For all conditions, the measurements were carried out at 1, 2, 4, 6, 24 h from the starting point.

Then, the stability of the RhB conjugation was performed by measuring the dye release in the same conditions (Figure 2A). After 24 h of incubation, the released RhB was below 15% in all cases, suggesting the system reliability for in vitro and in vivo NPs tracking. Additionally, as reported in Figure 2B, the fluorescence intensity of PLGA-PEG-RhB-NPs was not greatly affected by the incubation media showing that, once conjugated, the dye abolishes its pH-dependent emission properties [31].

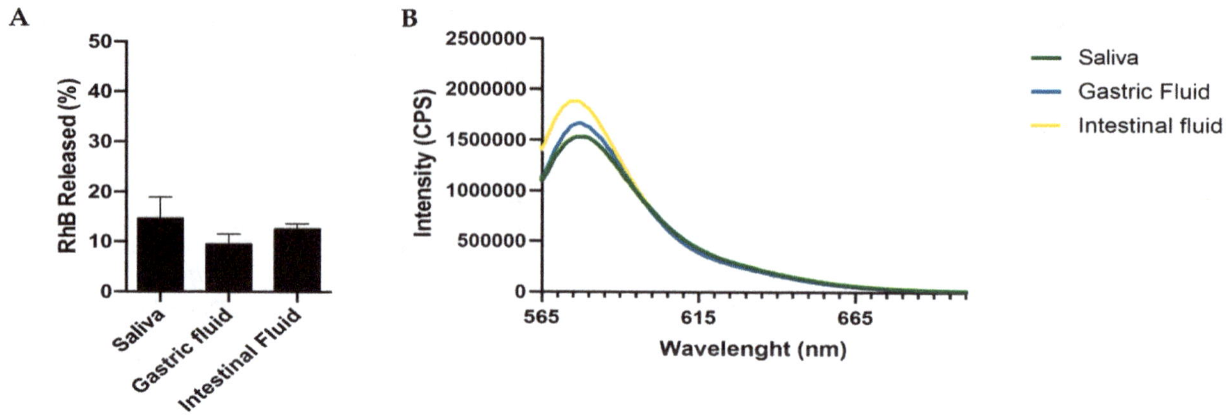

Figure 2. Graphics showing (**A**) the amount of RhB released from PLGA-PEG-RhB-NPs after 24 h incubation in artificial fluids mimicking the saliva, the gastric juice, or proximal intestinal fluid (mean ± SD; n = 5); (**B**) emission spectra of poly(lactic-*co*-glycolic acid)-polyethylene glycol-RhB-nanoparticles (PLGA-PEG-RhB-NPs) incubated in different media.

3.2. Pharmacokinetics

To understand the possible influence of the nanoformulate on the biodistribution of drugs, we performed a pharmacokinetic study of the well-known anti-cancer agent, paclitaxel, administered orally as a free drug (PTX) or loaded into NPs (PTX-PLGA-PEG-RhB-NPs). PTX release Figure 3 shows the levels of PTX measured in the stomach (A), in the duodenum (B) and in the colon (C) of mice sacrificed 30 min, 1 and 4 h after treatment with PTX free (blue bars) or with PTX-PLGA-PEG-RhB-NPs (red bars). The drug concentration in the samples collected at 24 h after treatment resulted under the limit of detection. Overall, the drug concentration measured in all the gastrointestinal tissues was comparable between the two formulations and higher in the stomach and duodenum compared to the colon. Despite the comparable tissue drug level, interestingly, the nano-formulation reduced the systemic absorption of the drug. The measurement of the plasmatic levels, in fact, showed a clear reduction of systemic absorption of PTX when administered as PTX-PLGA-PEG-RhB-NPs, leading to a consequent reduction of liver accumulation, as shown in Figure 3D,E. Similarly to previous results achieved by our group [32,33], no evidence of acute toxicity was observed in mice receiving the single administration of PTX-PLGA-PEG-RhB-NPs.

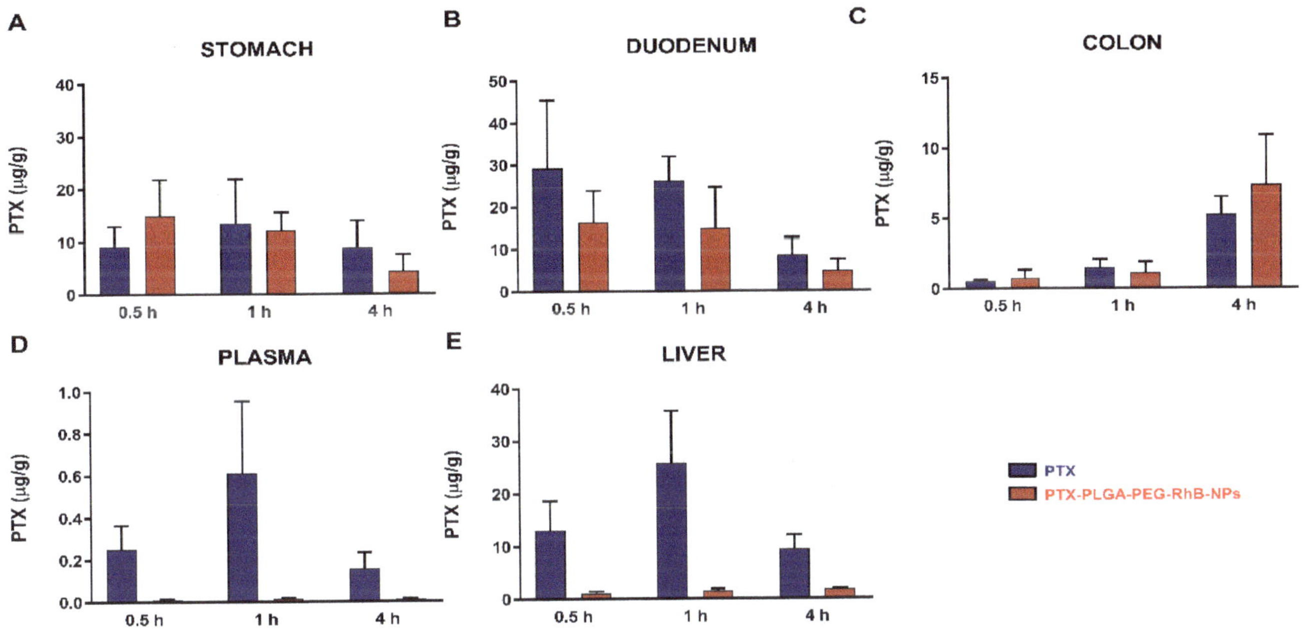

Figure 3. Comparison of the paclitaxel (PTX) distribution in (**A**) stomach, (**B**) duodenum, (**C**) colon, (**D**) plasma, and (**E**) liver of mice after administration of a single treatment of PTX or PTX-PLGA-PEG-RhB-NPs (20 mg/kg p.o.). The bars are the mean value ± SD (n = 4).

3.3. NPs Biodistribution and Nanosafety

To better understand the mechanisms that govern the different behavior of the free and NPs-encapsulated drug, we decided to monitor the NPs transit at the digestive tract level, the interactions with the gastric and intestinal structures, the possible transition to the bloodstream and penetration into filter organs by marking PLGA with a fluorescent molecule, RhB. Since the monitoring of biodegradable NPs through an indirect method, such as fluorescence analysis, presents the risk of artifacts caused by the dye release or degradation [34], all studies were carried out by comparing animals that received PLGA-PEG-RhB-NPs with those animals treated with the same dose of free RhB. As the in vitro studies suggested, the stability and reliability of this indirect approach (see Figure 2), enable us to obtain further evidence from the biodistribution study that explains the different behavior between an orally administered small molecule and our nanocarrier.

Figure 4A shows the distribution of the signal associated with the GI tract in animals sacrificed 1, 4, and 24 h after treatment with the vehicle (left) or RhB (upper blue panel), and PLGA-PEG-RhB-NPs (lower red panel), respectively. The power of the excitation laser was set in vehicle-treated mice to avoid any possible overlapping between RhB and tissue autofluorescence. In each panel, it is possible to see an upper region shaped like a sack, which represents the stomach. The small intestine is the snake-like shape in the middle. The enlargement in the last part of the intestine includes cecum, colon, and rectum and is called "large intestine". The signal associated with RhB is clearly detectable in both groups receiving the same amount of dye. As expected, in both groups, it is also possible to see a progressive decay of signal and a shift from the distal part of the GI tract. However, in mice treated with NPs, the presence of the dye was more persistent, in particular in the distal part of the small intestine and in the large intestine. The quantification of the signal (Figure 4B) confirmed this observational study: In particular, the levels of the signal in the intestine at the 4th hour after the treatment was markedly higher in animals receiving the nanoformulation.

To better understand the interaction between PLGA-PEG-RhB-NPs and the GI tract structures, histological evaluation was carried out, also exploiting the presence of RhB to track them along the anatomic path and their development in time. Even in this case, the same doses of RhB free were injected into a further group of mice to exclude any possible misinterpretation of the results due to the possible loss of NPs stability and the release of the dye.

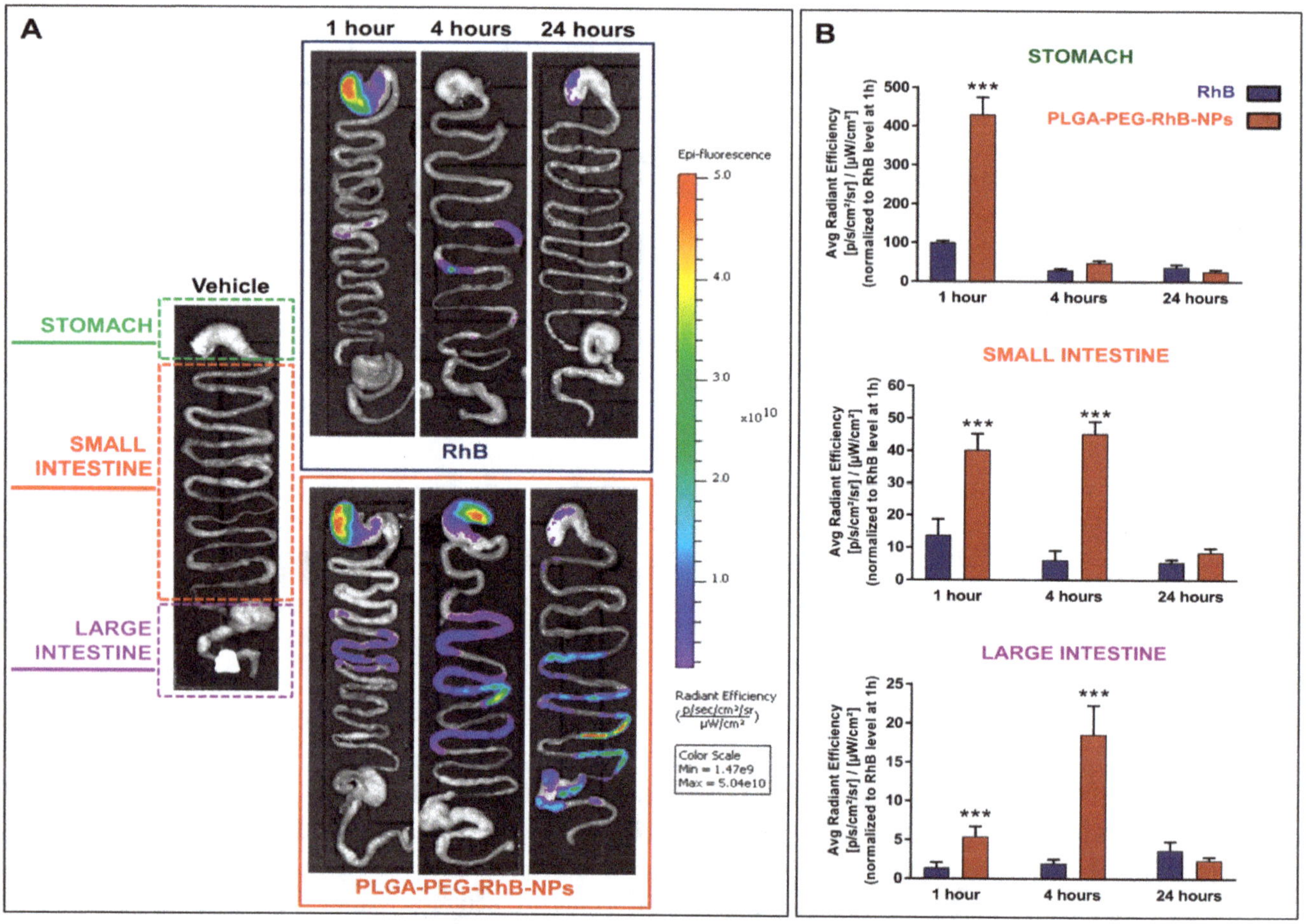

Figure 4. Signal distribution in the gastrointestinal (GI) tract of mice treated with RhB or PLGA-PEG-RhB-NPs. (**A**) Representative ex vivo scanning of the excised organs after washing with saline solutions to remove debris of feces. Animals were sacrificed at 1, 4, and 24 h after the treatment with the same dose of RhB. In the left column, a vehicle-treated mouse was shown to demonstrate the lack of the auto fluorescent component in this analysis. The interval of fluorescence signal intensity associated with the scale of colors is reported on the right. Five animals for each experimental group were used. (**B**) The quantification of the signal associated with the treatment was performed, dividing each sample into three tracts, as shown in the panel. The bars are the value of signal normalized to 100, considering the mean value measured in the stomach of mice treated with RhB alone and sacrificed 1 h after the oral administration. The bars are the mean value ± SD ($n = 5$). The Student's t-test was used to compare the levels between the two groups for each time point. *** $p < 0.0001$.

Figure 5A, upper panels, shows representative images taken from gastric sections of mice sacrificed 1, 4, and 24 h after PLGA-PEG-RhB-NPs administration. Although a progressive reduction of the signal can be seen, it is important to underline that the anatomical localization of the signal remains almost exclusively confined outside the gastric cells that are characterized by the intense blue staining due to the presence of the nuclear dye Hoechst 33258. Opposite, the RhB alone, Figure 5A lower panels, deeply penetrated inside the gastric parenchyma as clearly evidenced by the purple staining due to the merge between the red and the blue signal. This is more pronounced at the first hour and, interestingly, it does not involve the whole structure of the stomach, but it is almost confined to the superficial region of the gastric mucosa (left part of the picture at 1 h). At the 4th hour, the signal is lower but more penetrated and homogeneously spread in the parenchyma, whereas after one day, as already demonstrated by ex vivo quantification (Figure 4B), the fluorescent intensity strongly decreased. The different pattern of staining shown at the 4th and 24th hour strongly suggests that, in spite of the gastric activity, PLGA-PEG-RhB-NPs remain stable enough to avoid the release of the free dye. This is in line with the results reported in Figure 1A by DLS in solutions mimicking gastric juice.

The stability of the nanoparticles inside the stomach is essential to transport any encapsulated drug to the intestine. In Figure 4B, the signal measurement along the whole small intestine was evaluated, whereas histological analysis was focused on the more proximal part of the intestine, the duodenal region. The duodenum is one of the most critical portions of the GI for the absorption of metabolites and drugs. The active uptake by mucosae villi and Peyer's patches allows the absorption of many substances into the bloodstream and their consequent systemic distribution. Even if this process is required to provide energy and nutrients and to distribute therapeutic agents orally administered, it can be a hurdle for a localized gut delivery. In Figure 3, we have reported that the encapsulation in PLGA-PEG-RhB-NPs dramatically reduces the PTX absorption. This suggests that these kinds of NPs are able to pass through this first part of the intestine, maintaining their stability. Representative images from coronal sections of the duodenum from mice sacrificed 1 h after the treatment (lower panel on the left and higher magnification right in Figure 5B) shows that NPs are in the lumen and inside the intervilli space but are not absorbed by mucosa. A deeper interaction with villi can be seen at the 4th hour after treatment. However, even in this case, the red and blue signals are close but do not overlap. An overlapping was indeed clearly seen in distinction from mice treated with the same amount of RhB free at least up to the first 4 h after ingestion. A higher magnified picture furthermore confirms the restricted interaction between the red signal and the peripheral region of villi 1 h after treatment. As reported in the measurement of the intestinal levels by ex vivo scanning (Figure 4B), an almost complete disappearance of the red signal can be seen 24 h after the treatment in both experimental groups.

By histology, we found that RhB-free treated mice showed deep red staining in villi, whereas the red signal remained in the lumen of the intestinal tube in animals receiving RhB with NPs. Since enterocytes in villi are tightly connected to the vessels, it is, therefore, possible to hypothesize that RhB can easily penetrate the circulatory tree. To confirm that NPs can dramatically reduce the passage from the small intestine to the bloodstream, we compared the RhB levels both in plasma and in the liver of mice treated with PLGA-PEG-RhB-NPs or RhB free. Figure 6A, where plasmatic levels of RhB-related signals were normalized to the value measured in mice treated with RhB-free during the first hour of analysis, clearly reveals that the nanoformulation (red bars) leads to an almost complete abolishment of hematic absorption of RhB. This striking difference between the two groups supports the hypothesis that these NPs are stable and almost completely eradicate the absorption of themselves and of the relevant cargo by gastric and intestinal mucosae. The fast and quite elevated half-life of RhB in the blood led to an expected accumulation of the dye in the main filter organ, the liver, Figure 6B. Similar to the results obtained from the blood, the animals treated with RhB exclusively showed a well detectable red signal in liver sections (Figure 6C).

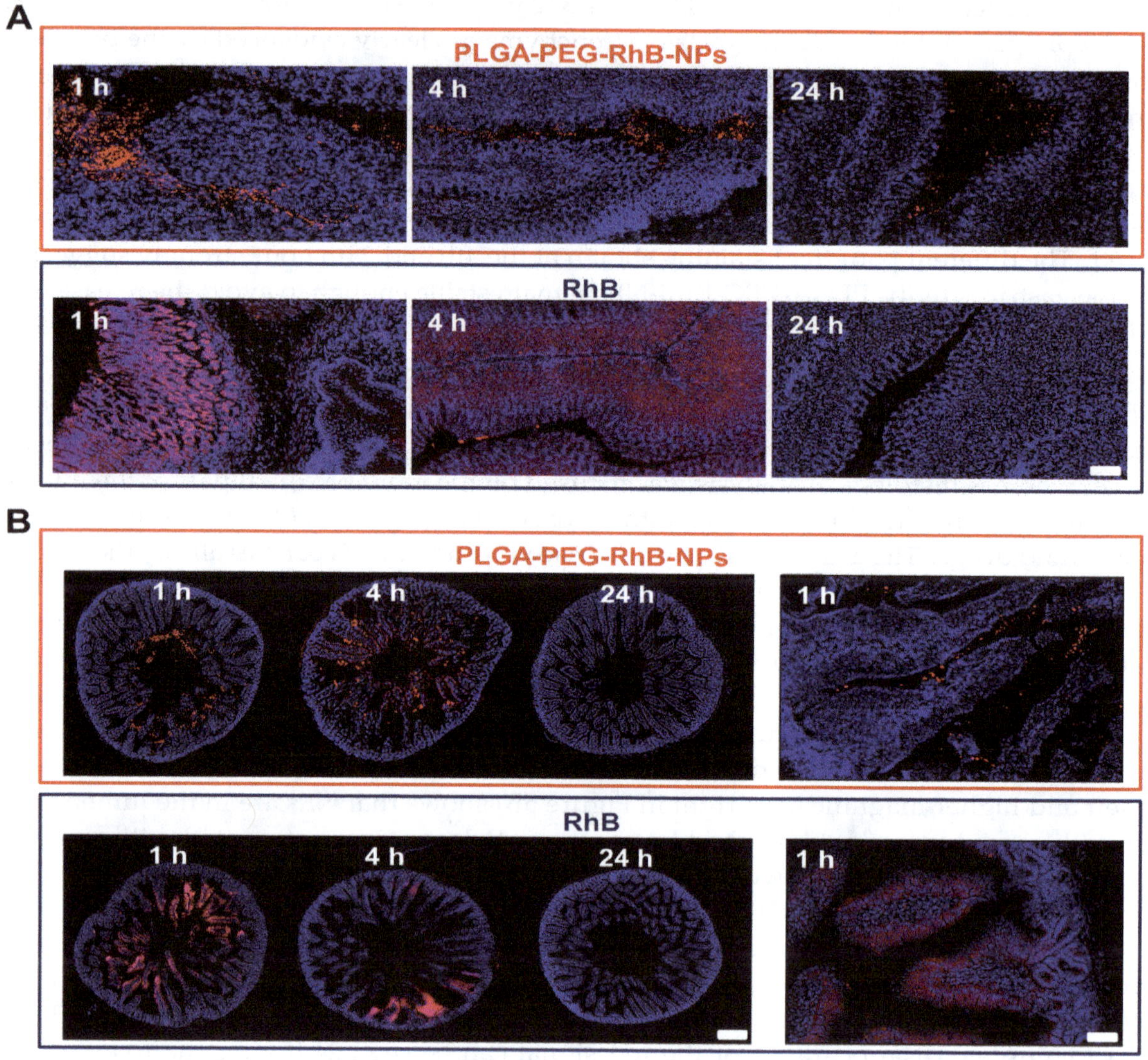

Figure 5. Representative images showing the distribution of RhB in (**A**) stomach and (**B**) duodenum of mice treated with either PLGA-PEG-RhB-NPs or RhB alone. (**A**) In the upper panels, the localization of signal (red) in gastric sections (blue) is shown 1, 4, and 24 h after the oral administration of PLGA-PEG-RhB-NPs. The same procedure has been used to track the presence of the dye in mice receiving the same amount of RhB (lower panels). Scale bar 100 μm. (**B**) Representative images of the duodenum are shown of PLGA-PEG-RhB-NPsand RhB-treated mice in upper and lower panels, respectively. Scale bar 200 μm. The thicker and more intense blue staining in the periphery of the sections represents the basal layer of the duodenum where the exchanges of tissue/blood occur. The red signal is more concentrated to the center, likely corresponding to the lumen close to the apical side of the villi. A higher magnified picture from a mouse sacrificed 1 h after the ingestion of NPs confirms the weak interaction between NPs and villi. In the duodenum of RhB-treated mice, a deep overlapping between the villi and the RhB was observed at both 1 and 24 h after treatment. A higher magnified image confirms the penetration of the dye into the external side of the villi. Scale bar 50 μm.

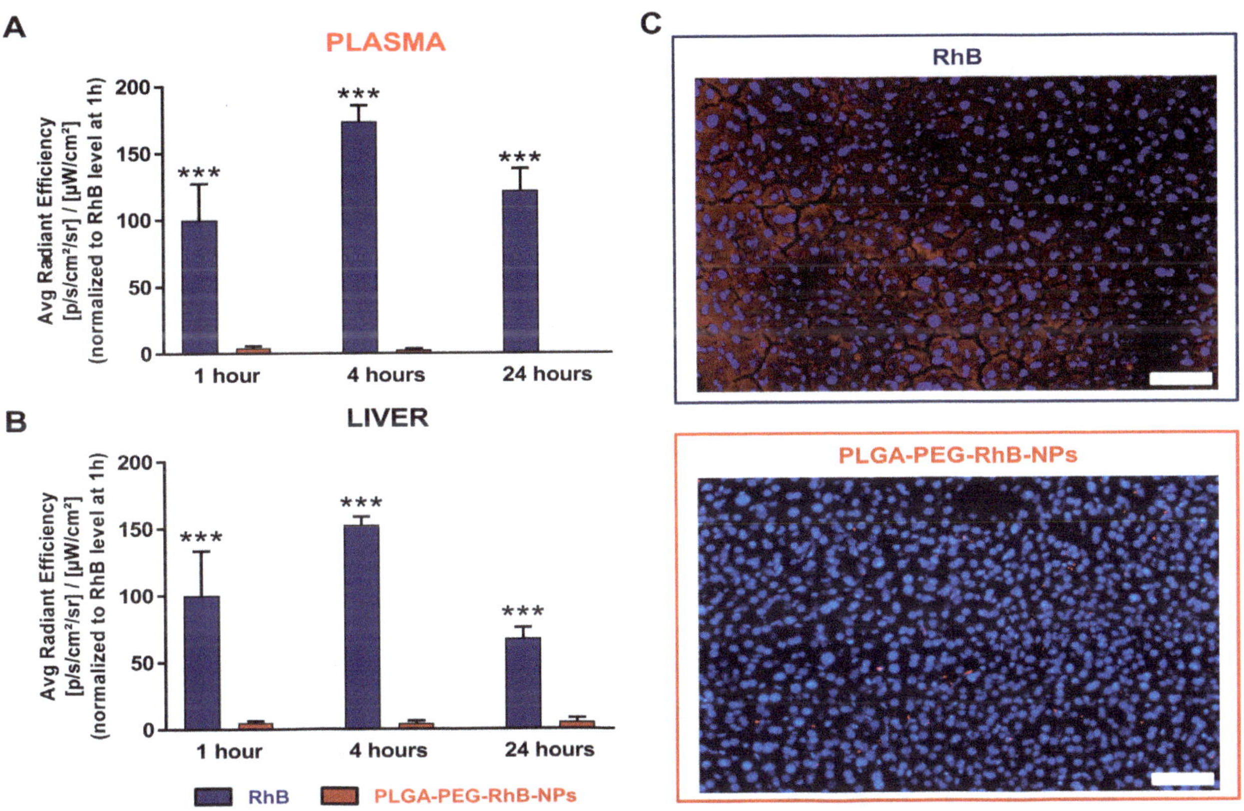

Figure 6. Signal measurement in (**A**) the plasma and (**B**) the liver of mice orally treated with RhB (blue bars) or PLGA-PEG-RhB-NPs (red bars). Animals were sacrificed at 1, 4, and 24 h after the treatment with the same dose of RhB. Five animals for each experimental group were used. In both graphics, quantification of the signal was normalized to the RhB level at 1 h and expressed as 100. The bars are the mean value ± SD ($n = 5$). The Student's t-test was used to compare the levels between the two groups for each time point. *** $p < 0.0001$. (**C**) Representative images of the signal related to the dye in a section of liver from mice treated with PLGA-PEG-RhB-NPs (upper panel) or RhB alone (lower panel), both sacrificed 1 h after the treatment. Scale bar 50 µm.

The last part of the study was carried out to investigate if these NPs were able to penetrate into $CaCo_2$ cells and where they localize inside the cells. This experiment was aimed at exploring the possible application of our results to future local treatment of colorectal cancer. Figure 7A shows the progressive process of internalization of NPs (orange spots). The quantification of the occupied area of NPs inside the cell cytoplasm is reported in Figure 7B. Progressive penetration of NPs occurs and, at the 4th hour after incubation, they already occupied the 2% to 3% of the whole cell area. Although relatively low, this percentage in terms of a potential release of a therapeutic cargo cannot be considered negligible. The red arrow in Figure 7A and the higher magnified picture in Figure 7D confirm that NPs are deeply penetrated (orange spots) and the deep internalization of NPs inside the cell cytoplasm starting from the 4th hour of incubation. Moreover, the cell viability assay confirmed the safety of the materials we selected for this study. Indeed, neither RhB nor PLGA-PEG-RhB-NPs alone modify the healthiness of the cells for the whole duration of the treatment (Figure 7C).

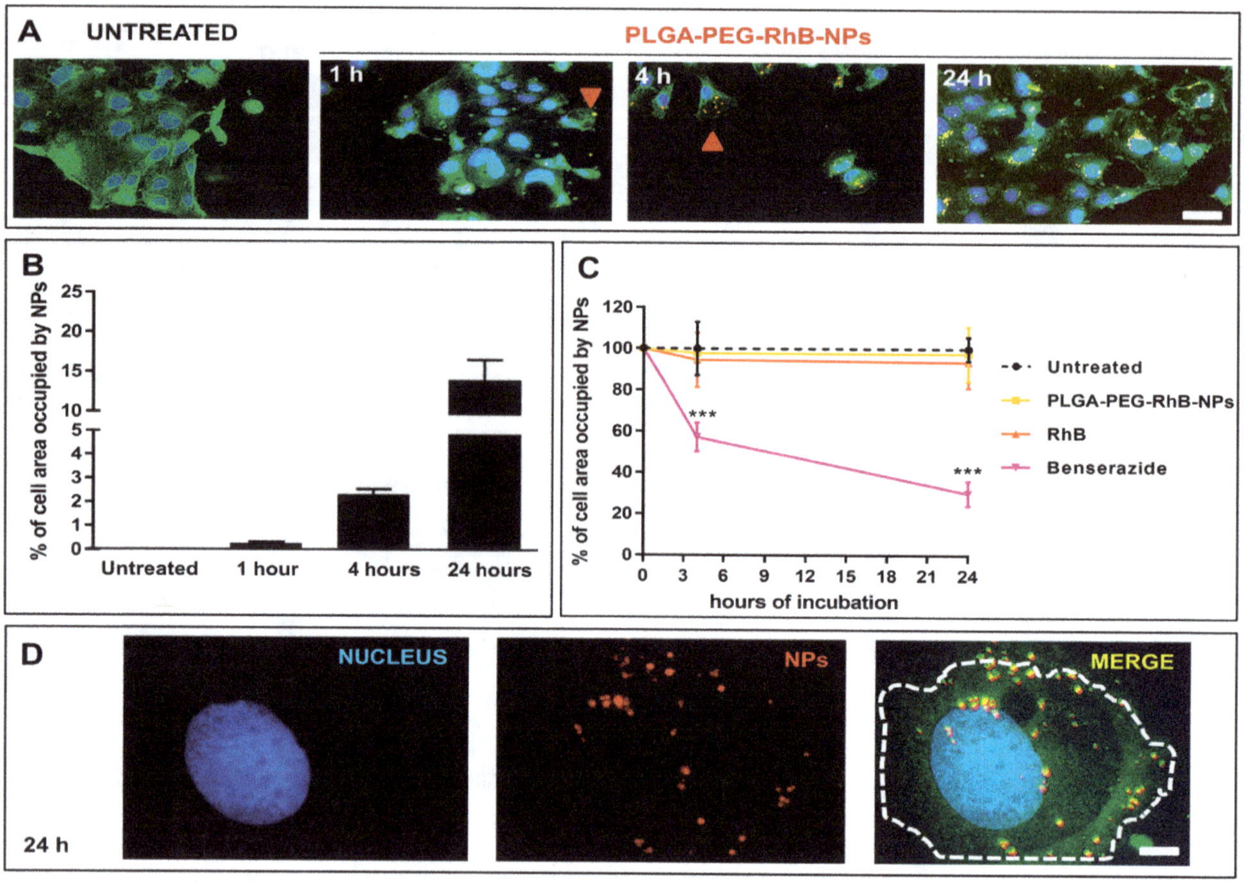

Figure 7. Longitudinal study to evaluate PLGA-PEG-RhB-NPs internalization in $CaCo_2$ cells. (**A**) Low magnified pictures showing the progressive penetration of NPs in cells. Representative images have been selected from non-treated cells (NT, left panel). For each image, the nuclei were stained with Hoechst 33258 (blue), whereas high excitation with the laser at the wavelength of 488 nm will allow unveiling the border of the cells by exploiting their auto fluorescent profile (green). Starting from the 1st hour, it is possible to see orange spots obtained by the merge between the red signal referred to the RhB and the green background. These spots became more evident 4 and 24 h after incubation. Scale bar 70 μm. (**B**) Quantification of the percentage of the area (pixels) occupied by NPs for every single cell at the different time-points. Data are expressed as mean value ± SD, $n = 10$. (**C**) Quantification of the viability of the cells of $CaCo_2$ after exposure to RhB (orange line), PLGA-PEG-RhB-NPs (yellow line), and Benserazide as inner control (purple line) measured by RealTime-Glo™ MT Cell Viability Assay (Promega kit) 4 and 24 h after incubation The values obtained from non-treated cells were normalized to 100 for each time point. Values are expressed as mean ± SD ($n = 6$). The Student's t-test was used to compare the levels among the two groups for each time point. *** $p < 0.0001$ compared to NT. (**D**) Higher magnification pictures showing the same field of view achieved 24 h after PLGA-PEG-RhB-NPs incubation. In the left panel, the cell nucleus, in the middle panel, the red spots associated with NPs, and in the right panel, the merge between the three channels. The dotted line is the border of the cell. Scale bar 15 μm.

4. Conclusions

The current study sought to evaluate the effect of the nanocarrier on the transport of a drug and its behavior within the gastrointestinal tract and absorption to the bloodstream. It is important to note, however, that although RhB was originally used as a tracer to visualize NPs. The results obtained by comparing the biodistribution in mice of the free fluorophore and linked to the NPs is of further relevance for future developments. It is, in fact, interesting how PLGA-PEG-NPs manage to preserve the gastroduodenal absorption by using chemically different molecules along with different loading approaches to the nanocarrier. The low systemic exposure and, at the same time, equivalent drug concentration at the intestinal level, with even a trend to increase in the colon 4 h after the treatment, could have a significant positive outcome on the safety of a wide range of drugs targeting inflammatory and neoplastic diseases.

Supplementary Materials:
Figure S1: STEM image of PTX-PLGA-PEG-RhB-NPs, Figure S2: Release kinetics of PTX loaded NPs in PBS containing 0.2 *v*/*v*% Tween 80. PTX-PLGA-PEG-RhB-NPs equivalent to 8.75 μg of PTX were suspended in 1 mL of release medium and incubated at 37 °C with constant agitation. At predetermined time points (0.5, 1, 2, 4, 6 and 24 h), the NPs were separated by centrifugation and the supernatant analyzed by HPLC. The results are the mean value ± SD ($n = 4$).

Author Contributions: L.M. (Lucia Morelli), L.S., M.G., B.C. performed nanoparticles synthesis, functionalization, and characterization; S.G., M.S. (Marta Sevieri), L.T., L.R., M.B.V. performed in vivo experiments; L.M. (Lavinia Morosi) performed pharmacokinetic analysis; L.P., A.F. did the data curation; D.P., M.S. (Mario Salmona) gave critical comments on the manuscript; D.P., M.C., P.B., M.Z. designed the research and provided funding; P.B., M.C. wrote the manuscript; all authors revised the manuscript critically.

Acknowledgments: We thank Tiziano Catalani for the STEM image.

References

1. Peer, D.; Karp, J.M.; Hong, S.; Farokhzad, O.C.; Margalit, R.; Langer, R. Nanocarriers as an emerging platform for cancer therapy. *Nat. Nanotechnol.* **2007**, *2*, 751–760. [CrossRef] [PubMed]
2. Heath, J.R. Nanotechnologies for biomedical science and translational medicine. *Proc. Natl. Acad. Sci. USA* **2015**, *112*, 14436–14443. [CrossRef] [PubMed]
3. Violatto, M.B.; Casarin, E.; Talamini, L.; Russo, L.; Baldan, S.; Tondello, C.; Messmer, M.; Hintermann, E.; Rossi, A.; Passoni, A.; et al. Dexamethasone Conjugation to Biodegradable Avidin-Nucleic-Acid-Nano-Assemblies Promotes Selective Liver Targeting and Improves Therapeutic Efficacy in an Autoimmune Hepatitis Murine Model. *ACS Nano* **2019**, *13*, 4410–4423. [CrossRef] [PubMed]
4. Bartneck, M.; Scheyda, M.K.; Warzecha, K.T.; Rizzo, Y.L.; Hittatiya, K.; Luedde, T.; Storm, G.; Trautwein, C.; Lammers, T.; Tacke, F. Fluorescent cell-traceable dexamethasone-loaded liposomes for the treatment of inflammatory liver diseases. *Biomaterials* **2015**, *37*, 367–382. [CrossRef] [PubMed]
5. Hoshyar, N.; Gray, S.; Han, H.; Bao, G. The effect of nanoparticle size on in vivo pharmacokinetics and cellular interaction. *Nanomedicine* **2016**, *11*, 673–692. [CrossRef]
6. Uziely, B.; Jeffers, S.; Isacson, R.; Kutsch, K.; Wei-Tsao, D.; Yehoshua, Z.; Libson, E.; Muggia, F.M.; Gabizon, A. Liposomal doxorubicin: Antitumor activity and unique toxicities during two complementary phase I studies. *J. Clin. Oncol.* **1995**, *13*, 1777–1785. [CrossRef]
7. Feng, S.; Mu, L.; Win, K.Y. Nanoparticles of Biodegradable Polymers for Clinical Administration of Paclitaxel. *Curr. Med. Chem.* **2004**, *11*, 413–424. [CrossRef]
8. Bhatt, P.; Lalani, R.; Vhora, I.; Patil, S.; Amrutiya, J.; Misra, A.; Mashru, R. Liposomes encapsulating native and cyclodextrin enclosed paclitaxel: Enhanced loading efficiency and its pharmacokinetic evaluation. *Int. J. Pharm* **2018**, *536*, 95–107. [CrossRef]
9. Venugopal, V.; Krishnan, S.; Palanimuthu, V.R.; Sankarankutty, S.; Kalaimani, J.K.; Karupiah, S.; Kit, N.S.; Hock, T.T. Anti-EGFR anchored paclitaxel loaded PLGA nanoparticles for the treatment of triple negative breast cancer.In-vitro and in-vivo anticancer activities. *PLoS ONE* **2018**, *13*, e0206109. [CrossRef]
10. Kamaly, N.; Yameen, B.; Wu, J.; Farokhzad, O.C. Degradable controlled-release polymers and polymeric nanoparticles: Mechanisms of controlling drug release. *Chem. Rev.* **2016**, *116*, 2602–2663. [CrossRef]
11. Colzani, B.; Pandolfi, L.; Hoti, A.; Iovene, P.A.; Natalello, A.; Avvakumova, S.; Colombo, M.; Prosperi, D. Investigation of antitumor activities of trastuzumab delivered by PLGA nanoparticles. *Int. J. Nanomed.* **2018**, *13*, 957–973. [CrossRef] [PubMed]
12. Park, J.; Fong, P.M.; Lu, J.; Russell, K.S.; Booth, C.J.; Saltzman, W.M.; Fahmy, T.M. PEGylated PLGA nanoparticles for the improved delivery of doxorubicin. *Nanomedicine* **2009**, *5*, 410–418. [CrossRef] [PubMed]
13. Ramezani, M.; Ebrahimian, M.; Hashemi, M. Current Strategies in the Modification of PLGA-based Gene Delivery System. *Curr. Med. Chem.* **2017**, *24*, 728–739. [CrossRef] [PubMed]
14. Li, J.; Sabliov, C.M. PLA/PLGA nanoparticles for delivery of drugs across the blood-brain barrier. *Nanotechnol. Rev.* **2013**, *2*, 241–257. [CrossRef]

15. Gamboa, J.M.; Leong, K.W. In vitro and in vivo models for the study of oral delivery of nanoparticles. *Adv. Drug Deliv. Rev.* **2013**, *65*, 800–810. [CrossRef]
16. Danhier, F.; Ansorena, E.; Silva, J.M.; Coco, R.; Le Breton, A.; Préat, V. PLGA-based nanoparticles: An overview of biomedical applications. *J. Control. Release* **2012**, *161*, 505–522. [CrossRef]
17. Wagner, A.M.; Gran, M.P.; Peppas, N.A. Designing the new generation of intelligent biocompatible carriers for protein and peptide delivery. *Acta Pharm. Sin. B* **2018**, *8*, 147–164. [CrossRef]
18. Santini, B.; Zanoni, I.; Marzi, R.; Cigni, C.; Bedoni, M.; Gramatica, F.; Palugan, L.; Corsi, F.; Granucci, F.; Colombo, M. Cream formulation impact on topical administration of engineered colloidal nanoparticles. *PLoS ONE* **2015**, *10*, e0126366. [CrossRef]
19. Musazzi, U.M.; Santini, B.; Selmin, F.; Marini, V.; Corsi, F.; Allevi, R.; Prosperi, D.; Cilurzo, F.; Colombo, M.; Minghetti, P. Impact of semi-solid formulations on skin penetration of iron oxide nanoparticles. *J. Nanobiotechnol.* **2017**, *15*, 14. [CrossRef]
20. Cunha, S.; Amaral, M.H.; Lobo, J.M.S.; Silva, A.C. Lipid Nanoparticles for Nasal/Intranasal Drug Delivery. *Crit Rev. Ther. Drug Carr. Syst.* **2017**, *34*, 257–282. [CrossRef]
21. Codullo, V.; Cova, E.; Pandolfi, L.; Breda, S.; Morosini, M.; Frangipane, V.; Malatesta, M.; Calderan, L.; Cagnone, M.; Pacini, C.; et al. Imatinib-loaded gold nanoparticles inhibit proliferation of fibroblasts and macrophages from systemic sclerosis patients and ameliorate experimental bleomycin-induced lung fibrosis. *J. Control. Release* **2019**, *310*, 198–208. [CrossRef] [PubMed]
22. Salvioni, L.; Fiandra, L.; Del Curto, M.D.; Mazzucchelli, S.; Allevi, R.; Truffi, M.; Sorrentino, L.; Santini, B.; Cerea, M.; Palugan, L.; et al. Oral delivery of insulin via polyethylene imine-based nanoparticles for colonic release allows glycemic control in diabetic rats. *Pharmacol. Res.* **2016**, *110*, 122–130. [CrossRef] [PubMed]
23. Suk, J.S.; Xu, Q.; Kim, N.; Hanes, J.; Ensign, L.M. PEGylation as a strategy for improving nanoparticle-based drug and gene delivery. *Adv. Drug Deliv. Rev.* **2016**, *99*, 28–51. [CrossRef] [PubMed]
24. Inchaurraga, L.; Martín-Arbella, N.; Zabaleta, V.; Quincoces, G.; Peñuelas, I.; Irache, J.M. In vivo study of the mucus-permeating properties of PEG-coated nanoparticles following oral administration. *Eur. J. Pharm. Biopharm.* **2015**, *97 Pt A*, 280–289. [CrossRef]
25. Aggarwal, S.; Gupta, S.; Pabla, D.; Murty, R.S.R. Gemcitabine-loaded PLGA-PEG immunonanoparticles for targeted chemotherapy of pancreatic cancer. *Cancer Nanotechnol.* **2013**, *4*, 145–157. [CrossRef]
26. Lazzari, S.; Moscatelli, D.; Codari, F.; Salmona, M.; Morbidelli, M.; Diomede, L. Colloidal stability of polymeric nanoparticles in biological fluids. *J. Nanopart. Res.* **2012**, *14*, 920. [CrossRef]
27. Fruscio, R.; Lissoni, A.A.; Frapolli, R.; Corso, S.; Mangioni, C.; D'Incalci, M.; Zucchetti, M. Clindamycin-paclitaxel pharmacokinetic interaction in ovarian cancer patients. *Cancer Chemother. Pharmacol.* **2006**, *58*, 319–325. [CrossRef]
28. Enlow, E.M.; Luft, J.C.; Napier, M.E.; DeSimone, J.M. Potent engineered PLGA nanoparticles by virtue of exceptionally high chemotherapeutic loadings. *Nano Lett.* **2011**, *11*, 808–813. [CrossRef]
29. Abouelmagd, S.A.; Sun, B.; Chang, A.C.; Ku, Y.J.; Yeo, Y. Release Kinetics Study of Poorly Water-Soluble Drugs from Nanoparticles: Are We Doing It Right? *Mol. Pharm.* **2015**, *12*, 997–1003. [CrossRef]
30. Gullotti, E.; Yeo, Y. Beyond the imaging: Limitations of cellular uptake study in the evaluation of nanoparticles. *J. Control. Release* **2012**, *164*, 170–176. [CrossRef]
31. Zhang, W.; Shi, K.; Shi, J.; He, X. Use of the fluorescence of rhodamine B for the pH sensing of a glycine solution. *Proc. SPIE* **2016**, 10155. [CrossRef]
32. Capasso Palmiero, U.; Morosi, L.; Lupi, M.; Ponzo, M.; Frapolli, R.; Zucchetti, M.; Ubezio, P.; Morbidelli, M.; D'Incalci, M.; Bello, E.; et al. Self-Assembling PCL-Based Nanoparticles as PTX Solubility Enhancer Excipients. *Macromol. Biosci.* **2018**, *18*, 1800164. [CrossRef]
33. Colombo, C.; Morosi, L.; Bello, E.; Ferrari, R.; Licandro, S.A.; Lupi, M.; Ubezio, P.; Morbidelli, M.; Zucchetti, M.; D'Incalci, M.; et al. PEGylated Nanoparticles Obtained through Emulsion Polymerization as Paclitaxel Carriers. *Mol. Pharm.* **2016**, *13*, 40–46. [CrossRef]
34. Tenuta, T.; Monopoli, M.; Kim, J.; Salvati, A.; Dawson, K.; Sandin, P.; Lynch, I. Elution of Labile Fluorescent Dye from Nanoparticles during Biological Use. *PLoS ONE* **2011**, *6*, e25556. [CrossRef]

6

PLGA-BMP-2 and PLA-17β-Estradiol Microspheres Reinforcing a Composite Hydrogel for Bone Regeneration in Osteoporosis

Patricia García-García [1], Ricardo Reyes [2,3], Elisabet Segredo-Morales [1], Edgar Pérez-Herrero [1,2], Araceli Delgado [1,2,*] and Carmen Évora [1,2,*]

1 Department of Chemical Engineering and Pharmaceutical Technology, University of La Laguna, 38206 La Laguna, Spain; patg0991@gmail.com (P.G.-G); esegredm@ull.edu.es (E.S.-M.); eperezhe@ull.edu.es (E.P.-H.)

2 Institute of Biomedical Technologies (ITB), University of La Laguna, 38206 La Laguna, Spain; rreyesro@ull.edu.es

3 Department of Biochemistry, Microbiology, Cell Biology and Genetics, University of La Laguna, 38206 La Laguna, Spain

* Correspondence: adelgado@ull.edu.es (A.D.); cevora@ull.edu.es (C.É.)

Abstract: The controlled release of active substances—bone morphogenetic protein 2 (BMP-2) and 17β-estradiol—is one of the main aspects to be taken into account to successfully regenerate a tissue defect. In this study, BMP-2- and 17β-estradiol-loaded microspheres were combined in a sandwich-like system formed by a hydrogel core composed of chitosan (CHT) collagen, 2-hidroxipropil γ-ciclodextrin (HP-γ-CD), nanoparticles of hydroxyapatite (nano-HAP), and an electrospun mesh shell prepared with two external electrospinning films for the regeneration of a critical bone defect in osteoporotic rats. Microspheres were made with poly-lactide-*co*-glycolide (PLGA) to encapsulate BMP-2, whereas the different formulations of 17β-estradiol were prepared with poly-lactic acid (PLA) and PLGA. The in vitro and in vivo BMP-2 delivered from the system fitted a biphasic profile. Although the in vivo burst effect was higher than in vitro the second phases (lasted up to 6 weeks) were parallel, the release rate ranged between 55 and 70 ng/day. The in vitro release kinetics of the 17β-estradiol dissolved in the polymeric matrix of the microspheres depended on the partition coefficient. The 17β-estradiol was slowly released from the core system using an aqueous release medium ($D_{eff} = 5.58{\cdot}10^{-16} \pm 9.81{\cdot}10^{-17} m^2 s^{-1}$) and very fast in MeOH-water (50:50). The hydrogel core system was injectable, and approximately 83% of the loaded dose is uniformly discharged through a 20G needle. The system placed in the defect was easily adapted to the defect shape and after 12 weeks approximately 50% of the defect was refilled by new tissue. None differences were observed between the osteoporotic and non-osteoporotic groups. Despite the role of 17β-estradiol on the bone remodeling process, the obtained results in this study suggest that the observed regeneration was only due to the controlled rate released of BMP-2 from the PLGA microspheres.

Keywords: BMP-2-microspheres; hydrogel system; 17-βestradiol release; bone regeneration; osteoporosis; poly-lactide-*co*-glycolide; polylactic acid

---

1. Introduction

Regeneration of bone critical defects is still a challenge in the orthopedic field. Local treatment with bone morphogenetic protein (BMP-2) incorporated in different biomaterial scaffolds has demonstrated to be efficient to induce new bone formation for critical bone defect in several animal models. Nowadays, collagen sponges loaded with recombinant BMP-2 are clinically available as bone graft substitutes for the treatment of nonunion and critical-sized bone defects. Although BMP-2 is a potent osteogenic agent, a controlled release profile is required for safety and efficacy. Thus, the scaffold to fill the bone defect should not only be designed to act as support and guide for tissue growth, but also to control the release rate of active substances. Although many materials and structures have been proposed to construct these scaffolds, the control of the release rate has not always been taken into account. In fact, in some cases the protein is incorporated in the material by incubation and, unless a material-protein interaction occurs, a burst release at an early period would be expected. Consequently, a high dose of BMP-2 would be in blood circulation, leading to a high risk of side effects and, at the same time, a significant loss of the protein in the site of action. In addition, some authors showed that BMPs in these cases might also stimulate bone resorption due to the high dose of BMP-2 associated to uncontrolled release [1]. To minimize the osteoclastic effect of BMPs, some authors proposed the addition of an anti-catabolic agent. The most frequently studied combination has been BMP-2 with bisphosphonates as anti-resorption agents such as alendronate [2,3] and zolendronate [4]. The results indicated good bone regeneration with improved bone quality and mineralization in different localizations compared to BMP-2 alone [5,6].

Among the several natural polymeric scaffolds prepared for bone regeneration, chitosan is a biomaterial frequently used for this purpose. In a recent extensive review [7] based on chitosan (CHT) applied in bone tissue regeneration, different advantageous aspects were showed and discussed such as biocompatibility, capacity for BMPs sustained release, improvement of cell proliferation, and increase of in vitro and in vivo differentiation and mineralization. However, bone graft materials to simulate bone structure, e.g., collagen, the major ECM of bone tissue, and hydroxyapatite (HAP), a mineral component of the bone, have also been widely studied [6,8–14].

Although the aforementioned studies indicated positive results, the mentioned strategies applied in osteoporosis (OP) conditions have not always been effective [15]. According to recent reports, the prolonged subcutaneous administration of alendronate and the low level of estrogen in OP alters the evolution of calvarial bone repair due to estrogen, Transforming Growth Factor beta 1 (TGF-β1), and α-estrogen receptor (α-ER) interaction [16]. Menopausal women are the population most affected by this disease due to estrogen deficiency. Previous reports revealed that local implantation of scaffolds loaded with combinations of BMP-2 and 17β-estradiol formulated in microspheres of polylactic acid (PLA) or PLGA, in rat calvaria critical defects increased the bone repair in OP rats, but the new bone that refilled the defect was less mineralized compared to non-OP groups [17,18].

As some biomaterials may promote bone regeneration, controlled release of the active substances is required for efficient and safe bone regeneration [19,20]. In this study, we propose a loaded BMP-2 and 17β-estradiol sandwich-like system, comprising two polymeric external films and a core of a biocomposite hydrogel containing microspheres, to provide sustained release of active substances. The core system composed of CHT, collagen, HAP nanoparticles (nano-HAP), polyethylene glycol (PEG-400) and 2-Hidroxipropil γ-Ciclodextrin HP-γ-CD was previously characterized in terms of composition, rheological behavior and mass-transfer using RITC-dextran as macromolecule model and 17β-estradiol in microspheres [21]. In the present study, we aim to study the influence of the release rate of 17β-estradiol on the osteogenic effect induced by BMP-2 released from PLGA microspheres within core system after sandwich-like system implantation in a OP rats critical size defect. Therefore, 17β-estradiol was incorporated into the system in 3 forms: free and dispersed in the core, encapsulated in microspheres prepared with a mixture of PLA and PLGA dispersed within the hydrogel and lastly encapsulated in the PLGA films shell prepared by electrospinning technique.

2. Materials and Method

2.1. Materials

PLGA 75:25 (Resomer® RG755-S), PLGA 50:50 (Resomer® RG504), PLGA 85:15 (Resomer® RG858-S), and PLA (Resomer® RG203-S) were supplied by Evonic Industries (Darmstadt, Germany). Chitosan

(Protasan® UP-CL-213) was purchased from NovaMatrix (Sandvika, Norway). 2-Hidroxipropil γ-Ciclodextrin (CAVASOL® W8 HP), was supplied by Wacker Chemical (Burghausen, Germany). The bovine collagen type I was purchased from CellSystems Biotechnologie (Vertrieb GmbH, Germany). Riboflavin (RB), Poly(ethylene glycol) 400, Poly(vinyl alcohol) (PVA, Mw 33–70 kDa; 87–90% hydrolyzed), 17β-estradiol, and all the other reagents were purchased from Sigma-Aldrich, (St. Louis, MO, USA). The recombinant human bone morphogenetic protein 2 (BMP-2) was bought from Biomedal Life Sciences (Sevilla, Spain). Citrate-coated carbonated apatite nanoparticles (nano-HAP) were kindly donated (Jaime Gómez-Morales, PhD, Laboratory of Crystallographic Studies, CSIC, Granada, Spain).

2.2. Microspheres Preparation and Characterization

The BMP-2 microspheres were prepared by the double emulsion method (w/o/w) previously described [22]. Briefly, 200 μL of an aqueous solution (0.2% PVA) of BMP-2 (260 μg) was emulsified with 1 mL of a PLGA mixture (150 mg) of RG504 and RG858 [4:1] in methylene chloride (DCM) by vortexing 1 min (position 10, Genie® Industries 2, Sciencies Industries Inc. USA). Then, this emulsion was poured into 10 mL of 0.2% PVA solution vortexed 15 s, then poured into 100 mL of 0.1% PVA and kept under magnetic stirring for 1 h for solvent evaporation.

The 17β-estradiol microspheres were prepared by a modified solvent evaporation method previously described [17]. Briefly a mixture of 17β-estradiol (4 mg), PLA-S RG203-S (160 mg) and PLGA RG858 (40 mg) dissolved in 0.6 mL of DCM:Methanol (DCM:MeOH) (80:20) was emulsified with 4 mL of 1% PVA aqueous solution by vortexing 1 min (position 10), and then added to 100 mL of 0.16% PVA solution, under magnetic stirring for organic solvent evaporation (1 h).

Both type of microspheres were collected by filtration (Pall Corporation, pore size 45 μm, Sigma-Aldrich, USA), lyophilized, and stored at 4 °C until use.

Microspheres were characterized in terms of size (Mastersizer 2000, Malver Instruments, Malvern, UK) and morphology (SEM, Jeol JSM-6300, Tokyo, Japan). To determine the BMP-2 encapsulation efficiency and to carry out the BMP-2 release assays, some batches were prepared with ^{125}IBMP-2. The BMP-2 was labeled with ^{125}INa (Perkin-Elmer) by the iodogen method [23]. The content of 17β-estradiol in the microspheres was determined spectrophotometrically at $\lambda = 280$ nm previous dissolution in a mix of DCM:MeOH (80:20).

To determine the solubility of 17β-estradiol in the polymer matrix of the microspheres, differential scanning calorimetry (DSC 025, TA Instruments, New Castle, DE, USA) was performed. 17β-estradiol and lyophilized microspheres were analyzed after drying in an oven at 37 °C overnight. In addition, samples of polymer blends (RG 203-S and RG 858, 4:1) and samples of the polymer blend with excess 17β-estradiol (8.5%) were dissolved in DCM:MeOH (80:20) and maintained in a hood for 24 h. Then, samples were placed 48 h more in a vacuum desiccator to complete the evaporation of the organic solvent. The analysis of all samples was performed with the same thermal program in two thermal cycles under a nitrogen atmosphere (50 mL/min). In the first cycle, temperature was increased to 40 °C (10 °C/min) and then cooled to −20 °C (5 °C/min) to avoid possible water interference. Once the samples were stabilized, they underwent a final heating cycle from −20 °C to 270 °C (10 °C/min).

2.3. Fabrication and Characterization of the Film

The film was fabricated by a previously described electrospinning method [24]. Briefly, 7 mg of 17β-estradiol and 300 mg of a mixture of PLGAs, RG755-S and RG858 [4:1] were dissolved in 2 mL of hexafluoroisopropanol (Sigma-Aldrich, Steinheim, Germany) and electrospun at 7kV; flow rate of 3.0 mL/h and 10 cm of distance from the collector.

The film quality was checked in terms of porosity, thickness and fiber diameter using helium pycnometer (AccuPyc 1330, Micromeritics, Norcross, GA, USA), stereo microscopy (Leica M205C, Leica Las, v3 sofware), and SEM (Jeol, JSM-6300, Tokyo, Japan), respectively.

2.4. Core System Preparation and Characterization

To prepare the core system, approximately 20 mg of microspheres were dispersed in 50 μL of the hydrogel composed by a mixture of collagen type I (5 mg/mL), HP-γ-CD (34 mg/mL), RB (0.4 mg/mL), CHT (5 mg/mL), PEG-400 (150 mg/mL), and 5 mg of nano-HAP. Then, the hydrogel was cross-linked with 5% *w/w* TPP sterile aqueous solution (0.5 μL/μL of hydrogel) and visible light blue at 468 nm (Dental device) for 3 min [21]. The dose of BMP-2 was 6 μg in microspheres and the total 17β-estradiol dose was 200 μg in three different forms: electrospun films, microspheres, or dispersed into the gel.

The quality of the core system was checked according to its rheological characteristics and porosity previously described [21]. In addition, water uptake and mass loss assays were carried out by incubation of aliquots of 300 μL of the core system in 5 mL of sterile MilliQ water (37 °C) under orbital agitation (25 rpm). At specific times, six samples were withdrawn, we then removed excess water, weighed, and freeze-dried the samples. Then, three samples were visualized by SEM (Jeol JSM-6300) to see the evolution of the internal structure after incubation. The other three samples were used to record the dried weight and calculate the percentage of mass loss and water uptake, applying Equations (1) and (2), respectively, where W_0 is the initial weight of the sample and W_w and W_d are the weights of the wet and dried sample, respectively, at the different times tested.

$$Mass\ loss(\%) = \frac{(W_0 - W_d)}{W_0} \times 100 \tag{1}$$

$$Water\ uptake(\%) = \frac{(W_w - W_d)}{W_d} \times 100 \tag{2}$$

To test the syringeability of the core system two syringes of 1 mL were loaded with a suspension of microspheres of 17β-estradiol in the hydrogel, up to 0.5 mL. Then, 4 doses of 50 μL each were unloaded from both syringes assayed for fluidity through a 20G needle and dose uniformity. For this, the discharged samples were lyophilized, and the 17β-estradiol content evaluated by spectrophotometry at 280 nm, after dissolution in DCM: MeOH (80:20).

2.5. In Vitro Release Assays

BMP-2 in vitro release assays were carried out by incubating an amount of ^{125}I-BMP-2 microspheres and an amount of core system with the same amount of ^{125}I-BMP-2 microspheres in sterile MilliQ water at 37 °C and 25 rpm. The amount of BMP-2 released was calculated by measuring the radioactivity of supernatant samples with a gamma counter (Cobra® II, Packard).

The in vitro release of 17β-estradiol from the different formulations (dispersed in the core system, microspheres, microspheres incorporated to the core system, and electrospun films) was carried out at 37 °C and 25 rpm using two release media: an aqueous solution of sodium lauryl sulfate (SLS) 1% [25] and MeOH:water (50:50) [26,27]. The released 17β-estradiol was measured in the supernatant using the spectrophotometric method. The effective diffusion coefficient, D_{eff} in the matrix of the microspheres and the mass transfer coefficient of the drug in the boundary layer h, were calculated according to the non-steady-state Fick law, as previously described in detail [21]. Whether or not the released fraction of 17β-estradiol from the microspheres dispersed in the core system was analyzed, and Equations (3)–(6) were applied for D_{eff} and h calculation.

$$\frac{M_t}{M_\infty} = 1 - \sum_{n=1}^{\infty} \frac{6\,L^2}{\beta_n^2\left(\beta_n^2 + L^2 - L\right)} exp\left(-\frac{\beta_n^2}{R^2} D_{eff}\, t\right) \tag{3}$$

where M_t and M_∞ are the total mass of drug released to the media at time t and at the end of the experiment, respectively. The β_ns are the infinite roots (eigenvalues) of the Equation (4):

$$\beta_n \cot \beta_n + L - 1 = 0 \tag{4}$$

L is the dimensionless mass transfer Biot number Equation (5):

$$L = \frac{h\,R}{D_{eff}} \tag{5}$$

For large values of L, the roots of Equation (4) are multiples of the number *pi* and Equation (3) can be simplified in the Equation (6), that is, a simplified solution of non-steady-state Fick law:

$$\frac{M_t}{M_\infty} = 1 - \frac{6}{\pi^2}\sum_{n=1}^{\infty}\frac{1}{n^2}exp\left(-\frac{n^2\,\pi^2}{R^2}\,D_{eff}\,t\right) \tag{6}$$

As stated previously, to minimize the residual sum of squares, "genetic algorithms" already implanted in R software (R Foundation for Statistical Computing, version 3.6.1., 2019, Vienna, Austria) were used [21].

2.6. Animal Experiments

All animal experiments were carried out in conformity with the European Directive (2010/63UE) on Care and Use in Experimental Procedures. Furthermore, the animal protocols were approved on 5 November 2014 by the Ethics Committee for Animal Cares of the University of La Laguna (CEIBA) with identification code CEIBA2014-0128. All surgical procedures were made under aseptic conditions.

2.6.1. Animal Models

Forty female adult Sprague-Dawley rats approximately 12 weeks old, weighing 200–250 g, were divided in 4 groups of 10 each. The experimental osteoporosis was induced in 3 groups by three different protocols, OVX, chronic administration of DEX and OD. The forth group was the sham, non-osteoporotic control group (non-OP). The bilateral ovariectomy was carried out under isoflurane anesthesia, via dorsal approach to the animals of OVX and OD groups. Analgesia consisted in buprenorphine administered subcutaneously (0.05 mg/kg) before surgery and paracetamol (70 mg/100 mL) in the water, for 3 days post-surgery. The DEX group received 0.3 mg/kg body weight of dexamethasone-21-isonicotinate (Deyanil retard, Fatro Ibérica, Barcelona, Spain) administered subcutaneously once ievery two weeks [28] up to the time of euthanasia. Then, two weeks after the ovariectomy, the rats of group OD were chronically treated with DEX as the DEX group. The 40 rats were sacrificed after 12 weeks and the calvaria and femurs were extracted to be histologically analyzed. The results of these analyzes were used to evaluate the 3 protocols tested to induce OP.

2.6.2. Animals Groups

Fifty female Sprague-Dawley rats (12 weeks old), weighing 200–250 g, were divided into 2 groups of 25 each: OP and non-OP. The rats of the OP group were ovariectomized and the rats of the non-OP group underwent similar surgery but the ovaries were not resected. Twelve weeks post-surgery, 8 mm critical size cranial defects were created surgically with a trephine burr in the rats under isoflurane and the systems were placed into the defects [20]. Analgesia treatment was administrated.

Female rats were divided into 5 groups of 10 rats each—5 OP and 5 non-OP—and the applied regenerative treatment is reflected in Table 1. The implantation of the systems was carried out following a two steps procedure. First, a layer of film (bottom film), previously soaked in the blood produced during the surgery, was placed in the defect then 50 μL of the hydrogel mixed with the microspheres and partially cross-linked with UV light, was discharged. Second, the hydrogel was completely cross-linked by dripping 25 μL of sodium tripolyphosphate (TPP) forming the core system, after 5 min, a second layer of film (soaked in blood) was placed on the top, like a sandwich, and the wound was then closed.

Table 1. Experimental groups to evaluate regenerative efficiency.

Group Designations	Treatment
Blank I (B)	System loaded with blank microspheres and blank films
Blank II (B-HAP)	System loaded with blank microspheres and 5 mg of nano-HAP and blank films
BMP+EF	System loaded with 6 μg of BMP-2 in microspheres and 200 μg of 17β-estradiol in the 2 films
BMP+EMs	System loaded with 6 μg of BMP-2 in microspheres and 200 μg of 17β-estradiol in microspheres, blank films
BMP+ED	System loaded with 6 μg of BMP-2 and 200 μg of 17β-estradiol dispersed, blank films

2.6.3. ^{125}I-BMP-2 in Vivo Release Assay

The BMP-2 release kinetics was monitored periodically by measuring the remaining ^{125}I-BMP-2 at the rat calvarial defect site (n = 5) using an external probe-type gamma counter (Captus ®, Capintec Inc., Ramsey, NJ, USA), as previously described and validated [29].

2.7. Rat Mesenchymal Stem Cells (rMSCs) Osteogenic Differentiation

The rMSCs were obtained by centrifugal isolation as previously described [30] from the bone marrow of the femur of OVX female Sprague-Dawley rats. Briefly, the cells were resuspended in high glucose DMEM (HyClone® Utah) supplemented with 10% fetal bovine serum (Biowest, South America Origin), 1% penicillin–streptomycin (PAA, Pasching, Austria), and 2 mM L-Glutamine stable (Biowest, France) (Complete Culture Medium, CCM). Then, cells were cultured in flasks of 75 cm^2 and subcultured by incubating at 37°C and 5% CO_2. The culture medium was changed every 2–3 days.

To test the osteogenic differentiation, 50,000 cells (passage 2) in 20 μL of CCM were added over aliquots of 300 μL of the core system (hydrogel with microspheres) with and without nano-HAP and incubated at 37 °C and 5% CO_2 for 1.5 h for cell adhesion. The homogeneous cell distribution was checked by light microscopy. Afterwards, 500 μL of CCM were added to each well, after 3 days incubation the medium was changed to CCM supplemented with 10 mM β-glycerol phosphate, 10^{-7} M dexamethasone and 50 μM ascorbate-2-phosphate. At 7, 14, and 21 days of culture, three wells of each time point were washed (2 times) with Hank's balanced salt solution (HBSS 1x) and cooled at 4 °C. Then, 500 μL of 0.1 M buffer Tris-HCl, 0.1M NaCl, and 0.05 M $MgCl_2$ (pH = 9.2–9.5) containing Nitro blue tetrazolium chloride (NBT, Roche Diagnostics, Mannheim, Germany) and 5-Bromo-4-chloro-3-indolyl phosphate (BCIP, Roche Diagnostics, Mannheim, Germany) were added and incubated at 37 °C and 5% CO_2 under soft agitation for 1.5 h. Then, the NBT/BCIP was removed and the cells were fixed with a solution of 3.7–4% p-formaldehyde buffered to pH = 7.0 (Panreac®, Barcelona, Spain) during 30 min. After this, the formaldehyde was removed, and the wells were washed 3 times with HBBS 1x. Immediately after this, cells were visualized by stereo microscopy (Leica M205C, Leica Las, v3 software). In addition, samples were dehydrated in a graded series of ethanol before being embedded in Paraplast® and microtome (Shandon Finesse 325, Thermo Fisher Scientific, Madrid, Spain) sections were observed by light microscopy (LEICA DM 4000B, Barcelona, Spain).

2.8. Histology, Immunohistochemical, and Histomorphometrically Evaluation

First, to check the osteoporotic-like condition, 12 weeks after the 12 rats undergone the different protocols were sacrificed and the femurs and calvaria were analyzed. The femurs and calvaria were fixed (4% paraformaldehyde solution), decalcified in Histofix® Decalcifier (Panreac, Barcelona, Spain) and prepared for histological analysis as previously described [20,22].

Bone morphology was analyzed by hematoxylin–erythrosin staining. The histomorphometric analyze was carried out in femurs by measuring the following parameters; thickness of the cortical bone (Ct.Wi) and number (Tb.N), width (Tb.Wi) and separation (Tb.Sp) of the trabeculae in cancellous bone. In the calvaria bone, the histomorphometric analysis was carried out by measuring the following parameters, cortical bone thickness (CBT) and intercortical space thickness (IST) occupied by trabecular bone in transversal sections of calvaria.

To determine the capacity of the bone active substances, so as to regenerate the critical size defect practiced in the calvaria of the rats, samples of the 10 groups of 5 rats each were examined.

Samples were processed as previously described [22]. New bone formation was identified by hematoxylin–erythrosin staining. Bone mineralization was assessed with VOF trichrome stain, in which red and brown staining indicates advanced mineralization, whereas less mineralized, newly formed bone stains blue [31]. Sections were analyzed by light microscopy (LEICA DM 4000B, Barcelona, Spain). Computer-based image analysis software (Leica Q-win V3 Pro-Image Analysis System, Barcelona, Spain) was used to evaluate all sections. A region of interest (ROI) within the defect (50 mm^2) for quantitative evaluation of new bone formation was defined. New bone formation was expressed as a percentage of repair with respect to the original defect area within the ROI. From the total bone repair, the areas of mature bone (MB) and immature bone (IB) were determined, and the MB/IB ratio for each experimental group as well as between non-osteoporotic and osteoporotic-like animals was calculated.

For immunohistochemical analysis, sections were deparaffined and rehydrated in Tris-buffered saline (TBS) (pH 7.4, 0.01 M Trizma base, 0.04 M Tris hydrochloride, 0.15 M NaCl), which was used for all further incubations and rinse steps. Sections were incubated in citrate buffer (pH 6) at 90 °C for antigen retrieval, followed by incubation in 0.3% hydrogen peroxide in TBS buffer for 20 min. After a rinse step, sections were blocked with 2% FBS in TBS–0.2% Triton X-100 (blocking buffer). The indirect immunohistochemical procedure was carried out by incubating the sections with osteocalcin (OCN) polyclonal antiserum (1/100) (Millipore, Barcelona, Spain) in blocking buffer overnight at 4 °C. Sections were rinsed three times, then incubated with biotin-SP-conjugated donkey anti-rabbit F(ab) fragment (1/200) (Millipore, Barcelona, Spain) in blocking buffer for 1 h followed, after another rinse step, by incubation in peroxidase-conjugated streptavidin (1/300) (Millipore, Barcelona, Spain) for 1 h. Peroxidase activity was revealed in Tris–HCl buffer (0.05 M, pH 7.6) containing 0.05% of 3,3′-diaminobenzidine tetrahydrochloride (Sigma, Poole, UK) and 0.004% hydrogen peroxide. Reaction specificity was confirmed by replacing the specific antiserum with normal serum or by pre-adsorption of the specific antiserum with the corresponding antigen.

OCN staining was evaluated using computer-based image analysis software (ImageJ, NIH, Bethesda, MD, USA). OCN staining was measured by applying a fixed threshold to select for positive staining within the ROI. Positive pixel areas were divided by the total surface size (mm^2) of the ROI. Values were normalized to those measured from blank scaffolds and are reported as relative staining intensities.

Statistical analysis was performed with SPSS.25 software. We compared the distinct treatments by means of a one-way analysis of variance (ANOVA) with a Tukey multiple comparison post-test. Significance was set at $p < 0.05$. Results are expressed as means ± SD.

3. Results

3.1. Sandwich-Like System Characterization

The characteristics of the microspheres, electrospun film, and core system are shown in Table 2.

Table 2. Characteristics of the component of the sandwich-like system. Microspheres: size and encapsulation efficiency. Electrospun film: thickness and porosity of the film and average diameter of the fibers). Core system: porosity freshly prepared and lyophilized and water uptake and mass loss after incubation in MilliQ water, 37 °C, and 25 rpm.

Microspheres	**Size (μm)**			**E.E. (%)**
17β-estradiol	101.4 (10% < 29.73, 90% < 198.31)			83.5 ± 1.84
BMP-2	112.1 (105 < 60.3, 905 < 174.8)			71 ± 7
Film	Thickness (μm)	Fiber diameter (μm)		Porosity (%)
	63.4 ± 4.3	1.2 ± 0.26		71.9 ± 0.41
Core system (Hydrogel + microspheres)	Porosity (%)	Incubation time	Water uptake (%)	Mass loss (%)
	72	7 days	135.9 ± 2.6	18.85 ± 7
		28 days	138.9 ± 11.0	29.19 ± 4.88

SEM image of the microspheres is shown in Figure 1A and the differential scanning calorimetry thermograms of the 17β-estradiol microspheres components are plotted in Figure 2. The glass transition temperature (Tg) of the mixture of polymers RG 203-S and RG 858 [4:1] was located at 52–58 °C, in the temperature range of the PLA (RG203-S) and PLGA (RG858). The DSC analysis of pure 17β-estradiol showed three endothermic peaks (Figure 2A), the first two at 118.1 °C and 174.4 °C, previously attributed to the partial and complete loss of hydrogen-bound water and reticular water, respectively. The third at 179.4 °C corresponds to the melting point [32]. This last peak, characteristic of the crystalline structure of 17β-estradiol, was not detected in the spectrum of the polymers and 17β-estradiol blend or in the thermogram of the microspheres (Figure 2B). These results indicated that 17β-estradiol was dissolved in the polymer by at least 8.5%.

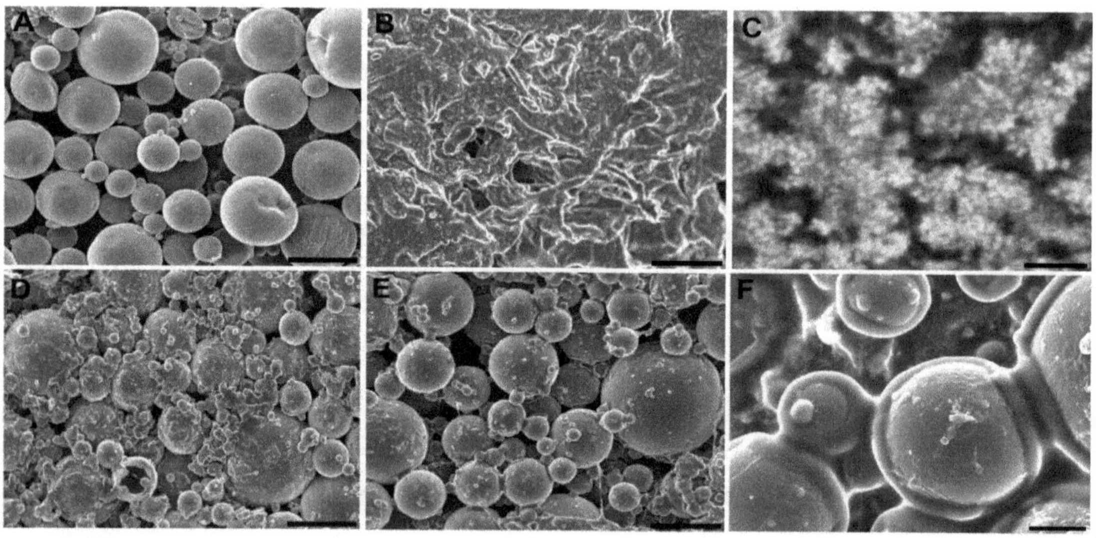

Figure 1. SEM images (**A**) microspheres, (**B**) hydrogel, (**C**) hydrogel high magnification detail, (**D**) core system freshly prepared, (**E**) internal structure of the core system after 4 weeks incubation in water at 37 °C and 25 rpm, and (**F**) high magnification detail of Figure 1E. Scale bars: (**A–E**) 100 μm, (**C**) 1 μm, (**F**) 20 μm.

The integrity of the system was assayed throughout the 4-week test duration. The SEM images of the internal structure of the hydrogel (Figure 1B,C), the freshly prepared core system (Figure 1D), and after 4 weeks incubation showed that the microspheres were homogeneously dispersed in the hydrogel and are trapped in the core system during incubation (Figure 1E,F). The core system absorbed a significant amount of water during the first days of incubation which was maintained over time.

Contrarily, the system lost little mass: less than 20% during the first week and approximately 35% after 4 weeks (Table 2). In addition, the core system flew well through the 20 G needle and the average dose discharged was 83.5 ± 6% of the loaded dose.

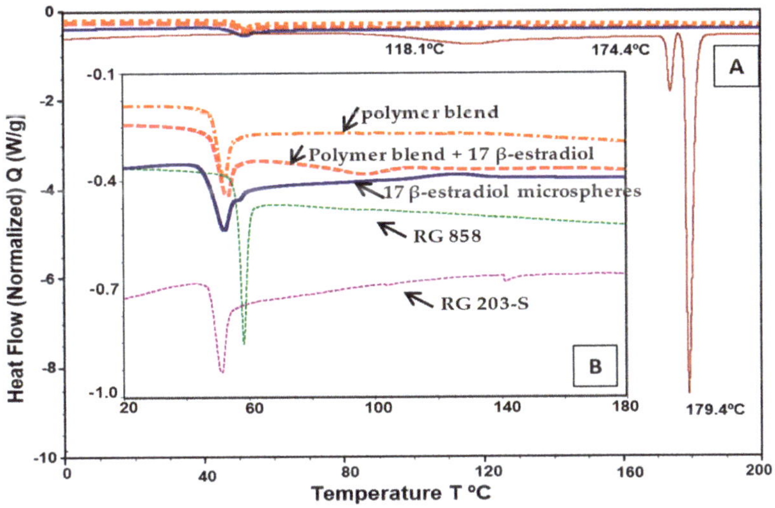

Figure 2. Differential scanning calorimetry thermograms. (**A**) Curve of pure 17β-estradiol. (**B**) Curves of PLA (RG203-S); PLGA (RG858), polymer blend (RG203-S:RG858, [4:1]), and polymer blend with 8.5% of 17β-estradiol, previously dissolved in DCM:MeOH (80:20) and the curve of the microspheres of 17β-estradiol (**B**).

3.2. Osteogenic Differentiation

The alkaline phosphatase positive (ALP+) cell count, in the hydrogels pre-seeded with rMSCs and cultured in the osteogenic differentiation culture medium, showed a discrete and progressive increase in the number of cells between 7 and 21 days of culture in the hydrogels without and with nano-HAP; the number being significantly higher in those containing nano-HAP (Figure 3). Likewise, qualitatively, the cells presented, in the scaffolds with nano-HAP, greater intensity of color, suggesting greater ALP activity (Figure 3) than without nano-HAP.

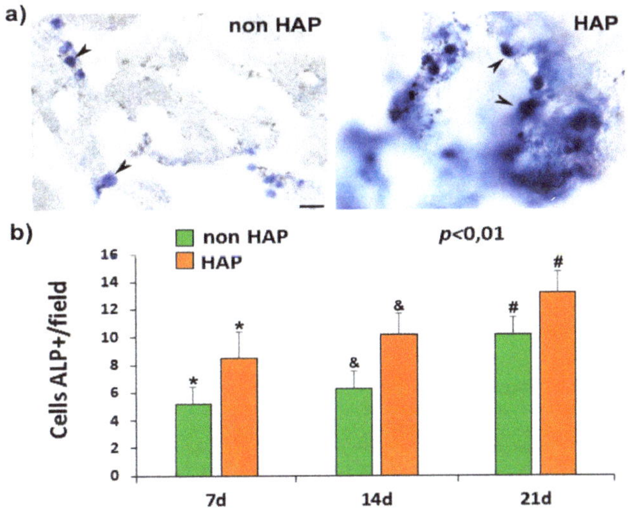

Figure 3. Alkaline phosphatase (ALP) activity in rMSCs cultures. (**a**) Representative images from hydrogels 20 days after cultured showing the AP-positive (ALP+) cells' morphology (arrowheads) in hydrogel without (non-HAP) and with nanohydroxyapatite (HAP). (**b**) Graphic showing the number of APL+ cells/ microscopic field at different time points of analyses (7, 14, and 21 days) after culture in each system. Scale bar = 20 μm. The identical symbol on different bars indicates significant differences.

3.3. Release Profiles of ^{125}I-BMP-2 and 17β-Estradiol.

Although the hydrogel provoked a strong reduction of the burst effect, the in vitro release of BMP-2 from the microspheres and from the core system showed a biphasic profile. During the first 24 h, approximately 7% of the protein was release from the core system versus 27% from the microspheres directly dispersed in the medium. Afterward, the release rate was kept in the range of 60 to 55 ng/day (Figure 4). The in vivo release profile was also biphasic, with a first phase that lasted up to 7 days whereas approximately 50% of the protein released. Then, the release rate was reduced to 70 ng/day, which is slightly higher than the in vitro rate.

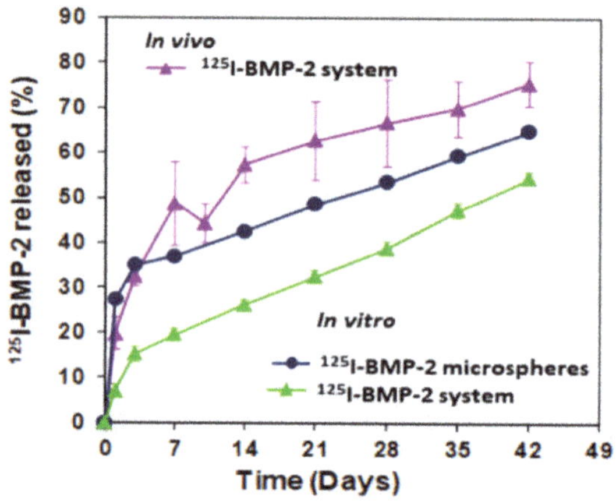

Figure 4. BMP-2 release assays. In vivo release profile of ^{125}I-BMP-2 from PLGA-microspheres in the system after implantation in the rat calvaria defect ($n = 5$). In vitro release of ^{125}I-BMP-2 (incubation in water at 37 °C and 25 rpm) from PLGA-microspheres and from the PLGA microspheres dispersed in the system.

The in vitro release rate of 17β-estradiol in the aqueous medium depended on the formulation (Figure 5B); 100% and 70% of the 17β-estradiol dispersed in the hydrogel and in the electrospun film were detected in the medium after 4 weeks incubation, respectively. The release profile was characterized by a high burst effect; approximately half of the dose was released during the first day. By contrast, the 17β-estradiol release rate was extremely slow from the microspheres alone and from the microspheres included in the hydrogel (core system). Both release profiles were similar: less than 20% was delivered in 4 weeks. However, in the MeOH: water (50:50) medium there were not differences in the transfer profiles. The presence of MeOH modifies the solubility of 17β-estradiol, showing a strong burst effect that varied in a range between 70 and 85% in the first 24 h (Figure 5A).

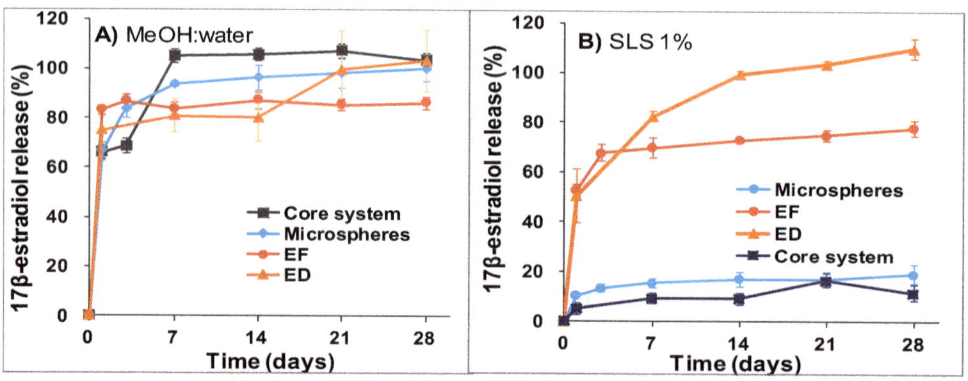

Figure 5. In vitro 17-β-estradiol release profiles in different release media at 37 °C and 25 rpm. (**A**) In MeOH:water (50:50). (**B**) In aqueous solution of SLS 1%. (ED) 17β-estradiol dispersed in the core system; (EF) 17β-estradiol in the electrospinned film; (microspheres) 17β-estradiol pre-encapsulated in microspheres and (core system) 17β-estradiol microspheres in the hydrogel.

The estimated values of D_{eff} and h for 17β-estradiol release in the different media are showed in Table 3. Although the value of D_{eff} of 17β-estradiol in SLS was significantly lower compared to the MeOH:water (50:50), there were not differences for h regardless of the release media used. h is the contribution of hydrogel, as part of the boundary layer, to the whole mass transfer process, and the value of this coefficient should not change by varying the release media. The values of R^2 (Table 3), together with the comparison of experimental and predicted values of the released fractions shows a good fit of the data to the proposed model for both release media.

Table 3. Estimated values of effective diffusion coefficient (D_{eff}) and mass transfer coefficient (h) for 17β-estradiol release in different media applying Equations (3)–(6).

Release Media	D_{eff} (m^2/s)	h (m/s)	R^2 (%) Value
MeOH:water (50:50)	$2.28 \cdot 10^{-15} \pm 5.00 \cdot 10^{-17}$	$7.56 \cdot 10^{-10} \pm 2.89 \cdot 10^{-10}$	95.47 ± 0.07
SLS 1%	$5.58 \cdot 10^{-16} \pm 9.81 \cdot 10^{-17}$	$4.01 \cdot 10^{-10} \pm 4.94 \cdot 10^{-10}$	92.49 ± 2.71

3.4. Histology, Immunohistochemical, and Histomorphometrically Evaluation

3.4.1. Osteoporotic Model

The osteoporotic model was assessed in both long bone (femur) and flat bone (calvaria). The histological analysis of calvaria showed evident changes in the structure and microarchitecture of the bone among the different experimental groups. Although the non-OP animals showed a normal bone structure in cortical bone (CB) and trabecular bone (TB), in the intercortical space (ICS), for the different OP models (DEX, OVX, and OD (Figure 6a), it was observed a progressive decrease in cortical bone thickness (CBT) and an increase in the intercortical space thickness (IST), being the group OD the one that presented greater alteration of the tissue bone structure (Figure 6b).

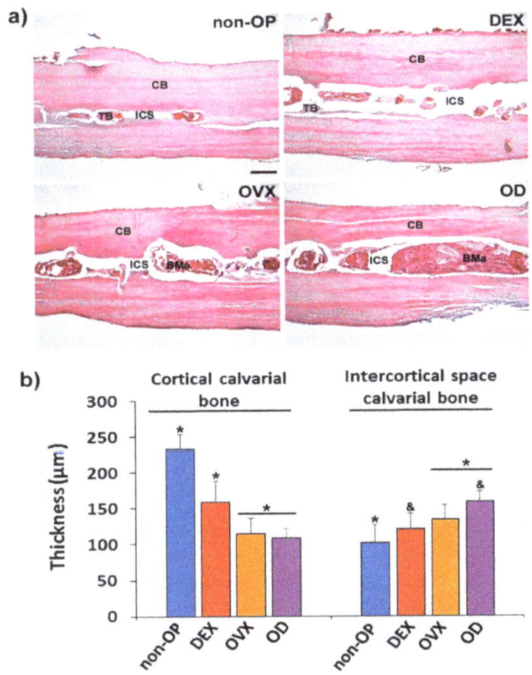

Figure 6. Validation of the OP model in calvarial bone. (**a**) Representative images in transversal section of calvaria in non-osteoporotic animals (non-OP) and in each of the different experimental models of osteoporosis tested showing the bone structure in each one. (**b**) Histomorphometric analysis of the cortical bone thickness and intercortical space thickness evaluated in calvaria in the different models of osteoporosis. CB: cortical bone; BMa: bone marrow; ICS: intercortical space; TB: trabecular bone. Scale bar = 100 µm. The identical symbol on different bars indicates significant differences.

The histological analysis of the femurs showed evident changes in the structure and microarchitecture of the bone among the different experimental groups. Although the non-OP animals showed a normal bone structure, in the different OP models (DEX, OVX and OD), structural changes were observed, both at the level of cortical and cancellous bone, showing a less compact bone and with a more porous structure (Figure 7a). The histomorphometric analysis revealed differences in the parameters measured in cancellous bone (Tb.N, Tb.Wi., and Tb.Sp.), with a significant reduction in all of them, in OVX and OD compared to the non-OP and DEX animals (Figure 7b–d). The cortical bone thickness (Ct.Wi.), although it showed a slight reduction in the groups (OVX and OD) with respect to the non-OP and DEX groups, was not significant (Figure 7e).

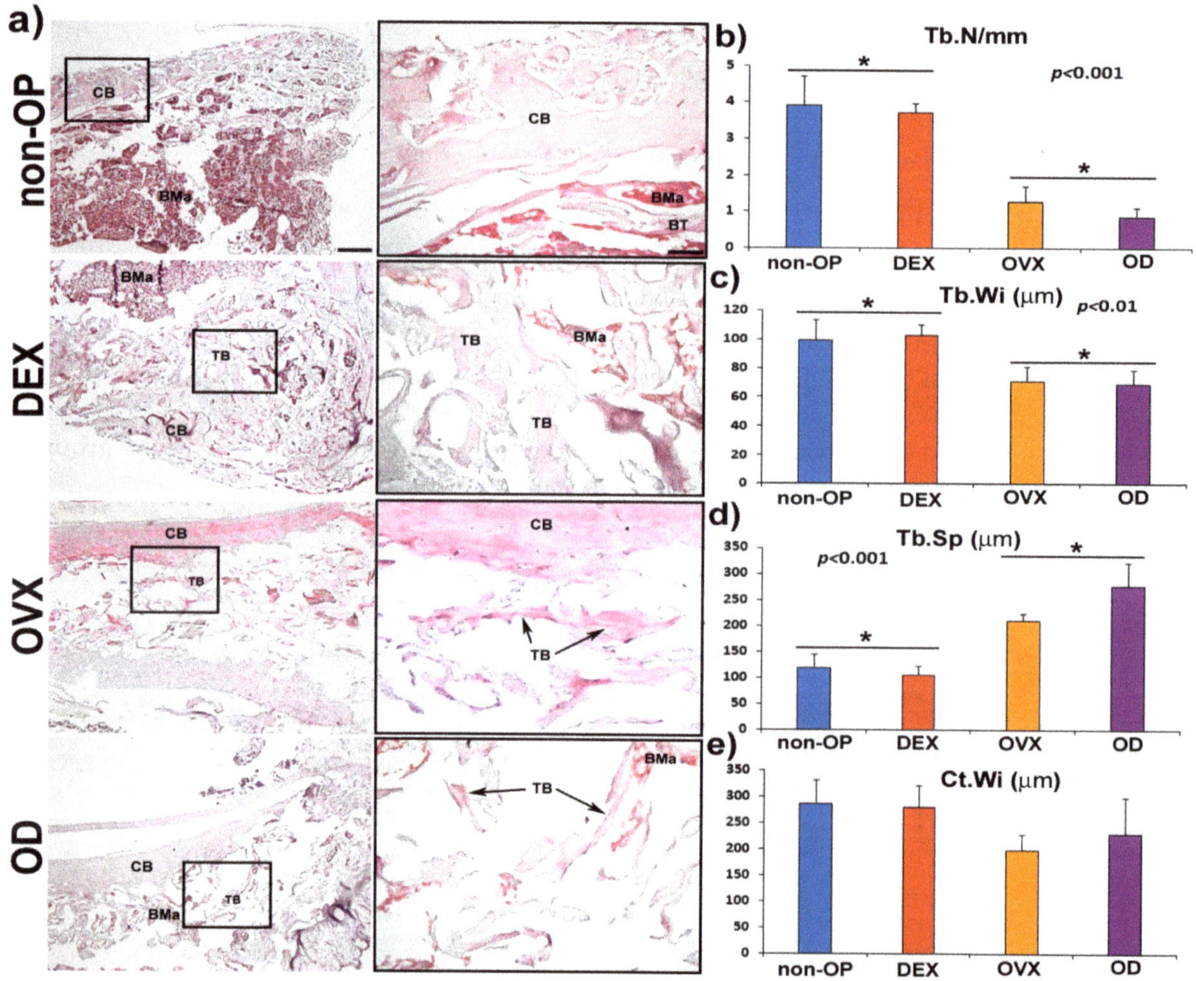

Figure 7. Validation of the OP model in long bone (femur). (**a**) The left column shows representative panoramic images in longitudinal section of rat femur in non-osteoporotic animals (non-OP) and in each of the different experimental models of osteoporosis tested. The right column shows high magnification images of the distal portion of the femur, showing differences in the microarchitecture of the bone in the different models. The column on the left shows detail of the boxed areas in which the structural characteristics of the compact and trabecular bone can be observed in each of the models. Histomorphometric analysis of the different parameters evaluated in femur in the different models of osteoporosis (**b**), Tb. N (mm), (**c**) Tb. Wi (μm), (**d**) Tb. Sp. (μm), and (**e**) Ct. Wi (μm). CB: cortical bone; TB: Trabecular bone; BMa: bone marrow. Scale bars: Left column 250 μm. Right column 50 μm. The identical symbol on different bars indicates significant differences.

3.4.2. Calvarial Critical Size Defect

The histological analysis at the level of the calvarial defect showed a few new bone formations in the blank groups (B and B HAP), being limited to the margins of the defect in both, non-OP, and OP groups (Figure 8a). The groups implanted with BMP-2 + 17β-estradiol in the three different formulations showed a greater area of newly formed bone in the defect area, not only in the margins, but also in inner zone of the defect (Figure 8a). The newly formed bone in the different experimental groups of non-OP and OP animals showed a normal morphology and VOF staining, revealing significant areas of mineralization, slightly higher in the groups of non-OP animals (Figure 8a).

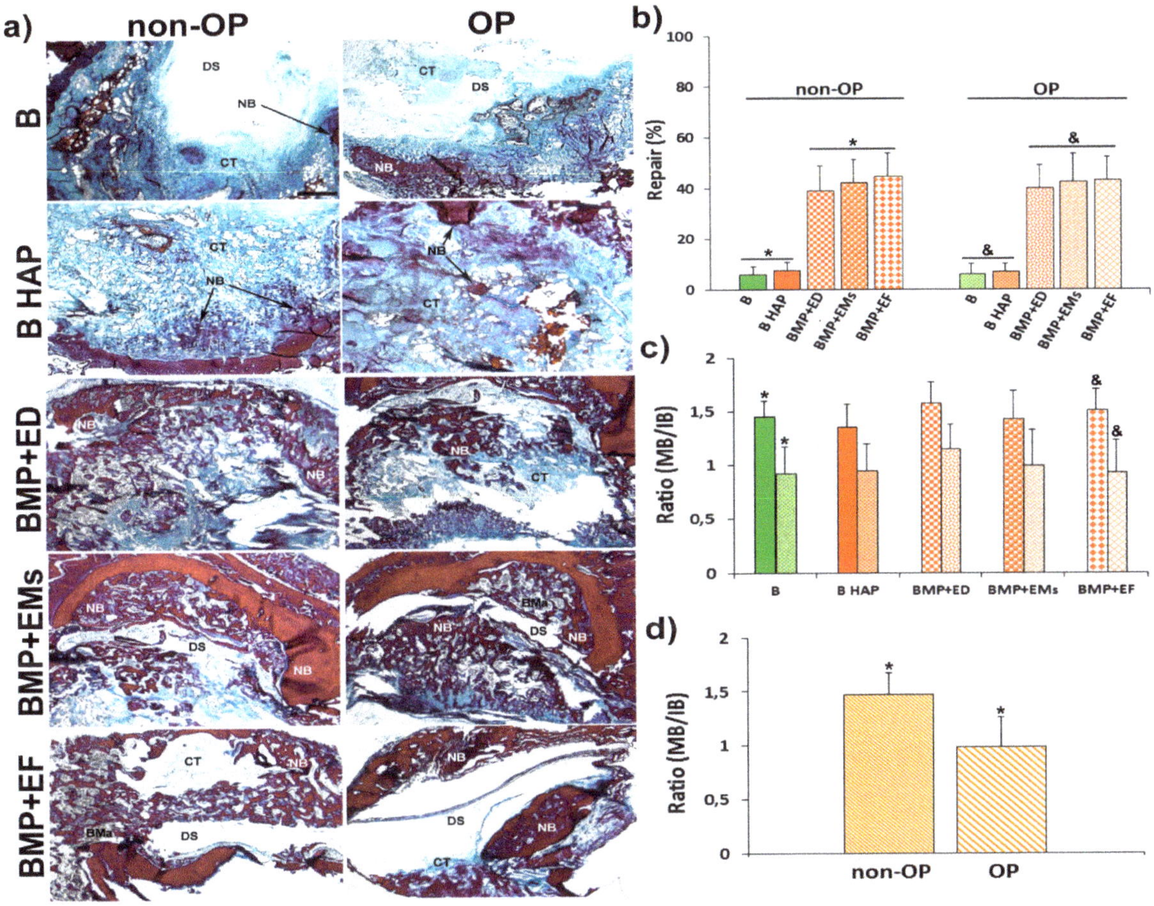

Figure 8. Repair process in calvarial defect. (**a**) Representative images in horizontal section of calvarial critical size defects in non-OP and OP rats showing the repair response at the defect level in the different experimental groups 12 weeks post-implantation. (**b**) Histomorphometrical analysis comparing of the degrees of repair (%) among the different experimental groups in non-OP and OP rats 12 weeks post-implantation. (**c**) Histomorphometric analysis showing the ratio between mature bone and immature bone (MB/IB) among the different experimental groups (**d**) and between non-OP and OP rats, estimated using VOF staining. Bars represent means ± SD ($n = 4$). The identical letter on different bars indicates significant differences. BMa: bone marrow; CT: connective tissue; NB: newly formed bone; DS: defect site. Scale bar = 1 mm. The identical symbol on different bars indicates significant differences.

The histomorphometric analysis showed little repair response in the blanks groups (B and B HAP) of non-OP and OP animals, with repair percent between 6 and 8%. The groups implanted with BMP-2 + 17β-estradiol in the three different formulations, on the contrary, showed a significantly higher repair response of 38–45%, with no differences being observed between non- OP and OP animals (Figure 8b).

The histomorphometric analysis of mature and immature bone showed a higher quantity of mature bone, and therefore with a greater degree of mineralization, in the experimental groups of non-OP with respect to OP animals. The ratio between mature and immature bone (MB/IB) showed individually higher values in all non-OP with respect to OP groups as well as on the whole, with values of 1.47 in non-OP animals and 0.99 in OP (Figure 8c,d).

The immunohistochemical analysis of osteocalcin (OCN), a marker of late osteogenesis and mineralization, showed a low immunoreaction in the blank groups (B and B HAP) in both non-OP and OP animals, with no differences between them (Figure 9a). In the groups implanted with BMP-2 + 17β-estradiol in the three different formulations, the immunoreaction was higher and more intense with respect to the blank groups, in this case being slightly higher in the non-OP animals (Figure 9a).

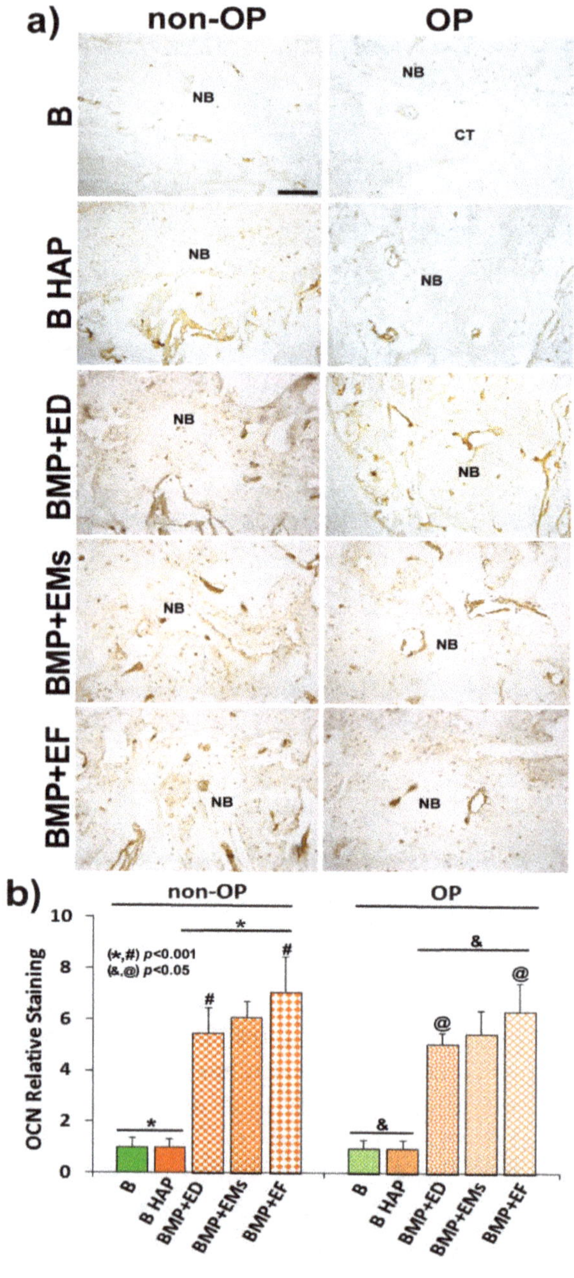

Figure 9. OCN relative expression. (**a**) Representative images in horizontal section of calvarial critical size defects in non-OP and OP rats showing OCN immunoreactivity in the different experimental groups 12 weeks post-implantation. (**b**) Histomorphometric analysis showing the relative staining values for OCN-ir. Bars represent means ± SD (n = 4). The identical letter on different bars indicates significant differences. CT: connective tissue; NB: newly formed bone. Scale bar = 100 µm. The identical symbol on different bars indicates significant differences.

The histomorphometric analysis confirmed the histological data, showing slightly higher relative staining values in the BMP-2 +17β-estradiol groups in non-OP animals (Figure 9b).

4. Discussion

In the present study, a BMP-2-17β-estradiol hydrogel system, with porosity of approximately 72%, was evaluated for regeneration of a critical size defect in rat calvaria. Although the system had already been characterized in terms of rheological behavior, porosity, interactions between components, mass transfer parameters, and cell viability, here the good injectability of the system was showed, and its characterization has been completed by testing the water uptake and mass loss as well as differentiation studies in cultures of osteoporotic rMSCs. In vitro release profiles of 17β-estradiol in two media and the in vitro and in vivo release profile of BMP-2 were also analyzed.

The osteogenic differentiation of osteoporotic rMSCs seeded on the system was assessed in order to test the effect of the incorporation of the nano-HAP on the cell behavior. The results showed greater ALP activity and a greater number of differentiated cells in the systems with nano-HAP. Therefore, nano-HAP systems were subsequently used in the in vivo experiments.

First, a histological evaluation of the femur and calvaria of rats suffering the three treatments for osteoporosis induction was carried out. OP is a systemic bone disease characterized by the increase of bone porosity, loss of bone mass and changes in the microstructure of the skeletal. Consequently, the OP population has an increased risk of fracture.

Despite the high number of OP studies and the several publications dedicated to tissue repair in non-OP specimens, very few reports devoted to bone defect regeneration in OP have been published. As OP might be primary post-menopausal or secondary, due to corticoid chronic administration, three animal models were used for OP induction: OVX, chronic glucocorticoid treatment, and the combination of both. In previous reports, a combination OD rat model was used. However, the high deterioration observed in the animals, the risk of induced additional disorders on the skeletal and the fact that bone loss reverses after corticoid stop [33] justify the bone histological study of the different treatment, in order to simplify the model and improve animal welfare. In general, OP condition is established through the analysis of long bones and lumbar spine but few data of the effect on the calvaria of the animals used as OP models are available [34]. Most of the publications on the regeneration of calvaria critical size defect in OP animals do not report the effects of OP in the calvaria [35,36]. In the present study, the data comparing the response of the femurs and calvarias to the three treatments revealed that the effect of OVX was similar to OD combination, consequently the fabricated system was tested in OVX rats.

As some authors have observed a delay in bone consolidation of OVX rats [37] and as this combination of BMP-2 and 17β-estradiol, formulated in microspheres, when applied to a critical calvaria defect, improved bone healing in OP rats, but the new bone was less mineralized [17,18], we tried to prolong the release of active substances to cover this delay. The drugs were incorporated to the hydrogel system pre-encapsulated in microspheres for prolonged controlled release. To reduce the release rate of the active substances the microspheres were prepared with a mixture of polymers, 25% of the RG 858 was incorporated to the RG 504 for BMP-2 microspheres as well as to the RG203-S for 17β-estradiol microspheres. RG 858 is a PLGA 85:15, of high molecular weight with a degradation rate lower than that of RG 504 and RG203-S. The BMP-2 release profiles showed a two-phase behavior with a weak burst effect that coincides with the period in which the system loses mass and uptakes a high amount of water. However, the burst effect of BMP-2 that can be seen from the microspheres was damped by the hydrogel, probably due to the interaction of the protein with the chemical groups of the HAP [6,13]. Afterwards, the second phases were practically parallel, which indicated a mass transfer process controlled by the access of water inside the microspheres, dissolution and diffusion of the protein throughout the porous of the polymeric matrix.

The release profile of 17β-estradiol as liposoluble drug in a MeOH:water (60:40) release medium was previously characterized [21]. By contrast, here two release media were used, MeOH:water (50:50) and an aqueous solution of SLS, because we suspected that the solvent affected the release rate of the lipophilic substance. In fact, the release of 17β-estradiol in MeOH:water was fast regardless of the formulations. However, the in vitro release of 17β-estradiol was formulation-dependent when an aqueous medium was used; a high decrease of the release rate of the drug from the microspheres was observed. As DSC results indicated, 17β-estradiol formed a solid solution in the microspheres, which indicates that the release process takes place by molecular diffusion of 17β-estradiol within the microspheres, governed by the partition coefficient, and consequently the aqueous medium dissolved it very slowly. In addition, the higher estimated values of D_{eff} in the MeOH:water compared with the aqueous medium, confirmed the dependency on the release media. The calorimetric analysis of the electrospun sheet was not carried out because the amount of 17β-estradiol would have had to be increased to be detected and its characteristics would have been modified. Although 17β-estradiol is expected to also be dissolved in the polymer of the film, the large specific surface area that microfibers expose to the medium causes the drug to release rapidly. Similarly, 17β-estradiol dispersed in the hydrogel was very little retained. Obviously, neither media are physiological, but it seems more correct to use an aqueous medium to predict release in vivo. Although, with reservations, one would also expect a slightly faster release rate in vivo as the biological components present in the tissue could accelerate the drug release from the system.

Despite the beneficial role of the nano-HAP controlling the BMP-2 burst effect as well as its positive effect on the proliferation and osteogenic differentiation of rMSC, which justifies the use of nano-HAP in the system, the reparative effect of the blank scaffolds with and without nano-HAP was not enough to be considered useful. Unlike that observed in this study, other authors showed better bone repair in different bone defects practiced in osteoporotic goats implanted with a system of type I collagen containing nano-HAP than without [38]. By contrast, another study [6] found, as in the present study, that the use of nano-HAP and calcium sulfate bone substitute scaffolds in rat critical calvaria defect showed no effect on repair and mineralization at 8 and 12 weeks with respect to the empty defect. In both studies, the systems were loaded with BMP-2 combined with 17β-estradiol or zolendronic acid [6] that might abolish the effect of the HAP observed in vitro.

Although previously our group reported [17,18] a better result in bone regeneration of OP animals combining BMP-2 and 17β-estradiol, in this study, the repair effect observed has been similar to that observed in non-OP groups. The three combinations of BMP-2 with 17β-estradiol in each of the three formulations used showed the same effect at 12 weeks. However, the ratios of mature and immature bone in normal and osteoporotic animals showed significant differences, indicating that the quality of the repaired bone, at least after 12 weeks, was better in normal animals.

Although these results coincide with previous work, in the present study it seems that the mineralization of the bone formed slightly improved in the OP animals. The difference in the relative osteocalcin expression was not statistically significant. These results might suggest that a longer release of BMP-2 together with the composition of the system, presence of collagen and nanoHAP favor the mineralization process. In any case, it would be necessary in future to conduct studies aimed at discerning the role of each of these components in the process. However, we have not been able to reproduce the positive effect of 17β-estradiol combined with BMP-2 in a hydrogel composed of Pluronic, Tetronic and, cyclodextrin, with other scaffolds of different composition [18]. In addition, according to the present study, the fact that the different release profiles of 17β-estradiol had no effect on the repair of the defect indicates that 17β-estradiol, when applied locally, and regardless of the release rate (available dose) and of the obvious role that it plays on bone remodeling, does not justify its inclusion as active substance in the repair of bone defects neither in normal animals nor in osteoporotic ones. Therefore, new strategies and alternative drugs are currently being designed trying to accelerate mineralization of new bone in OP groups.

5. Conclusions

The prepared hydrogel system resulted to be easily injectable and solidified fast due to crosslinking of collagen and chitosan chains. The system helps control the burst effect of BMP-2 pre-encapsulated in PLGA microspheres, probably due to the nano-HAP. Release of 17β-estradiol from PLA-PLGA microspheres was more complex and is governed by the partition coefficient of the drug which is in solid dissolution in the microspheres. The system was biocompatible both in vivo and in vitro. However, the regenerative effect detected in the critical bone defect of both OP and non -OP rats was mainly due to the osteogenic effect of BMP-2 released in a controlled rate for 6 weeks. A delay in the mineralization of the new bone which fills the defect in OP animals was observed. 17β-estradiol released from different formulations and included in the system does not improve bone repair.

Author Contributions: Conceptualization, E.P.-H., A.D., and C.É.; methodology, E.P.-H., A.D., C.É., R.R., E.S.-M., P.G.-G; validation, R.R.; formal analysis, E.P.-H., A.D., C.É., R.R., P.G.-G.; investigation, E.P.-H., A.D., C.É., R.R. and P.G.-G.; resources, A.D. and C.É.; writing—original draft preparation, R.R., A.D., and C.É.; writing—review and editing, A.D. and C.É.; supervision, A.D. and C.É.; funding acquisition, A.D. and C.E. All authors have made a substantial contribution to the work.

References

1. Murphy, C.M.; Schindeler, A.; Gleeson, J.P.; Yu, N.Y.; Cantrill, L.C.; Mikulec, K.; Peacock, L.; O'Brien, F.J.; Little, D.G. A collagen–hydroxyapatite scaffold allows for binding and co-delivery of recombinant bone morphogenetic proteins and bisphosphonates. *Acta Biomater.* **2014**, *10*, 2250–2258. [CrossRef] [PubMed]
2. Cho, T.H.; Kim, I.S.; Lee, B.; Park, S.N.; Ko, J.H.; Hwang, S.J. Early and Market Enhancement of New Bone Quality by alendronate-Loaded Collagen Sponge Combined with Bone Morphogenetic Protein-2 at High Dose: A Long-Term Study in Calvarial Defects in Rat Model. *Tissue Eng. Part A* **2017**, *23*, 1343–1360. [CrossRef] [PubMed]
3. Kim, H.C.; Son, J.M.; Kim, C.J.; Yoon, S.Y.; Kim, I.R.; Park, B.S.; Shin, S.H. Effect of bisphosphonate and recombinant human bone morphogenetic protein 2 on bone healing of rat calvarial defects. *Maxillofac. Plast. Reconstr. Surg.* **2015**, *37*, 16. [CrossRef] [PubMed]
4. Horstmann, P.F.; Raina, D.B.; Isaksson, H.; Hettwer, W.; Lidgren, L.; Petersen, M.M.; Tägil, M. Composite Biomaterial as a Carrier for Bone-Active Substances for Metaphyseal Tibial Bone Defect Reconstruction in Rats. *Tissue Eng. Part A* **2017**, *23*, 1403–1412. [CrossRef]
5. Raina, D.B.; Isaksson, H.; Teotia, A.K.; Lidgren, L.; Tägil, M.; Kumar, A. Biocomposite macroporous cryogels as potential carrier scaffolds for bone active agents augmenting bone regeneration. *J. Control Release* **2016**, *10*, 365–378. [CrossRef]
6. Teotia, A.K.; Raina, D.B.; Singh, C.; Sinha, N.; Isaksson, H.; Tägil, M.; Lidgren, L.; Kumar, A. Nano-Hydroxyapatite Bone Substitute Functionalized with Bone Active molecules for Enhanced Cranial Bone Regeneration. *Appl. Mater. Interfaces* **2017**, *1*, 6816–6828. [CrossRef]
7. Venkatesan, J.; Anil, S.; Kim, S.K.; Shim, M.S. Chitosan as a vehicle for growth factor delivery: Various preparations and their applications in bone tissue regeneration. *Int. J. Biol. Macromol.* **2017**, *104*, 1383–1397. [CrossRef]
8. Ma, X.; He, Z.; Han, F.; Zhong, Z.; Chen, L.; Li, B. Preparation of collagen/hydroxyapatite/alendronate hybrid hydrogels as potential scaffolds for bone regeneration. *Colloids Surf. B Biointerfaces* **2016**, *1*, 81–87. [CrossRef]
9. Cholas, R.; Kunjalukkal Padmanabhan, S.; Gervaso, F.; Udayan, G.; Monaco, G.; Sannino, A.; Licciulli, A. Scaffolds for bone regeneration made of hydroxyapatite microspheres in a collagen matrix. *Mater. Sci. Eng. C Mater. Biol. Appl.* **2016**, *63*, 499–505. [CrossRef]
10. Zhang, P.; Hong, Z.; Yu, T.; Chen, X.; Jing, X. In vivo mineralization and osteogenesis of nanocomposite scaffold f poly(lactide-co-glycolide) and hydroxyapatite surface-grafted wit poly(L-lactide). *Biomaterials* **2009**, *30*, 58–70. [CrossRef]
11. Zhang, B.; Zhang, P.B.; Wang, Z.L.; Lyu, Z.W.; Wu, H. Tissue-engineered composite scaffold of poly(lactide-co-glycolide) and hydroxyapatite nanoparticles seeded with autologous mesenchymal stem cells for bone regeneration. *J. Zhejiang Univ. Sci. B* **2017**, *18*, 963–976. [CrossRef] [PubMed]
12. Gupta, V.; Lyne, D.V.; Barragan, M.; Berkland, C.J.; Detamora, M.S. Microsphere-Based Scaffolds Encapsulating

Tricalcium Phosphate and Hydroxyapatite for Bone Regeneration. *J. Mater. Sci. Mater. Med.* **2016**, *27*, 121. [CrossRef] [PubMed]
13. Quinlan, E.; López-Noriega, A.; Thompson, E.; Kelly, H.M.; Cryan, S.A.; O'Brien, F.J. Development of collagen-hydroxyapatite scaffolds incorporating PLGA and alginate microparticles for the controlled delivery of rhBMP-2 for bone tissue engineering. *J. Control. Release* **2015**, *28*, 71–79. [CrossRef] [PubMed]
14. Wang, X.; Wu, X.; Xing, H.; Zhang, G.; Shi, Q.; E, L.; Liu, N.; Yang, T.; Wang, D.; Qi, F.; et al. Porous Nanohydroxyapatite/Collagen Scaffolds Loading Insulin PLGA Particles for Restoration of Critical Size Bone Defect. *ACS Appl. Mater. Interfaces* **2017**, *5*, 11380–11391. [CrossRef] [PubMed]
15. Segredo-Morales, E.; García-García, P.; Évora, C.; Delgado, A. BMP delivery systems for bone regeneration: Healthy vs osteoporotic population. Review. *J. Drug Deliv. Sci. Tec.* **2017**, *42*, 107–118. [CrossRef]
16. Giovanini, A.F.; de Sousa Passoni, G.N.; Göhringer, I.; Deliberador, T.M.; Zielak, J.C.; Storrer, C.L.M.; Costa-Casagrande, T.A.; Scariot, R. Prolonged use of alendronate alters the biology of cranial repair in estrogen-deficients rats' associated simultaneous immunohistochemical expression of TGF-β1 + α-ER+, and BMPR1B. *Clin. Oral Investig.* **2018**, *22*, 1959–1971. [CrossRef]
17. Segredo-Morales, E.; Reyes, R.; Arnau, M.R.; Delgado, A.; Évora, C. In situ gel-forming system for dual BMP-2 and 1717β-estradiol controlled release for bone regeneration in osteoporotic rats. *Drug Deliv. Transl. Res.* **2018**, *8*, 1103–1113. [CrossRef]
18. Segredo-Morales, E.; García-García, P.; Reyes, R.; Pérez-Herrero, E.; Delgado, A.; Évora, C. Bone regeneration in osteoporosis by delivery BMP-2 and PRGF from tetronic-alginate composite thermogel. *Int. J. Pharm.* **2018**, *30*, 160–168. [CrossRef]
19. Seo, B.B.; Koh, J.T.; Song, S.C. Tuning physical properties and BMP-2 release rates injectable hydrogel systems for an optimal bone regeneration effect. *Biomaterials* **2017**, *122*, 91–104. [CrossRef]
20. Rodríguez-Évora, M.; Delgado, A.; Reyes, R.; Hernández-Daranas, A.; Soriano, I.; San Román, J.; Évora, C. Osteogenic effect of local, long versus short term BMP-2 delivery from a novel SPU-PLGA-βTCP concentric system in a critical size defect in rats. *Eur. J. Pharm. Sci.* **2013**, *16*, 873–884. [CrossRef]
21. Pérez-Herrero, E.; García-García, P.; Gómez-Morales, J.; Llabrés, M.; Delgado, A.; Évora, C. New injectable two-step forming hydrogel for delivery of bioactive substances in tissue regeneration. *Regen. Biomater.* **2019**, *6*, 149–162. [CrossRef] [PubMed]
22. Hernández, A.; Reyes, R.; Sánchez, E.; Rodríguez-Évora, M.; Delgado, A.; Évora, C. In vivo osteogenic response to different ratios of BMP-2 and VEGF released from a biodegradable porous system. *J. Biomed. Mater. Res.* **2012**, *100*, 2382–2391. [CrossRef] [PubMed]
23. Fraker, P.J.; Speck, J.C. Proteion and cell membrane iodinations with a spraringly soluble chloroamide, 1,3,4,6-tetrachloro-3a,6a-diphenylglycoluril. *Biochem. Biophys. Res. Commum.* **1978**, *80*, 849–857. [CrossRef]
24. García-García, P.; Reyes, R.; Pérez-Herrero, E.; Arnau, M.R.; Évora, C.; Delgado, A. Alginate-hydrogel versus alginate-solid system. Efficacy in bone regeneration in osteoporosis. *Eur. J. Pharm. Biopharm.*. Manuscript submitted.
25. *Pharmaceutical Compounding–Estradiol Tablets*; The United States Pharmacopeial Convention: Baltimore, MD, USA, 2014.
26. Birnbaum, D.T.; Kosmala, J.D.; Henthorn, D.B.; Brannon-Peppas, L. Controlled release of b-estradiol from PLAGA microparticles:The effect of organic phase solvent on encapsulation and release. *J. Control Release* **2000**, *65*, 375–387. [CrossRef]
27. Zaghloul, A.A. *β*-Estradiol biodegradable microspheres: Effect of formulation parameters on encapsulation efficiency and in vitro release. *Pharmazie* **2006**, *61*, 775–779.
28. Govindarajan, P.; Khassawna, T.; Kampschulte, M.; Böcker, W.; Huerter, B.; Dürselen, L.; Faulenbach, M.; Heiss, C. Implications of combined ovariectomy and glucocorticoid (dexamethasone) treatment on mineral, microarchitectural, biomechanical and matrix properties of rat bone. *Int. J. Exp. Pathol.* **2013**, *94*, 387–398. [CrossRef]
29. Delgado, J.; Évora, C.; Sánchez, E.; Baro, M.; Delgado, A. Validation of a method for non-invasive in vivo measurement of growth factor release from a local delivery system in bone. *J. Control Release* **2006**, *114*, 223–229. [CrossRef]
30. Dobson, K.R.; Reading, L.; Haberey, M.; Marine, X.; Scutt, A. Centrifugal isolation of bone marrow from bone: An improved method for the recovery and quantitation of bone marrow osteoprogenitor cells from rat tibiae and femurae. *Celcif. Tissue Int.* **1999**, *65*, 411–413. [CrossRef]

31. Martínez-Sanz, E.; Ossipov, D.A.; Hilborn, J.; Larsson, S.; Jonsson, K.B.; Varghese, O.P. Bone reservoir: Injectable hyaluronic acid hydrogel for minimal invasive bone Augmentation. *J. Control Release* **2011**, *152*, 230–240. [CrossRef]
32. Turek, A.; Olakowska, E.; Borecka, A.; Janeczek, H.; Sobota, M.; Jaworska, J.; Kacmarczyk, B.; Jarzabek, B.; Gruchlik, A.; Libera, M.; et al. Shape-Memory Terpolymer Rods with 17-17β-estradiol for the Treatment of Neurodegenerative Diseases: An In Vitro and In Vivo Study. *Pharm. Res.* **2016**, *33*, 2967–2978. [CrossRef] [PubMed]
33. Zhang, Z.; Ren, H.; Shen, G.; Qiu, T.; Liang, D.; Yang, Z.; Yao, Z.; Tang, J.; Jiang, X.; Wei, Q. Animal models for glucocorticoid-induced postmenopausal osteoporosis: An updated review. *Biomed. Pharmacother.* **2016**, *84*, 438–446. [CrossRef] [PubMed]
34. Calciolari, E.; Mardas, N.; Dereka, X.; Kostomitsopoulos, N.; Petrie, A.; Donos, N. The effect of experimental osteoporosis on bone regeneration: Part 1, histology findings. *Clin. Oral. Impl.* **2017**, *28*, 101–110. [CrossRef] [PubMed]
35. Durão, S.F.; Gomes, P.S.; Colaço, B.J.; Silva, J.C.; Fonseca, H.M.; Duarte, J.R.; Felino, A.C.; Fernandes, M.H. The biomaterial-mediated healing of critical size bone defects in the ovariectomized rat. *Osteoporos Int.* **2014**, *25*, 1535–1545.
36. Engler-Pinto, A.; Siéssere, S.; Calefi, A.; Oliveira, L.; Ervolino, E.; Souza, S.; Furlaneto, F.; Messora, M.R. Effects of leukocyte- and platelet-rich fibrin associated or not with bovine bone graft on the healing of bone defects in rats with osteoporosis induced by ovariectomy. *Clin. Oral Impl. Res.* **2019**, *30*, 962–976. [CrossRef]
37. Cortet, B. Bone repair in osteoporosic bone: Postmenopausal and cortione-induced osteoporosis. *Osteoporos Int.* **2011**, *22*, 2007–2010. [CrossRef]
38. Alt, V.; Cheung, W.H.; Chow, S.K.; Thormann, U.; Cheung, E.N.; Lips, K.S.; Shenettler, R.; Leung, K.S. Bone formation and degradation behavior of nanocrystalline hydroxyapatite with or without collagen-type 1 in osteoporotic bone defects—An experimental study in osteoporotic goats. *Injury* **2016**, *47*, 58–65. [CrossRef]

7

Dry Tablet Formulation of PLGA Nanoparticles with a Preocular Applicator for Topical Drug Delivery to the Eye

Woo Mi Ryu [1,†], Se-Na Kim [2,†], Chang Hee Min [1] and Young Bin Choy [1,2,3,*]

1 Interdisciplinary Program in Bioengineering, College of Engineering, Seoul National University, Seoul 08826, Korea; wmryu@snu.ac.kr (W.M.R.); ddf5209@snu.ac.kr (C.H.M.)
2 Institute of Medical & Biological Engineering, Medical Research Center, Seoul National University, Seoul 03080, Korea; ksn777@snu.ac.kr
3 Department of Biomedical Engineering, Seoul National University College of Medicine, Seoul 03080, Korea
* Correspondence: ybchoy@snu.ac.kr
† These authors contributed equally to this work.

Abstract: To enhance ocular drug bioavailability, a rapidly dissolving dry tablet containing alginate and drug-loaded poly(lactic-*co*-glycolic acid) (PLGA) nanoparticles was proposed. For hygienic and easy administration of an accurate drug-dose with this tablet, the use of a preocular applicator was suggested. Herein, a dry tablet was prepared by embedding dexamethasone-loaded PLGA nanoparticles in alginate, which was deposited on the tip of the applicator. The nanoparticles were loaded with 85.45 μg/mg drug and exhibited sustained drug release for 10 h. To evaluate in vivo efficacy, dexamethasone concentration in the aqueous humor was measured after topical administration of the dry tablet, with the applicator, to rabbit eyes and was compared to that achieved with Maxidex®, a commercially-available dexamethasone eye drops. When applied with the preocular applicator, the dry tablet containing alginate could be fully detached and delivered to the eye surface. In fact, it showed up to 2 h of nanoparticle retention on the preocular surface due to tear viscosity enhancement, causing an estimated 2.6-fold increase in ocular drug bioavailability compared to Maxidex®. Therefore, the preocular applicator combined with a dry alginate tablet containing PLGA nanoparticles can be a promising system for aseptically delivering an accurate dose of ophthalmic drug with enhanced bioavailability.

Keywords: PLGA; nanoparticles; alginate; ophthalmic drug delivery; dexamethasone

1. Introduction

Topical drug administration is an easy route for ocular drug delivery. However, an ophthalmic drug, prepared as a solution and suspension, is known to clear very rapidly from the eye surface (<3 min), leading to a short preocular residence time, ultimately limiting drug bioavailability [1,2]. Less than 5% of a topically-applied drug can reach the interior target tissue of the eye [3,4]. Micro- or nano-particles have thus been suggested as ophthalmic drug carriers to achieve prolonged preocular residence time as well as sustained drug release [5]. Nevertheless, when formulated in the aqueous suspension, an additional fluid added to the eye would accelerate tear clearance, which would also expedite the drainage of the drug-loaded particles [6]. Therefore, an alternative strategy has been suggested and it includes a dry tablet formulation, where the drug-loaded particles are embedded in a tablet medium of a rapidly-dissolving polymer [7]. When applied to the eye surface, the tablet medium would dissolve in the tear fluid to free the drug-loaded particles on the preocular surface. The dissolution of the tablet medium would thus increase tear viscosity to delay tear clearance, which in turn would improve the preocular retention of drug-loaded particles. However, applying a dry tablet to the sensitive eye may not be convenient for patients. In addition, this administration route might not be hygienic, as the tablet would be retrieved with the bare fingers [8,9].

Herein, a combined system of a preocular applicator and a rapidly-dissolving dry tablet containing drug-loaded nanoparticles was proposed. The applicator was designed to contain two compartments (i.e., a handle plus a tip to hold the dry tablet). Thus, for administration, a dry tablet on the tip could approach and touch the eye surface while the handle is held by one's fingers. The tablet would then be separated from the tip and its medium would be dissolved in the tear fluid to free the drug-loaded nanoparticles. This would provide an easy way to topically administer the dry tablet and importantly, allow tablets to remain aseptic during administration.

To test the system and strategy, a preocular applicator using the biocompatible polydimethylsiloxane (PDMS) was prepared in this study. The shape and dimension of the applicator herein was designed to be similar to that of the commercially-available, one-time use applicator of artificial tear fluid based on patients' familiarity [10]. The commercially-available applicator is basically a container of liquid; however, a dry tablet formulation was loaded at the tip of the applicator proposed in this work. For the formulation, poly(lactic-*co*-glycolic acid) (PLGA) nanoparticles were prepared to be loaded with dexamethasone, a widely used corticosteroid drug for the treatment of eye inflammation [11,12], to achieve sustained drug release. The nanoparticles were then suspended in a solution containing a mixture of water-soluble polymers, polyvinyl alcohol (PVA), and alginate, which was then freeze-dried on top of the applicator tip to produce a rapidly-dissolving dry tablet. PLGA has been widely used for sustained drug delivery due to its high biocompatibility and degradability to non-toxic by-products [13,14]. PVA has already been approved for clinical use in various ophthalmic applications [15,16]. In the present study, alginate was also employed in the tablet medium as a viscosity enhancer of tear fluids. Alginate is a highly-biocompatible polymer [17] that can form a gel in the presence of the multivalent cation, Ca^{2+}, which is abundant in the tear fluid [18,19]. Due to this unique property, when dissolved in the tear fluid, alginate can further increase tear viscosity, thereby synergistically improving the preocular retention of the drug-loaded nanoparticles.

Dexamethasone-loaded PLGA nanoparticles (DX/NP) were prepared by the solid-in-oil-in-water (S/O/W) emulsion method and characterized by scanning electron microscopy (SEM) and dynamic light scattering (DLS), which were employed to assess nanoparticle size and morphology. The cytotoxicity of DX/NP was examined using human corneal epithelial cells (HCECs). To examine the effect of alginate on tear viscosity enhancement, two distinct tablet formulations containing DX/NP were prepared with media containing both PVA and alginate (DX/NP AL_TAB) and PVA alone (i.e., without alginate) (DX/NP TAB), respectively. For in vivo experiments, these tablet formulations were applied to rabbit eyes, and drug concentration in the aqueous humor was assessed and compared to the commercially-available ophthalmic dexamethasone medication, Maxidex®, (i.e., an aqueous suspension of dexamethasone itself).

2. Materials and Methods

2.1. Materials

PLGA (lactic acid:glycolic acid = 50:50; i.v. = 48,000) was purchased from Evonik Industry (Essen, Germany). Dexamethasone and Nile red were purchased from Tokyo Chemical Industry (Tokyo, Japan). PVA (87–89% hydrolyzed), phosphate buffered saline (PBS) tablets, tween 80, trifluoroacetic acid (TFA; >99%), and calcium chloride dihydrate (>99%) were obtained from Merck (St. Louis,

MO, USA). Dichloromethane (DCM; >99.5%), *N*,*N*-dimethylformamide (DMF; >99.5%), and acetone (>99.5%) were supplied by DaeJung (Siheung-si, Korea). Acetonitrile (ACN; >99.9%) was purchased from J.T. Bakers (Phillisburg, NJ, USA). PDMS (Sylgard 184) was obtained from Sewang Hitech Silicone (Bucheon-si, Korea). Alcaine® (0.5% proparacaine hydrochloride ophthalmic solution) and Maxidex® (0.1% dexamethasone ophthalmic suspension) were purchased from Alcon-Couvreur (Fort Worth, TX, USA).

2.2. Preparation of Drug-Loaded Nanoparticles

DX/NP was prepared via S/O/W emulsification [20]. Briefly, 300 mg PLGA and 100 mg dexamethasone were dissolved in 7 mL DCM. The resulting solution was then added to 8 mL of 1% *w/v* PVA solution, which was emulsified with a sonicator (Sonic Dismembrator Model 500, Fisher Scientific, Illkirch-Graffenstaden, France) at 160 W for 10 min. The emulsion was transferred into 100 mL of 1% *w/v* PVA solution at room temperature and stirred at 400 rpm under vacuum (−10 psi) for 60 min for solvent evaporation. The final suspension was then centrifuged at 200 rpm for 10 min, where the precipitates were eliminated and only the suspension at the top was collected. The collected suspension was then washed with deionized (DI) water three times via centrifugation at 13,000 rpm for 10 min. Thereafter, the suspension was lyophilized for 20 h to obtain dry DX/NP. PLGA nanoparticles loaded with Nile red (NR/NP) instead of dexamethasone were also prepared to evaluate its in vivo preocular retention properties. As such, 5 mg Nile Red and 500 mg PLGA were dissolved in 7 mL DCM for emulsification.

2.3. Preparation of Tablet-Loaded Preocular Applicators

A preocular applicator with a dry tablet on the tip was prepared, as depicted in Figure 1. To prepare a preocular applicator, two different molds were first made to fabricate a handle and tip (Figure 1a). In the molds, a mixture of a PDMS base and its curing agent (10:1, *v/v*) was poured and cured slightly at 80 °C for 2 h. Then, each of the constituent pieces was assembled and cured further at 80 °C for another 2 h to allow for their bonding. In this work, two different tablets, with media containing both PVA and alginate, and PVA alone, were produced to yield DX/NP AL_TAB and DX/NP TAB, respectively. To prepare the DX/NP AL_TAB, 20 mg/mL DX/NP were suspended in a solution containing 0.1% *w/v* PVA and 2% *w/v* alginate. Above this alginate concentration, the solution became too viscous to properly distribute the DX/NP. To prepare the DX/NP TAB, 20 mg/mL DX/NP were suspended in a solution of 0.1% *w/v* PVA only. Twenty μL of the resulting suspension was then poured in the reservoir that was made by tightly fitting a cylindrical connector with open ends to a tip of the applicator (Figure 1b). The whole piece was then rapidly frozen using liquid nitrogen, which was then lyophilized for 5 h at 0.01 mbar with the collector temperature set at −80 °C (FreeZone 6 Dryer system, Labconco, Kansas City, MO, USA) [21–23]. After that, a connector was carefully removed to produce the preocular applicator loaded with the tablet formulation. To evaluate the in vivo preocular retention properties, NR/NP was embedded instead of DX/NP to produce tablets of NR/NP AL_TAB and NR/NP TAB, prepared under the same condition employed for DX/NP AL_TAB and DX/NP TAB, respectively.

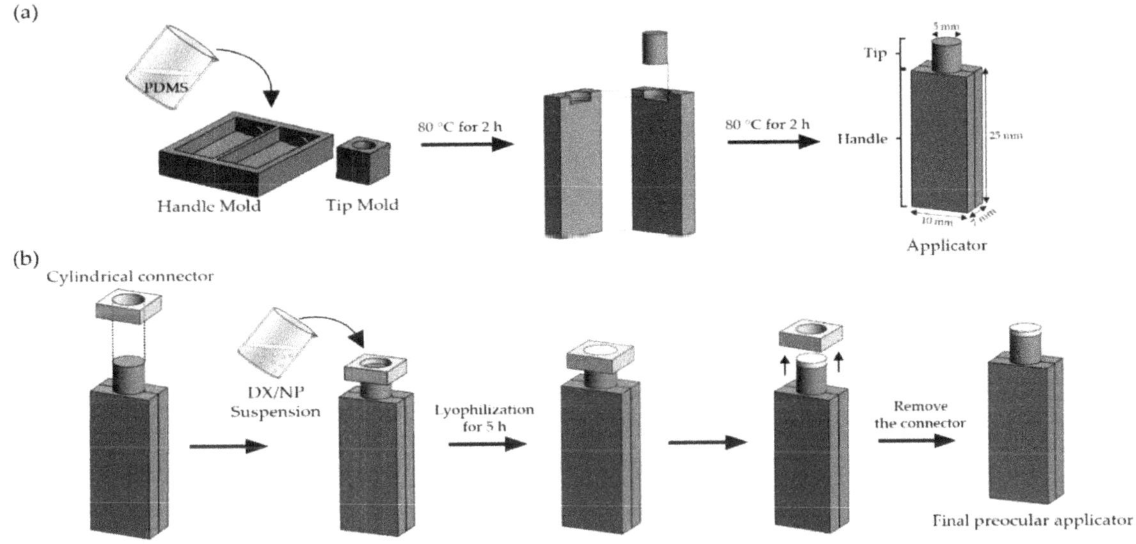

Figure 1. Schematic illustration of the fabrication of the DX/NP tablet-loaded applicator. (**a**) Fabrication of the PDMS applicator. (**b**) Tablet preparation on the tip of the applicator.

2.4. *Characterization*

The morphology of DX/NP was examined by SEM (JSM-7800F Prime, JEOL, Tokyo, Japan). Its size distribution was determined using DLS (ELS-2000ZS, Otsuka Electronics, Osaka, Japan) and a zetasizer (Nano ZS, Malvern, UK) with a particle suspension prepared in DI water [24]. To measure the drug loading amount, the solution of dexamethasone that was fully extracted from the DX/NP and tablet was respectively prepared. Briefly, 4 mg of DX/NP was completely dissolved in 4 mL DMF. The tablet at the applicator tip was fully immersed in 1 mL DMF, sonicated for 2 h, and centrifuged at 13,000 rpm. The supernatant was then diluted with ACN in a 1:1 ratio. Drug concentration in each resulting solution was measured using high-performance liquid chromatography (HPLC; Agilent 1260 series, Agilent Technologies, Santa Clara, CA, USA) with a Diamonsil C_{18} column (5 μm, 150 × 4.6 mm). Column temperature and absorbance wavelength were set at 37 °C and 240 nm, respectively. Injection volume and flow rate were 20 μL and 1.5 mL/min, respectively. The mobile phase was comprised of 0.1% TFA and ACN mixed in a 65:35 ratio. Given with the loading amount of the DX/NP, the encapsulation efficiency (EE) was calculated by the equation.

$$\text{EE}\ (\%) = \frac{\text{Amount of drug loaded in nanoparticles}}{\text{Initial amount of drug}} \times 100 \tag{1}$$

The thicknesses of the tablets herein were measured using a caliper (ABSOLUTE Digimatic Caliper, Mitutoyo, Kanagawa, Japan). To assess the particle distribution in the tablet, the NR/NP TAB and NR/NP AL_TAB were imaged with a fluorescence microscope (Leica DMI4000 B, Leica Microsystems, Wetzlar, Germany). To examine the effect of the tablet medium, DX/NP AL_TAB and DX/NP TAB were each immersed in 1 mL of the medium mimicking tear fluid, i.e., PBS containing Ca^{2+} (10 mM, pH 7.4, $[Ca^{2+}]$ = 39.4 μg/mL) [25], for 10 min at 37 °C. The viscosity of the resulting solution was then measured using a rheometer (Advanced Rheometric Expansion System, Rheometric Scientific, New Castle, DE, USA), where gap separation, temperature, and shear rate were set at 0.8 mm, 25 °C, and 100 s^{-1}, respectively.

2.5. *In Vitro Drug Release Study*

To examine the in vitro drug release profiles, 400 μg DX/NP, two different tablets containing the DX/NP (i.e., DX/NP TAB and DX/NP AL_TAB) and Maxidex®, all of which contained the same amount of about 35 μg DX were each placed in a dialysis membrane bag (SnakeSkin™ Dialysis Tubing, 10 kDa,

Thermo Scientific, USA). The bag was then immersed in 5 mL pH 7.4 PBS containing 39.4 μg/mL Ca^{2+} and 0.5% *w/v* Tween 80 to meet the sink condition of DX [26]. While being incubated at 37 °C, at scheduled times, 1 mL of the release medium was collected and the same volume of fresh PBS was added back. The amount of released dexamethasone was measured using HPLC as described above.

2.6. Cytotoxicity Evaluation

The in vitro cytotoxicity of DX/NP was evaluated using HCECs (PCS-700-010, ATCC, Manassas, VA, USA). HCECs were grown in a corneal epithelial cell basal medium (PCS-700-030, ATCC, USA) with supplements (PCS-700-040, ATCC) at 37 °C in a humidified environment with 5% CO_2. Prior to the assay, HCECs were seeded in a 96-well plate at 1×10^5 cells/well and grown for 24 h. Subsequently, 100 μL of the DX/NP suspension, which was prepared in the cell growth medium at concentrations of 5, 10, 25, 50, 100, 250, 500, and 1000 μg/mL, was added to each well and incubated at 37 °C for 24 h. The medium was then completely removed and replaced with 100 μL of fresh medium. Thereafter, 10 μL of an EZ-Cytox solution was added to each well and incubated at 37 °C for 2 h under dark conditions. Cell viability was measured using a microplate reader, with absorbance and reference wavelengths of 450 nm and 600 nm, respectively (VersaMax ELISA Microplate Reader; Molecular Devices, San Jose, CA, USA).

2.7. Animal Experiments

In vivo experiments were conducted with the healthy eyes of male New Zealand White rabbits (weight 2.1–2.5 kg). Rabbits were granted free access to food and water and were housed in a controlled environment: temperature; 21 ± 1 °C, humidity; 55 ± 1%, and light/dark cycle; 12 h/12 h. The in vivo experimental protocols were approved by the Institutional Animal Care and Use Committee at Seoul National University Hospital (IACUC No. 19–0133, date: 30 July 2019).

First, the in vivo preocular retention properties of the nanoparticles were evaluated after topical administration to the eye. The preocular retention properties were assessed as reported in our previous studies, with slight modifications [27,28]. Briefly, the NR/NP AL_TAB or NR/NP TAB on the applicator tip was applied on the lower cul-de-sac of the left eye of rabbits. At scheduled times, the rabbit eye was anesthetized by topical administration of a drop of Alcaine® and the entire preocular surface was thoroughly wiped with a surgical sponge (PVA spear; Sidapharm, Thessaloniki, Greece) to collect the NR/NP. The sponge was then fully immersed in 5 mL DMF and sonicated for 2 h to fully dissolve the NR/NP. The amount of Nile red in the sample was measured using HPLC-mass spectroscopy (LC-MS) with a Polaris 5 C_{18}-A (2.7 μm pore size, 4.6 × 150 mm) and the following conditions: column temperature, 30 °C; absorbance wavelength, 243 nm; injection volume, 20 μL; and flow rate, 0.45 mL/min. The mobile phase was prepared by mixing 0.1% formic acid and ACN in the ratio, 55:45. For statistics, four animals (i.e., one left eye for each rabbit) were assigned per time point for each formulation. With the NR/NP AL_TAB and NR/NP TAB, the in vivo profile of tablet disintegration was also assessed. For this, the eye was imaged using a digital camera (Galaxy S10, Samsung, Seoul, Korea) at 0 and 30 s after topical administration of the tablet to rabbit eyes.

To assess the in vivo ocular drug bioavailability, each of the three formulations (i.e., the DX/NP AL_TAB and DX/NP TAB in the applicator, and 35 μL Maxidex®) with the same dose of dexamethasone (ca. 35 μg dexamethasone) was administered onto the lower cul-de-sac of rabbit eyes. At scheduled times, the rabbit was anesthetized with a subcutaneous injection of a cocktail containing 20 mg/kg ketamine and 10 mg/kg xylazine. Thereafter, approximately 100 μL of aqueous humor (AH) was collected using a 31 G needle (BD Ultra-Fine II, Becton Dickinson and Company, Franklin Lakes, NJ, USA). Drug concentration in AH was analyzed by LC-MS as described above. For statistics, three animals (i.e., the left eye of each rabbit) were assigned per time point for each formulation.

2.8. Statistical Analysis

Statistical analysis was performed using the amount of particles remaining on the preocular surface and drug concentration in AH by the Mann–Whitney U-test. A p-value < 0.05 was considered to indicate statistical significance (SPSS version 22, IBM, Armonk, NY, USA).

3. Results

3.1. Characterization of the Formulations

DX/NP was prepared using the emulsion method. As a result, the drug-loaded nanoparticles were found to display a spherical shape, as shown in Figure 2a. Particle diameter was 336.92 ± 5.56 nm (Figure 2b) while drug-loading amount was 85.45 ± 5.44 μg/mg (i.e., EE = c.a. 25.6%). The size and shape of NR/NP were similar to those of DX/NP (Figure S1 in the Supplementary Information). As shown in Figure 2c, the zeta potential of the blank PLGA nanoparticles was measured to be −3.9 mV, which was shifted to −27.2 mV with the DX/NP due to a negative charge of the encapsulated drug, DX [29]. Figure 3a shows the tablets prepared in the present experiment (i.e., the DX/NP TAB and DX/NP AL_TAB). They displayed a cylindrical shape and were well attached at the tip applicator. As shown in Figure 3b, the tablets loaded with the NR/NP exhibited a evenly-distributed fluorescent signal throughout the medium, implying a homogenous distribution of the particles in the tablet. As the same amount of DX/NP was embedded during tablet preparation, the drug loading amount per tablet was similar between DX/NP TAB and DX/NP AL_TAB (34.11 ± 0.48 and 34.89 ± 0.28 μg, respectively). For the same reason, the thicknesses of the DX/NP TAB and DX/NP AL_TAB were also similar, which were measured to be 1.02 ± 0.03 and 1.02 ± 0.06 mm, respectively. When tablets were dissolved in Ca^{2+}-containing PBS, the solution with DX/NP AL_TAB (i.e., the tablet containing 400 μg alginate) had a higher viscosity of 0.93 Pa s than that with DX/NP TAB (i.e., the tablet without alginate) of 0.01 Pa s. However, both tablets herein were observed to be disintegrated in 30 s by dissolution in tear fluid when topically administered to rabbit eyes (Figure 3c).

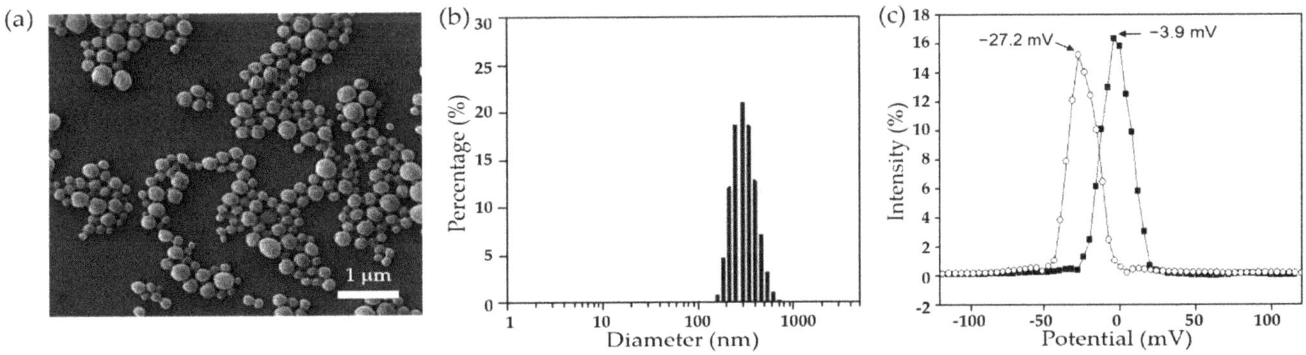

Figure 2. Characterization of DX/NP. (**a**) Representative scanning electron micrographs of DX/NP. (**b**) Particle size distribution of DX/NP measured by the dynamic light scattering (DLS) method; Polydispersity index = 0.056. (**c**) Zeta potentials of the blank PLGA nanoparticles (■) and DX/NP (○).

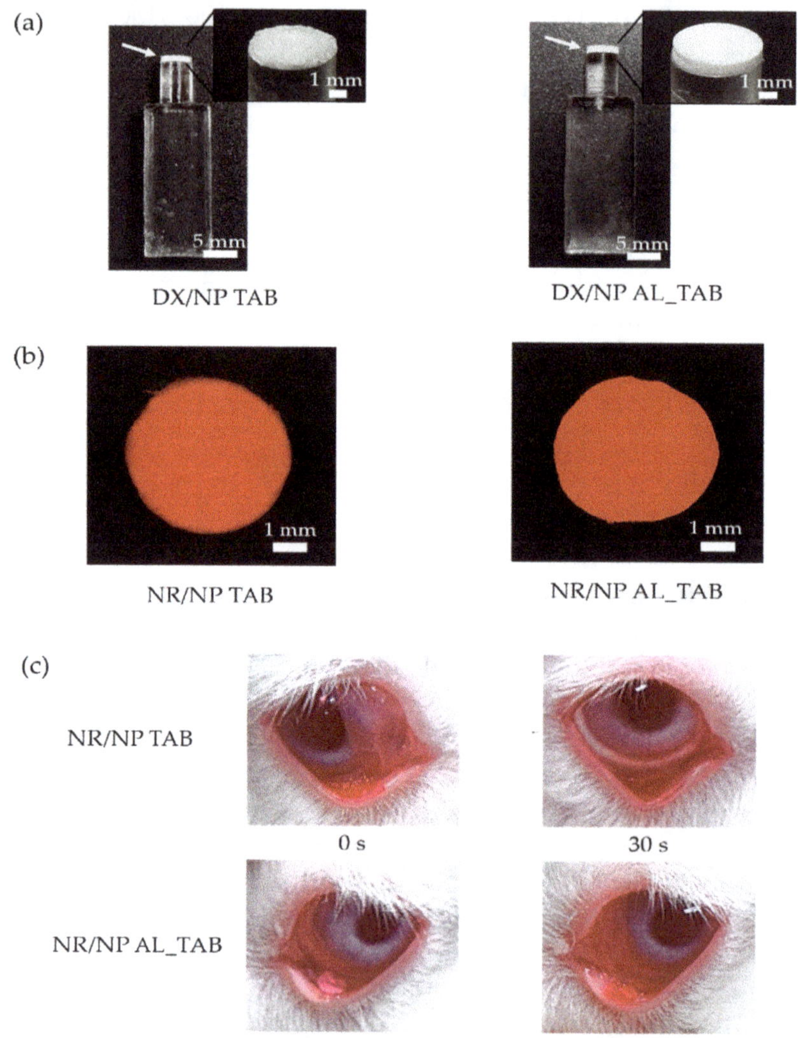

Figure 3. Characterizations of tablets. (**a**) Representative optical images of the applicator with the DX/NP TAB and DX/NP AL_TAB. White arrows indicate the dry tablets prepared on the applicator tip. (**b**) Representative fluorescence images of the NR/NP TAB and NR/NP AL_TAB. (**c**) Disintegration profiles of the NR/NP TAB and NR/NP AL_TAB administered topically to rabbit eyes.

3.2. *In Vitro Evaluation Results*

Figure 4 shows the in vitro drug release profiles of DX/NP and the tablet formulations, which displayed sustained drug release for up to 10 h. The release profiles did not differ among the formulations as the tablet medium dissolved rapidly to achieve almost instantaneous freeing of DX/NP. Drug release was slightly more suppressed with DX/NP AL_TAB, which could be due to a slight increase in the viscosity of the release medium in a dialysis membrane bag owing to the interaction between algnate and Ca^{2+}. On the other hand, Maxidex®, which is basically a suspension of DX, exhibited almost complete dissolution of the drug in 2 h. When tested with HCECs, the DX/NP exhibited a cell viability greater than 90% at all testing concentrations (Figure 5), suggesting that the DX/NP was non-cytotoxic.

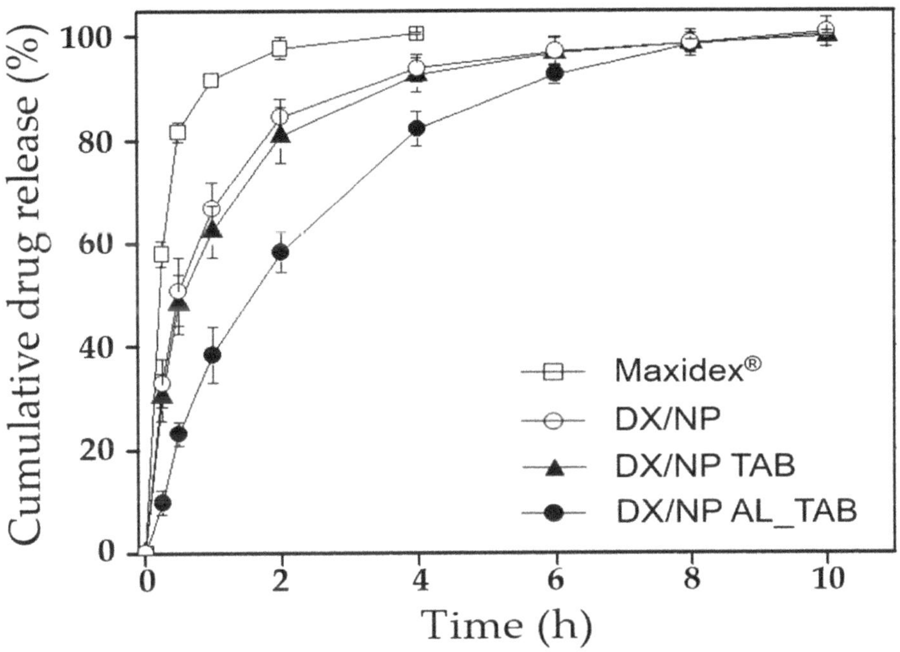

Figure 4. In vitro drug release profiles of Maxidex® (□), DX/NP (○), DX/NP TAB (▲), and DX/NP AL_TAB (●).

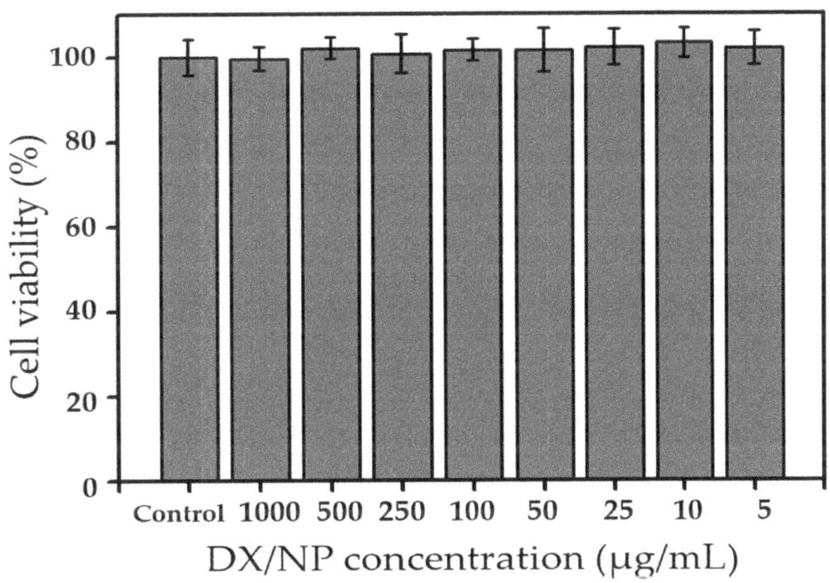

Figure 5. In vitro cytotoxicity of DX/NP on human primary corneal epithelial cells.

3.3. In Vivo Experimental Results

To examine the effect of alginate on preocular retention of the nanoparticles, two different tablets embedded with the Nile red-loaded nanoparticles (i.e., NR/NP TAB and NR/NP AL_TAB) were employed for in vivo evaluation. As shown in Figure 6, by incorporating alginate in the tablet, the amount of nanoparticles remaining at the preocular surface increased. For the tablet without alginate, the average percent of remaining particles was relatively low (i.e., 4.8 and 0.2% at 15 min and 1 h, respectively). However, owing to the presence of alginate in the tablet, 33 and 12% of particles remained at 15 min and 1 h, respectively, and could still be detected until 2 h. As conventional eye drops are known to completely disappear in 5 min [1], such findings suggest a greater improvement in drug retention at the eye surface. For the tablet with alginate, there was a high variability in particle retention observed at 1 h. Right after the tablet medium dissolved in the tear fluid to interact with Ca^{2+} ions, the tear viscosity increased to allow for an evident retention of the NP at the preocular surface. However, as the time progressed, the tear fluid with alginate would be continuously diluted with a newly-generated fresh tear, which would vary greatly depending on the subject. After 2 h, almost all particles would be cleared from the preocular surface.

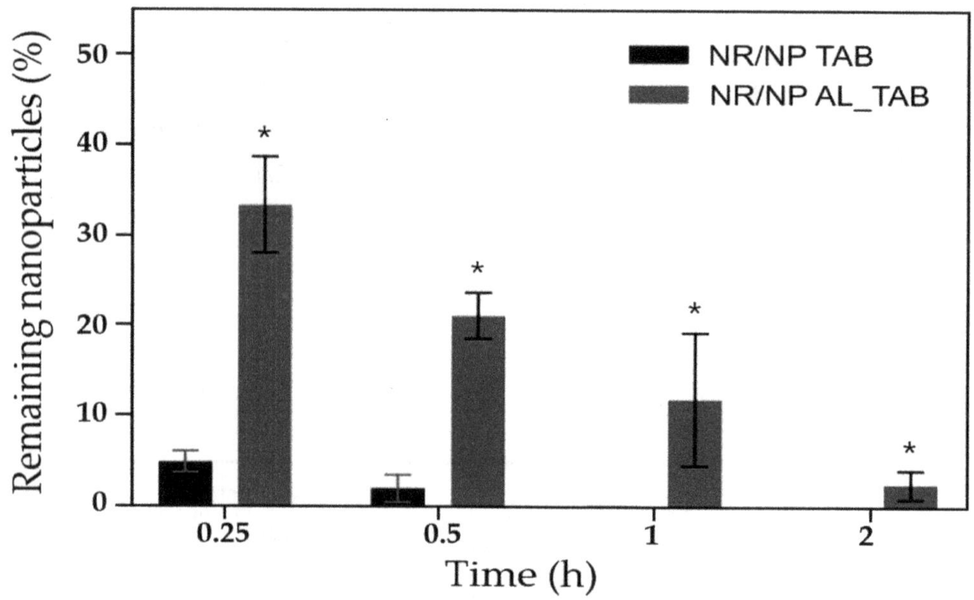

Figure 6. In vivo preocular retention profiles of NR/NP TAB (■) and NR/NP AL_TAB (■) on rabbit eyes. * indicated statistical significance between the formulations at each time point ($p < 0.05$).

The pharmacokinetic profiles of the tablet formulations were assessed and compared with that of the commercially-available dexamethasone eye drops, Maxidex®. Figure 7 and Table 1 display the drug concentration profiles in the AH and their pharmacokinetic parameters, respectively. At 30 min, Maxidex® had a C_{max} of 285.93 ng/mL; however, this value rapidly decreased to an undetectable level at 6 h after the administration. Interestingly, albeit formulated in a dry tablet, the DX/NP TAB without alginate exhibited a much lower drug bioavailability. In addition, its area under the drug concentration-time curve (AUC) and Cmax were less than a half of those with Maxidex®. Such finding could be due to a lower amount of drug exposure at the eye surface, where the DX/NP disappeared relatively rapidly and only a small portion of drug within the particles was actually released during the early period post-administration. On the other hand, 100% drug would be exposed right after a bolus administration with Maxidex®.

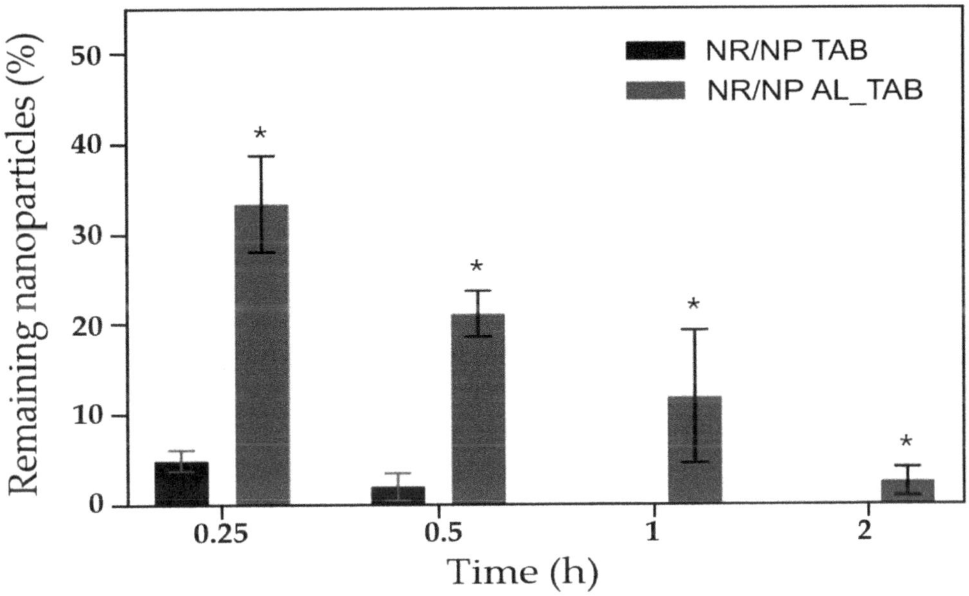

Figure 7. Dexamethasone concentration in the AH of rabbit eyes after the administration of Maxidex® (○), DX/NP TAB (□), and DX/NP AL_TAB (▲). * DX/NP AL_TAB was significantly different from Maxidex®.

Table 1. Pharmacokinetic parameters of dexamethasone in the AH.

Formulations	T_{max} (h)	C_{max} (ng·mL^{-1})	AUC [a] (ng·h·mL^{-1})
Maxidex®	0.5	285.93	388.51
DX/NP TAB	1	62.18	165.93
DX/NP AL_TAB	2	370.33	981.23

[a] calculated using the trapezoidal rule.

The highest drug bioavailability was observed with the DX/NP AL_TAB. In fact, its AUC was 2.5-fold greater than that of Maxidex®. By incorporating alginate in the tablet, it appeared to increase the viscosity of the tear fluid, enabling a larger amount of DX/NP to be retained in the preocular space for a longer period. During this period, the DX/NP would release and expose a significant amount of dexamethasone in a sustained manner. As a result, the drug concentration in tear would gradually increase before being absorbed into the AH to shift the time to reach C_{max} (T_{max}) to a later point (i.e., 2 h) and further increase the value of C_{max} itself, compared to that of Maxidex®. Due to prolonged retention and sustained drug release, drug clearance from the AH was delayed, demonstrating that drug concentration in the AH was statistically significantly higher than that of Maxidex® at 4–10 h ($p < 0.05$). All tablets tested in this experiment were almost instantaneously fully detached and released from the applicator tip to the preocular surface when they were in contact with the lower cul-de-sac of rabbit eyes (Figure S2 in Supplementary Information).

4. Discussion

Topical drug administration is considered to be an easy route for ophthalmic drug delivery. However, for conventional formulations of drops and suspensions, the additional liquid accelerates tear clearance to further lower drug bioavailability in the eye [30,31]. To overcome this, a dry tablet loaded with microparticles had been proposed as topical drug-delivery formulations [7]. The tablet was prepared by compressing the medium of mannitol together with drug-loaded microparticles composed of PLGA and a mucoadhesion promoter, PEG. Thus, dissolution of mannitol increased the tear viscosity to allow for a prolonged time of interaction between PEG in particles and mucin in the preocular surface. However, the tablet with a high density appeared to dissolve in tear fluid in minutes, during which a relatively large tablet could cause eye irritation. Therefore, the formulation was upgraded to be able to dissolve rapidly in tear fluid and for this, the dry tablet was prepared by freeze-drying [7]. In this way, the tablet medium could possess a porous structure and thus, after administration, it dissolved almost instantaneously in tear fluid to free the drug-loaded particles in the preocular surface. With this strategy, the particles still maintained a preocular retention property, as well as showing sustained drug release, hence improved drug bioavailability in the eye.

Herein, a rapidly-dissolving dry tablet formulation embedded with drug-loaded PLGA nanoparticles (i.e., the DX/NP) was proposed again for topical drug delivery to the eye. Owing to the presence of alginate in the tablet medium, tear viscosity increased because of the interaction between alginate and Ca^{2+}. This hampered tear clearance, leading to a higher preocular retention of DX/NP (Figure 6). Therefore, in addition to residing longer in the preocular space, DX/NP could continuously release the drug to tear fluids, providing more time for drug diffusion into the eye and eventually improving ocular drug bioavailability (Figure 7).

In the present study, the tablets were prepared by freeze-drying the DX/NP suspension; this allowed the tablet medium of the water-soluble polymers to be highly porous for rapid dissolution of the tablet in the tear fluid. Considering commercialization, the moisture content in the tablet may need to be minimized further to provide with an appropriate shelf-life of the product. Owing to the nano-sizes of DX/NP, the sensitive eye surface would not be irritated [32]. Therefore, with the alginate content employed for the tablet herein, any sign of eye irritation or discomfort was observed during in vivo experiments. By using the applicator, the tablet could be delivered without being touched, thereby achieving a hygienic application. PDMS was employed as the constituent material for the applicator because of its biocompatibility, should the applicator touch the eye surface. More importantly, PDMS is inherently hydrophobic and it is known to possess a low surface release energy [33]. Therefore, the dry tablet composed of hydrophilic polymers could be separated almost instantaneously without loss when wet with tear fluids (Figure S2), thereby enabling the delivery of an accurate drug dose to the eye using the tablet formulation.

5. Conclusions

Herein, a formulation consisting of a dry tablet containing alginate and drug-loaded PLGA nanoparticles is derived to improve the bioavailability of drugs that are topically delivered to the eye. Owing to the ease and hygienic administration of the developed tablet formulation, the use of a preocular applicator is suggested. Based on the hydrophobicity and low surface release energy of the constituent material, PDMS, the applicator could almost instantaneously cause full separation of the dry tablet composed of hydrophilic polymers when applied to the eye surface. After topical delivery, the tablet medium dissolved rapidly to free the drug-loaded nanoparticles in the tear fluid, where alginate could react with Ca^{2+} to increase its viscosity. Such findings suggest that the drug-loaded PLGA nanoparticles can be better retained in the preocular space and the drug can be subsequently released in a sustained manner, ultimately enhancing ocular drug bioavailability. Therefore, it is concluded that the combination of a dry tablet formulation with an alginate medium, drug-loaded PLGA nanoparticles, and a preocular applicator is a promising strategy to achieve patient-friendly, topical drug delivery to the eye, with enhanced drug availability.

Author Contributions: Conceptualization, Y.B.C.; Methodology, Y.B.C., W.M.R., and S.-N.K.; Validation, W.M.R. and S.-N.K.; Animal experiments, W.M.R, S.-N.K., and C.H.M.; Formal analysis, W.M.R. and S.-N.K.; Investigation, W.M.R. and S.-N.K.; Writing—original draft preparation, W.M.R. and S.-N.K.; Writing—review and editing, W.M.R., S.-N.K., and Y.B.C.; Visualization, W.M.R. and S.-N.K.; Supervision, Y.B.C.; Project administration, Y.B.C.; Funding acquisition, Y.B.C.

References

1. Lee, V.H.; Robinson, J.R. Topical ocular drug delivery: Recent developments and future challenges. *J. Ocul. Pharmacol.* **1986**, 2, 67–108. [CrossRef]

2. Lang, J.C. Ocular drug delivery conventional ocular formulations. *Adv. Drug Deliv. Rev.* **1995**, *16*, 39–43. [CrossRef]
3. Sigurdsson, H.H.; Konráðsdóttir, F.; Loftsson, T.; Stefansson, E. Topical and systemic absorption in delivery of dexamethasone to the anterior and posterior segments of the eye. *Acta Ophthalmol. Scand.* **2007**, *85*, 598–602. [CrossRef]
4. Järvinen, K.; Järvinen, T.; Urtti, A. Ocular absorption following topical delivery. *Adv. Drug Deliv. Rev.* **1995**, *16*, 3–19. [CrossRef]
5. Tsai, C.H.; Wang, P.Y.; Lin, I.; Huang, H.; Liu, G.S.; Tseng, C.L. Ocular Drug Delivery: Role of Degradable Polymeric Nanocarriers for Ophthalmic Application. *Int. J. Mol. Sci.* **2018**, *19*, 2830. [CrossRef]
6. Zhu, H.; Chauhan, A. A mathematical model for ocular tear and solute balance. *Curr. Eye Res.* **2005**, *30*, 841–854. [CrossRef]
7. Choy, Y.B.; Patel, S.R.; Park, J.H.; McCarey, B.E.; Edelhauser, H.F.; Prausnitz, M.R. Mucoadhesive Microparticles in a Rapidly Dissolving Tablet for Sustained Drug Delivery to the Eye. *Investig. Ophthalmol. Vis. Sci.* **2011**, *52*, 2627–2633. [CrossRef]
8. Dart, J.K.G.; Stapleton, F.; Minassian, D. Contact lenses and other risk factors in microbial keratitis. *Lancet* **1991**, *338*, 650–653. [CrossRef]
9. Radford, C.F.; EWoodward, G.; Stapleton, F. Contact lens hygiene compliance in a universitypopulation. *J. Br. Contact Lens Assoc.* **1993**, *16*, 105–111. [CrossRef]
10. Refresh. REFRESH®Classic. Available online: https://www.refreshbrand.com/Products/refresh-classic (accessed on 15 October 2019).
11. Graham, R.O.; Peyman, G.A. Intravitreal injection of dexamethasone: Treatment of experimentally induced endophthalmitis. *Arch. Ophthalmol.* **1974**, *92*, 149–154. [CrossRef]
12. Tan, D.T.; Chee, S.P.; Lim, L.; Lim, A.S. Randomized clinical trial of a new dexamethasone delivery system (Surodex) for treatment of post-cataract surgery inflammation. *Ophthalmology* **1999**, *106*, 223–231. [CrossRef]
13. Makadia, H.K.; Siegel, S.J. Poly Lactic-*co*-Glycolic Acid (PLGA) as Biodegradable Controlled Drug Delivery Carrier. *Polymers* **2011**, *3*, 1377–1397. [CrossRef] [PubMed]
14. Jain, R.A. The manufacturing techniques of various drug loaded biodegradable poly(lactide-*co*-glycolide) (PLGA) devices. *Biomaterials* **2000**, *21*, 2475–2490. [CrossRef]
15. Lee, S.S.; Hughes, P.; Ross, A.D.; Robinson, M.R. Biodegradable implants for sustained drug release in the eye. *Pharm. Res.* **2010**, *27*, 2043–2053. [CrossRef]
16. Davis, J.; Gilger, B.; Robinson, M. Novel approaches to ocular drug delivery. *Curr. Opin. Mol. Ther.* **2004**, *6*, 195–205.
17. Draget, K.I.; Skjåk-Bræk, G.; Smidsrød, O. Alginate based new materials. *Int. J. Biol. Macromol.* **1997**, *21*, 47–55. [CrossRef]
18. Braccini, I.; Pérez, S. Molecular Basis of Ca^{2+}-Induced Gelation in Alginates and Pectins: The Egg-Box Model Revisited. *Biomacromolecules* **2001**, *2*, 1089–1096. [CrossRef]
19. Fu, S.; Thacker, A.; Sperger, D.M.; Boni, R.L.; Buckner, I.S.; Velankar, S.; Munson, E.J.; Block, L.H. Relevance of rheological properties of sodium alginate in solution to calcium alginate gel properties. *Aaps Pharmscitech* **2011**, *12*, 453–460. [CrossRef]
20. Villanueva, J.R.; Bravo-Osuna, I.; Herrero-Vanrell, R.; Martínez, I.T.M.; Navarro, M.G. Optimising the controlled release of dexamethasone from a new generation of PLGA-based microspheres intended for intravitreal administration. *Eur. J. Pharm. Sci.* **2016**, *92*, 287–297. [CrossRef]
21. Labconco. FreeZone 6 Liter -84C Console Freeze Dryer. Available online: https://www.labconco.com/product/freezone-6-liter-84c-console-freeze-dryer-11/6303 (accessed on 26 November 2019).
22. Loan, T.; Easton, C.; Alissandratos, A. DNA amplification with in situ nucleoside to dNTP synthesis, using a single recombinant cell lysate of *E. coli*. *Sci. Rep.* **2019**, *9*, 1–8. [CrossRef]
23. Ojha, T.; Pathak, V.; Drude, N.; Weiler, M.; Rommel, D.; Rütten, S.; Lammers, T. Shelf-Life Evaluation and Lyophilization of PBCA-Based Polymeric Microbubbles. *Pharmaceutics* **2019**, *11*, 433. [CrossRef]
24. Sun, C.; Wang, X.; Zheng, Z.; Chen, D.; Wang, X.; Shi, F.; Wu, H. A single dose of dexamethasone encapsulated in polyethylene glycol-coated polylactic acid nanoparticles attenuates cisplatin-induced hearing loss following round window membrane administration. *Int. J. Nanomed.* **2015**, *10*, 3567.
25. Bright, A.M.; Tighe, B.J. The composition and interfacial properties of tears, tear substitutes and tear models. *J. Br. Contact Lens Assoc.* **1993**, *16*, 57–66. [CrossRef]

26. Kim, J.; Peng, C.-C.; Chauhan, A. Extended release of dexamethasone from silicone-hydrogel contact lenses containing vitamin E. *J. Control. Release* **2010**, *148*, 110–116. [CrossRef]
27. Park, C.G.; Kim, M.J.; Park, M.; Choi, S.Y.; Lee, S.H.; Lee, J.E.; Choy, Y.B. Nanostructured mucoadhesive microparticles for enhanced preocular retention. *Acta Biomater.* **2014**, *10*, 77–86. [CrossRef]
28. Kim, S.N.; Park, C.G.; Huh, B.K.; Lee, S.H.; Min, C.H.; Lee, Y.Y.; Choy, Y.B. Metal-organic frameworks, NH2-MIL-88(Fe), as carriers for ophthalmic delivery of brimonidine. *Acta Biomater.* **2018**, *79*, 344–353. [CrossRef]
29. Araújo, J.; Gonzalez, E.; Egea, M.A.; Garcia, M.L.; Souto, E.B. Nanomedicines for ocular NSAIDs: Safety on drug delivery. *Nanomed. Nanotechnol. Biol. Med.* **2009**, *5*, 394–401. [CrossRef]
30. Doane, M.G. Blinking and the Mechanics of the Lacrimal Drainage System. *Ophthalmology* **1981**, *88*, 844–851. [CrossRef]
31. Garaszczuk, I.K.; Montes Mico, R.; Iskander, D.R.; Expósito, A.C. The tear turnover and tear clearance tests—A review. *Expert Rev. Med. Devices* **2018**, *15*, 219–229. [CrossRef]
32. Choy, Y.B.; Park, J.-H.; Prausnitz, M.R. Mucoadhesive microparticles engineered for ophthalmic drug delivery. *J. Phys. Chem. Solids* **2008**, *69*, 1533–1536. [CrossRef]
33. Jin, X.; Strueben, J.; Heepe, L.; Kovalev, A.; Mishra, Y.K.; Adelung, R.; Staubitz, A. Joining the Un-Joinable: Adhesion Between Low Surface Energy Polymers Using Tetrapodal ZnO Linkers. *Adv. Mater.* **2012**, *24*, 5676–5680. [CrossRef]

8

Vitamin E-Loaded PLA- and PLGA-Based Core-Shell Nanoparticles: Synthesis, Structure Optimization and Controlled Drug Release

Norbert Varga [1], Árpád Turcsányi [1], Viktória Hornok [1,2] and Edit Csapó [1,3,*]

1 Interdisciplinary Excellence Centre, Department of Physical Chemistry and Materials Science, University of Szeged, Rerrich B. square 1, H-6720 Szeged, Hungary

2 Department of Physical Chemistry and Materials Science, MTA Premium Post Doctorate Research Program, University of Szeged, Rerrich B. Square 1, H-6720 Szeged, Hungary

3 MTA-SZTE Biomimetic Systems Research Group, Department of Medical Chemistry, University of Szeged, Dóm square 8, H-6720 Szeged, Hungary

* Correspondence: juhaszne.csapo.edit@med.u-szeged.hu

Abstract: The (±)-α-Tocopherol (TP) with vitamin E activity has been encapsulated into biocompatible poly(lactic acid) (PLA) and poly(lactide-*co*-glycolide) (PLGA) carriers, which results in the formation of well-defined nanosized (d ~200–220 nm) core-shell structured particles (NPs) with 15–19% of drug loading (DL%). The optimal ratios of the polymer carriers, the TP active drug as well as the applied Pluronic F127 (PLUR) non-ionic stabilizing surfactant, have been determined to obtain NPs with a TP core and a polymer shell with high encapsulation efficiency (EE%) (69%). The size and the structure of the prepared core-shell NPs as well as the interaction of the carriers and the PLUR with the TP molecules have been determined by transmission electron microscopy (TEM), dynamic light scattering (DLS), infrared spectroscopy (FT-IR) and turbidity studies, respectively. Moreover, the dissolution of the TP from the polymer NPs has been investigated by spectrophotometric measurements. It was clearly confirmed that increase in the EE% from ca. 70% (PLA/TP) to ca. 88% (PLGA65/TP) results in the controlled release of the hydrophobic TP molecules (7 h, PLA/TP: 34%; PLGA75/TP: 25%; PLGA65/TP: 18%). By replacing the PLA carrier to PLGA, ca. 15% more active substance can be encapsulated in the core (PLA/TP: 65%; PLGA65/TP: 80%).

Keywords: vitamin E; tocopherol; PLA; PLGA; core-shell nanoparticles; drug delivery; controlled drug release

---

1. Introduction

The encapsulation of the pharmaceutical ingredients in a macro- or a nanocarrier is a key factor in nanomedicine developments [1–3]. Utilization of drug delivery systems can increase and prolong the efficiency of the active drugs. Due to the good biocompatibility and structural properties, several materials such as proteins and mostly biodegradable polymers, e.g., chitosan, alginate, hyaluronic acid, poly(lactide) or poly(lactic acid) (PLA), polycaprolactone (PCL), poly(trimetilene-carbonate) (PTMC), etc., have been widely used as potential carriers of the nanosized drug delivery systems [4–12]. Many types of PLA copolymers, such as poly(lactide-*co*-glycolide) (PLGA), polylactide-poly(ethylene glycol) (PLA-PEG), poly(caprolactone-ethylene glycol-lactide) (PCELA), etc., are also well-known as drug carriers [13–17]. As a result of copolymerization, the hydrophilicity of the PLA can be remarkably tuned, which opens the possibility of encapsulating active ingredients that have hydrophilic or hydrophobic character into the polymer matrix.

The (±)-α-Tocopherol (TP) is one of the highest biological activity fat-soluble vitamins from the vitamin E family and is composed of eight tocopherols and tocotrienols (alpha (α), beta (β), gamma (γ)

and delta (δ) isomers for both cases) [18]. Several studies focus on the encapsulation of the TP, because vitamin E can prevent and treat many chronic and age-related diseases, e.g., Alzheimer's disease [19]. Furthermore, the TP is described as functioning as an antioxidant, and the higher vitamin E content is associated with a lower risk of several cancer diseases (kidney, lung, bladder, etc.).

Alqahtani et al. synthesized TP-loaded PLGA50 NPs with an average size of ca. 130 nm using Polyvinyl alcohol (PVA) as a stabilizer, but only 4–4.5% of drug loading (in mg drug/100 mg PLGA) was achieved [20]. However, Zigoneanu and coworkers increased the TP loading to 8–16% using the PLGA50 carrier and PVA and sodium dodecyl sulphate (SDS) surfactant stabilizing agents, but it was confirmed that the 86% of the drug dissolved for NPs (d ~220–280 nm) with 8% TP loading, while 36% of the TP drug released from the NPs when the loading was 16% after 1 h [19]. However, Astete et al. synthesized Span80-stabilized TP-containing PLGA50-based nanosized particles in the range of 150–200 nm and the effect of salt concentration on the size and morphology of the NPs has been interpreted, but data for the drug loading and release were not presented [21]. Murugeshu and coworkers also synthesized chitosan/PLGA50-based TP-containing NPs with 8%, 16% and 24% initial loading, but the EE% was only 45–50% and the release studies were carried out in gastrointestinal conditions (pH ~1.50) [22]. Simon et al. successfully encapsulated the TP into PLGA50 using PVA, but only 2.5 mg drug/100 mg NPs can be obtained [23].

In our previous work, the TP as well as the water-soluble derivative of TP (D, α-Tocopherol polyethylene glycol 1000 succinate (TPGS)) and the non-steroidal anti-inflammatory ketoprofen (KP) have been successfully encapsulated into PLA and PLGA75 (lactide:glycolide ratio 75:25) and PLGA65 (lactide:glycolide ratio 65:35) nanocarriers [13]. Instead of the commonly used and above mentioned PLGA50, the PLGA65 and PLGA75 derivatives have been firstly used as carriers for the encapsulation of TP, and the hydrophilicity properties of the carriers and the model drugs on the EE% have been studied in detail. The release measurements of nanocomposites including hydrophobic drugs are very difficult to carry out. In order to facilitate the above-mentioned studies, stabilizing agents such as surfactants have been widely used [5,19]. Non-ionic poloxamer Pluronic F127 was applied previously, which stabilized the drug-containing polymeric NPs by increasing the biocompatibility. The optimal ratios of the carrier, the drug and the stabilizing agent have a dominant effect on the structure and the EE%, as well as the controlled drug release process of the nanosized drug delivery systems, which were not studied previously.

In the present work, the results of the TP-containing nanocomposites, using PLA, PLGA65 and PLGA75 carriers, have been completed and the determinative role of the concentration of the polymer, the TP and the PLUR stabilizing agent on the structure of the drug-containing nanocomposites has been investigated. Moreover, the drug release studies of the prepared TP-containing PLA, PLGA65 and PLGA75 core-shell NPs have also been interpreted.

2. Materials and Methods

2.1. Materials

Polylactide (PLA, Mw = 72,200 ± 15,000 Da) and two poly(lactide-*co*-glycolide) (PLGA) derivatives with a lactide to glycolide ratio at 75:25 (PLGA75, Mw = 69,900 ± 4000 Da) and at 65:35 (PLGA65, Mw = 93,000 ± 1000 Da) were synthetized according to the previously published procedure [13]. Pluronic F127 (PLUR), (±)-α-tocopherol (TP) and sodium phosphate monobasic monohydrate ($NaH_2PO_4 \cdot H_2O$, ≥99%) were obtained from Sigma Aldrich (Budapest, Hungary). Sodium phosphate dibasic anhydrous (Na_2HPO_4, ≥99%) and sodium chloride (NaCl, ≥99%) were purchased from Molar Chemicals (Halásztelek, Hungary). All other reagents and solvents were of analytical grade and used without further purification. The deionized water was obtained by Millipore purification apparatus (18.2 MΩ cm at 25 °C).

2.2. *Preparation of TP-Loaded PLA/PLGA NPs*

The TP-loaded PLA/PLGA NPs were prepared by nanoprecipitation method (Figure 1). The detailed experimental conditions were presented previously [13]. Briefly, the PLA/PLGA and TP with increasing concentrations (see Table 1) were dissolved in 1.5 mL of acetone, which was dropped slowly (10 μL/5 s) into the aqueous solution of the PLUR stabilizer (15 mL) under room temperature using magnetic stirring with 1000 rpm. In the interest of the evaporation of acetone, the prepared samples were further stirred (350 rpm) for two days. The dispersion was centrifugated with 40 mL MQ water at 12,000 rpm (t = 15 min, T = 25 °C). After the supernatant was removed, the NPs were redispersed in MQ water and the washing methods were repeated two times. The obtained NPs samples were freeze-dried by liquid nitrogen and lyophilized (by Christ Alpha 1-2 LDplus apparatus).

Table 1. The concentration of the components, the average particle diameter, the polydispersity index (PI), the encapsulation efficiency (EE%) and the drug loading (DL%) of the TP-loaded PLA NPs.

	Acetone Phase		Aqueous Phase				
Sample	c_{PLA} (mg·mL^{-1})	c_{TP} (mg·mL^{-1})	c_{PLUR} (mg·mL^{-1})	d_{DLS} ± SD [1] (nm)	PI ± SD	EE%	DL%
PLA concentration dependence	1.25	2.5	0.1	120 ± 33	0.120 ± 0.043	–	–
	2.5	2.5	0.1	156 + 28	0.039 ± 0.012	–	–
	5.0	2.5	0.1	179 ± 35	0.082 ± 0.049	–	–
	10.0	2.5	0.1	201 ± 38	0.095 ± 0.026	69.11	14.73
TP concentration dependence	10.0	0	0.1	188 ± 37	0.092 ± 0.059	–	–
	10.0	0.5	0.1	189 ± 34	0.048 ± 0.028	91.28	4.36
	10.0	1.0	0.1	192 ± 30	0.062 ± 0.032	75.61	7.02
	10.0	2.5	0.1	201 ± 38	0.095 ± 0.026	69.11	14.73
	10.0	5.0	0.1	252 ± 53	0.073 ± 0.033	66.15	24.85
PLUR concentration dependence	10.0	2.5	0	179 ± 40	0.315 ± 0.040	72.19	15.29
	10.0	2.5	0.05	178 ± 21	0.304 ± 0.095	98.34	19.73
	10.0	2.5	0.1	201 ± 38	0.095 ± 0.026	69.11	14.73
	10.0	2.5	0.5	206 ± 36	0.089 ± 0.065	57.94	12.65
	10.0	2.5	1.0	212 ± 36	0.066 ± 0.029	40.75	9.24

[1] The experimental error of the peak maximum is below 2.5%.

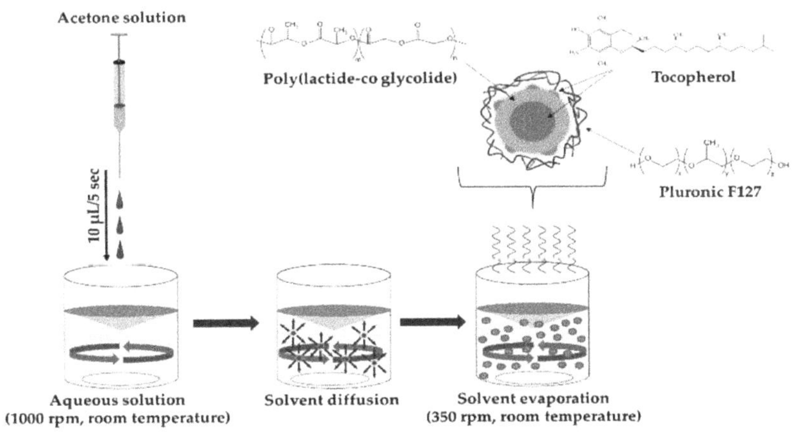

Figure 1. Schematic representation of the preparation of TP-loaded PLGA NPs stabilized by PLUR using nanoprecipitation technique.

2.3. *Characterization Methods*

The particle size was determined by dynamic light scattering (DLS) with Horiba Sz-100 (HORIBA Jobin Yvon, Longjumeau, France) equipped with a diode pumped frequency doubled (532 nm, 10 mW) laser. The measurements were carried out at 25 ± 0.1 °C with 90° of detection angle in every case.

The transmission electron microscopy (TEM) images were obtained by Jeol JEM-1400plus equipment (JEOL Ltd., Tokyo, Japan) at 120 keV accelerating voltage. The Fourier transform infrared (FT-IR) spectra of the PLA/PLGA-TP NPs were registered by a Jasco FT/IR-4700 with ATR PRO ONE Single-reflection accessory (ABL&JASCO, Budapest, Hungary). The experiments were performed at room temperature from 600 cm^{-1} to 3600 cm^{-1}. The resolution of the spectra was 2 cm^{-1}, which was determined by 128 interferograms.

The particles were dissolved in 1,4-dioxane to determine the EE% and DL% of the composites. The absorbance spectra of the prepared solutions were measured by a Shimadzu UV-1800 UV-Vis double beam spectrophotometer. The spectra were registered in the range of 200–500 nm using 1 cm quartz cuvette at room temperature. The characteristic absorbance band of the TP appeared at 294 nm. The concentration of the encapsulated drug was determined from the calibration curve (Figure S1). The data of the EE% in *w/w*% were calculated by the total drug mass used in the synthesis of the NPs (Equation (1)), while DL% was calculated by the mass of the NPs (Equation (2)).

$$EE\% = \frac{encapsulated\ mass\ of\ drug}{total\ mass\ of\ drug\ in\ synthesis} \times 100 \quad (1)$$

$$DL\% = \frac{encapsulated\ mass\ of\ drug}{total\ mass\ of\ the\ nanoparticles} \times 100 \quad (2)$$

2.4. Determination of the Solubility Properties of TP Drug

In order to determine the solubility of TP, 100 μL of acetone solutions of TP (5 mg·mL^{-1}) was added dropwise to 10 mL of PLUR solutions (0.1–1.2 mg·mL^{-1}), and the turbidity was followed with a Precision Bench Turbidity Meter LP2000 (Hanna Ins. Service Kft., Szeged, Hungary). The experiments were performed in a pure aqueous medium and in a phosphate (PBS) buffer (pH = 7.4, 0.9% NaCl) solution at 25 °C and 37 °C.

2.5. Critical Micelle Concentration (cmc) Studies

The critical micelle concentration (cmc) of the applied PLUR was determined by inverse titration method in Krüss K100MK2 type surface tension equipment. The computer-controlled apparatus was supplied with a thermostat and an automatic burette. The Wilhelmy-plate method was applied. A volume of 50 mL of a 1.6 mM surfactant solution was titrated with MQ water or PBS in an aliquot of 10 mL in 40 steps. Each experimental point was the average of at least 5 measurements.

2.6. In Vitro Release Study

The in vitro studies of the different TP-loaded PLA/PLGA NPs were carried out by a UV-Vis spectrophotometer (500–200 nm). The release experiments were performed at 37 °C and a PBS buffer (pH = 7.4, NaCl 0.9%) containing 1 mg·mL^{-1} of PLUR was used, which facilitated the easier feasibility of the release studies [5]. The TP-loaded samples were placed into the cellulose membrane (Sigma Aldrich) with 5 mL of PLUR/PBS medium inserted into 35 mL of a dissolution phase. During the measurements, 3 mL of the release media were taken at specified intervals to measure the released concentration of TP at 268 nm.

The release curves of the TP can be fitted by different kinetic models, such as the first order, Korsmeyer–Peppas, Peppas–Sahlin and Weibull models [24–27]. The measured points were fitted with a nonlinear regression by the QtiPlot 0.9.8.9 svn 2288 program. During the calculation session, the program finds the best fitting function for the measured points. The results consist of the fitted parameters, their standard deviation and the goodness of fitting (root mean squared error).

Depending of the release chemical condition (such as temperature, buffer solution, ionic strength, etc.), the shape of the polymers and the solubility of the drugs, the dissolution curves can be described with different kinetic models. For our calculation, the following kinetic models were used.

First order equation is a frequently used kinetic model. This formula is well applicable for drugs where the dissolution is continuously changing over time and depends only on the concentration.

$$c_t = ce^{-kt} \tag{3}$$

where c_t is the concentration of the solid drug in the matrix of the carried system at t time, c_0 is the initial concentration of the drug and k is the first order release constant.

The Korsmeyer–Peppas kinetic formula is a semi-empirical power law equation where the shape of the polymer matrix (such as film, cylinder or sphere) can be taken into account in the release curve.

$$\frac{c_t}{c_0} = k_m t^n \tag{4}$$

where c_t is the concentration of the dissolved drug at t time, c_0 is the initial concentration of drug, k_m is the kinetic constant and n is the diffusion dissolution index (for sphere shaped particles $n = 0.42$ for the diffusion-controlled mechanism, $n = 1$ for the Case II relaxation controlled mechanism and $0.42 \leq n \leq 1$ for both of them).

The Weibull equation is a general empirical formula which can be used for all release profiles.

$$c_t = 1 - exp\left(\frac{-(t - T_i)^b}{a}\right) \tag{5}$$

where c_t is the concentration of the released component in t time, T_i is the lag time between the initial of measurement and the release of drug (in most cases $T_i = 0$), a is the time scale of the process and b is the shape parameter (shape of the release curve is exponential if $b = 1$, parabola if $b < 1$ or sigmoid if $b > 1$).

The kinetic formula reported by Peppas and Sahlin specifies the diffusion and the relaxation contribution in the drug dissolution process.

$$\frac{c_t}{c_0} = k_1 t^m + k_2 t^{2m} \tag{6}$$

where c_t is the concentration of the dissolved drug in the t time, c_0 is the initial concentration of the drug and k_1, k_2 and m are constants: k_1 is the Fick diffusion contribution, k_2 is the Case II relaxation contribution and m is the diffusion exponent (sphere shaped: $m = 0.43$, Fick diffusion mechanism; $m = 0.85$, Case II relaxation transport mechanism; $0.43 \leq m \leq 0.85$, anomalous transport mechanism).

3. Results

3.1. *Effect of the Component Concentrations on the Core-Shell Structure*

In order to determine the role of the component quantities of the nanocomposites on the size and the structure, as well as on the EE% the concentration, only one building block (polymer carrier, drug or stabilizing agent) has been modified during the synthesis while the other parameters have been kept constant. The average particle diameters of the NPs were measured by DLS, and the results are summarized in Table 1. In case of PLA concentration dependence, regardless of the amount of the TP ($c = 2.5$ mg·mL^{-1}), the diameter of the NPs permanently increases from 120 nm ($c_{PLA} = 1.25$ mg·mL^{-1} in aceton phase) to ca. 200 nm ($c_{PLA} = 10$ mg·mL^{-1} in the acetone phase). The morphology and the structure of the NPs have been investigated by TEM images as well (Figure 2). The images clearly represent that the structure of the TP/PLUR NPs in the absence of a polymer shows less amorphous structures and TP crystal-like objects are observed. Moreover, we established that an increase in the polymer concentration results in the formation of a well-defined core-shell structure at $c_{PLA} = 10.0$ mg·mL^{-1}. At lower polymer concentrations, this structure is not formed, and because of the low polymer concentration, the purification (centrifugation) of the NPs is impracticable; thus, the determination of the EE% was not possible. For TP that is concentration-dependent, the diameters show a slightly increasing tendency to 2.5 mg·mL^{-1}, but for a 5 mg·mL^{-1} amount of TP, a higher size is obtained (d_{DLS} = 252 nm) (Table 1). The TEM images also confirm this observation (Figure 2). The well-defined core-shell structure is formed at 2.5 mg·mL^{-1} of TP quantity. With a further increase in the TP amount, the core, including the drug, shows a rather crystallized structure instead of the previously confirmed amorphous form. The EE% and the drug loading were determined for all composites. We obtained that the value of the EE% decreased from 91.28% (c_{TP} = 0.5 mg·mL^{-1}) to 66.15% (c_{TP} = 5 mg·mL^{-1}), while the DL% increased from 4.36% (c_{TP} = 0.5 mg·mL^{-1}) to 24.85% (c_{TP} = 5 mg·mL^{-1}). Considering the expected size of the NPs for optimal nanosized drug delivery systems (ca. 200 nm) as well as the crystallization of the core, the 2.5 mg·mL^{-1} amount of TP will be used for further studies at 10.0 mg·mL^{-1} of PLA polymer concentration. Besides optimizing the amount of carrier and active drug, the ratio of the stabilizing PLUR surfactant was also studied. It was clearly confirmed that in the absence of PLUR, the TP molecules were not capsulated into the polymer core, only the binding of the TP drugs onto the surface of the polymer shell is observed (Figure 2). Furthermore, it was established that the smallest particle diameter (d = 178 nm), as well as the highest DL% (ca. 20%), is obtained at 0.05 mg·mL^{-1} of PLUR concentration. Increase in the PLUR amount resulted in a higher particle size (212 nm) as well as a lower DL% values (9%). Most probably, the increase in the PLUR concentration facilitated the solubility of the hydrophobic TP, thus hindering the encapsulation process. In order to confirm the above-mentioned phenomena, turbidity measurements were carried out (Figure S2). According to the TEM images (Figure 2) and the turbidity studies (Figure S2), we can conclude that a low quantity (0.1 mg·mL^{-1}) of PLUR surfactant is advantageous for the formation of PLA-based core-shell NPs, but the presence of a higher amount of PLUR (>0.1 mg·mL^{-1}) results in the decrease of the EE%. Moreover, the presence of a higher amount of stabilizer (≥1.0 mg·mL^{-1}) causes aggregation (Figure 2).

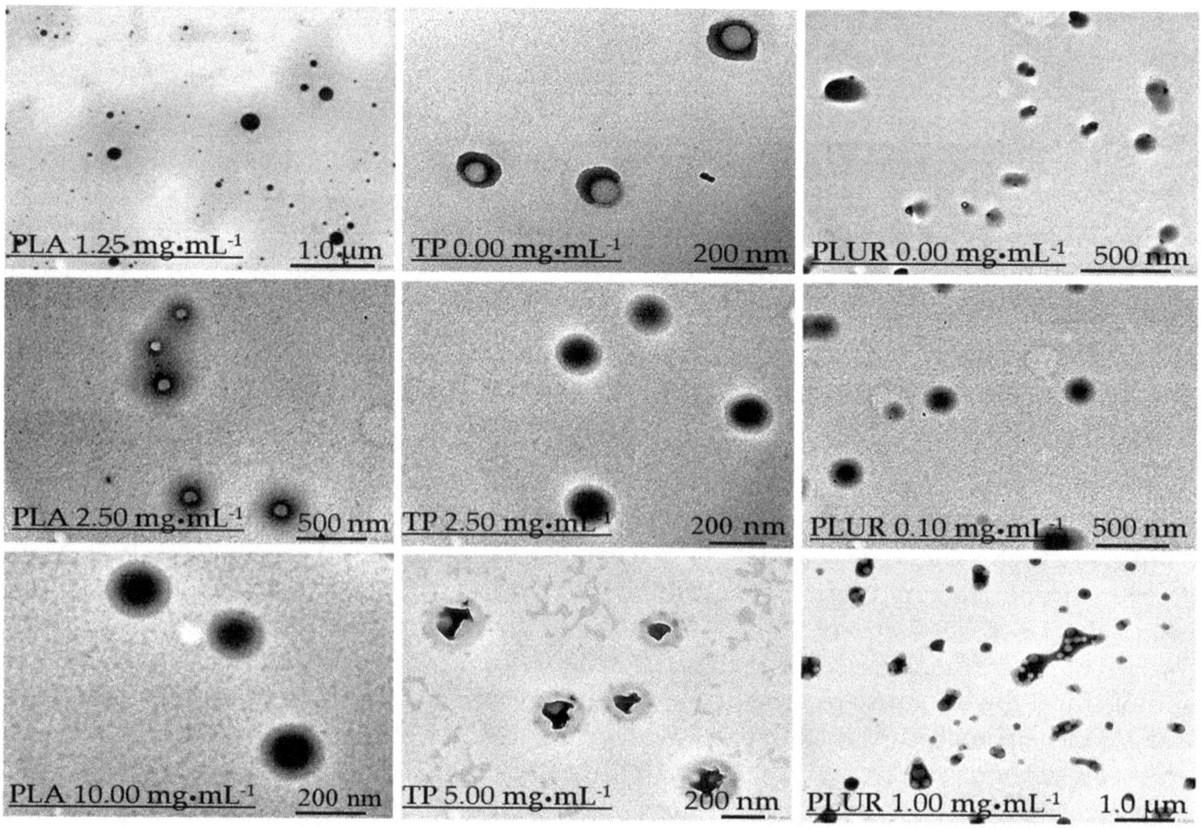

Figure 2. Representative TEM images of the TP-containing PLA NPs using different component concentrations (PLA: 1.25–10.0 mg·mL^{-1}; TP: 0–5.0 mg·mL^{-1} and PLUR: 0–1.0 mg·mL^{-1}).

Besides the determination of the optimal ratio of the composite building blocks, the TP was encapsulated in PLGA75 and PLGA65 copolymers that have increasing hydrophilicity. During the NPs synthesis, the previously optimized concentrations of the polymer carrier (10.0 mg·mL^{-1}), the PLUR (0.1 mg·mL^{-1}) and the TP (2.5 mg·mL^{-1}) were used. Based on DLS studies, we established that the particle size increases from 203 nm to 226 nm with a decrease of the lactide part in the polymer (Figure 3A). Using the optimized component quantities, the core-shell structure was confirmed for PLGA75 and PLGA65-based TP-containing NPs (Figure 3B). The EE% and DL% has been determined for the PLGA75 and PLGA65-based system as well, and we observed that the replacement of the PLA carrier to PLGA75 and PLGA65 polymers resulted in the increase in the EE% to 75.72% and 87.69%, respectively. In addition, the drug loading also increased from 14.73% (PLA) to 15.92% (PLGA75) and to 17.98% (PLGA65) with decreasing lactide content. The higher EE% and DL% can be explained by the fact that the precipitation of the more hydrophilic PLGA carriers is slower than that for PLA and TP, which helps the formation of the well-defined core-shell structure [13].

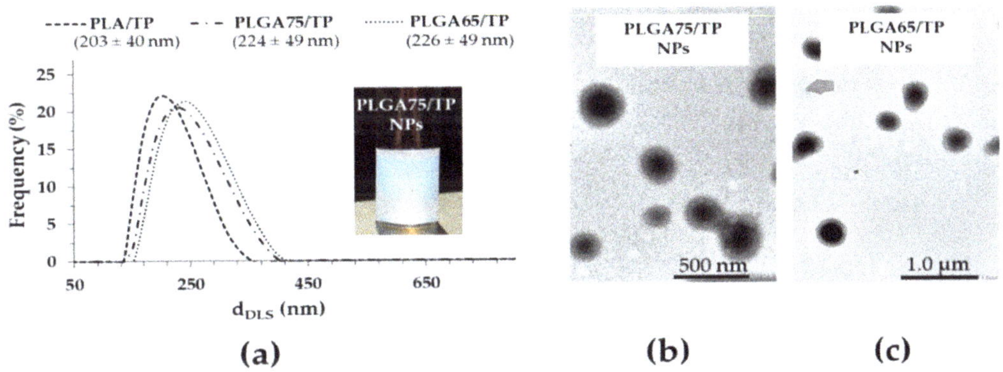

Figure 3. The particle size distribution of the TP-loaded PLA and PLGA NPs (**a**), and representative TEM images of the PLGA75–(**b**) and PLGA65–(**c**) based composites.

3.2. Structural Characterization of the TP-Loaded PLA and PLGA Core-Shell NPs

To determine the interaction between the PLA and TP, the composites have been examined by infrared spectroscopy measurements. Figure 4 displays the spectra of the PLA-based NPs in the absence (Figure 4A) and in the presence of TP at different concentrations (Figure 4B,C). The TP-sensitive bands appear in the range of 3050–2800 cm^{-1} and 1150–1000 cm^{-1}. It is obvious that the intensity of all the determinative bands systematically increase by increasing TP content. At 2994, 2944 and 2968 cm^{-1}, the asymmetric and symmetric CH stretching vibrations of the –CH_2 and –CH_3 groups of the drug appear. Due to the increasing TP concentration, these bands become more intense, indicating the presence of TP molecules in the polymer NPs. The carbonyl group of the PLA appears at 1750 cm^{-1} [28,29]. The TP does not contain a C=O group, thus this band could originate only from the polymer. In the fingerprint region ($\nu \leq 1500$ cm^{-1}), the deformation and bending vibration of the –CH_3 and –CH_2 groups appear at 1453, 1381 and 1267 cm^{-1}, while the band at 1181 cm^{-1} attributes to the stretching mode of the C–O–C (ester). At around 1086 cm^{-1}, further bands of the C–O–C stretching vibration can be observed, which have shoulders (symmetric and asymmetric stretching vibrations). Because of the Ar–O–C group in the TP, the intensity of this C–O–C symmetric stretching vibration at around 1050 cm^{-1} is increased. The band at 865 cm^{-1} and 751 cm^{-1} is characteristic of the polymer carrier, and no shift is observed. The IR measurements performed for PLGA75 and PLGA65 resulted in similar spectra. A strong irreversible interaction between the PLA (or PLGA75, PLGA65) and the TP cannot be discovered (Figures S3 and S4), which facilitates the spontaneous release of the TP active drug from the polymer NPs, but the presence of the TP in the different composites were definitely confirmed by IR.

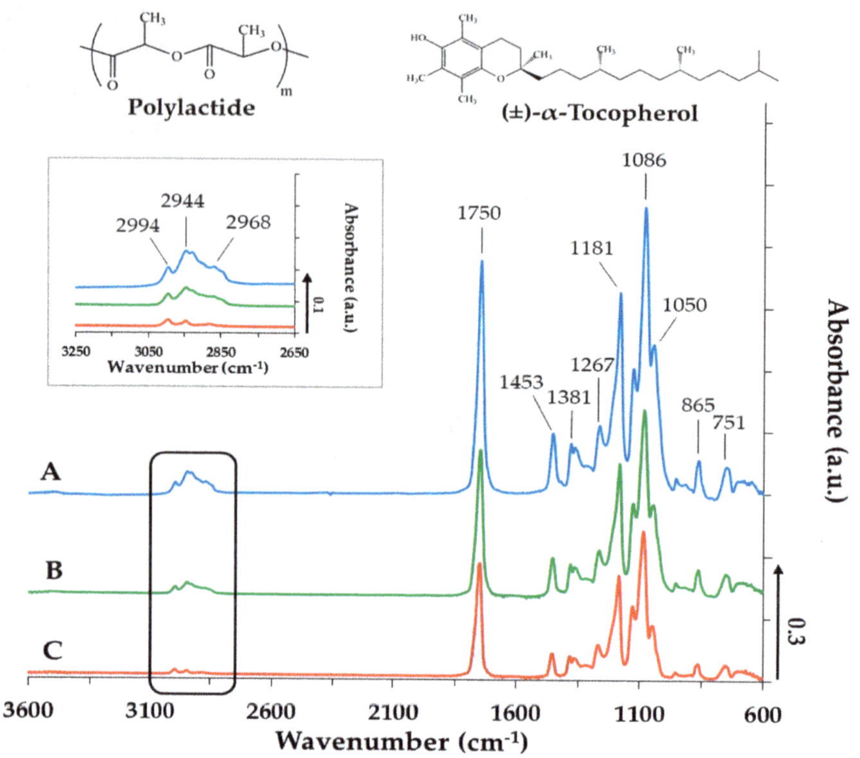

Figure 4. IR spectra of the TP-loaded PLA NPs (A: c_{TP} = 0 mg·mL^{-1}; B: c_{TP} = 2.5 mg·mL^{-1}; C: c_{TP} = 5 mg·mL^{-1}, c_{PLA} = 10 mg·mL^{-1} and c_{PLUR} = 0.1 mg·mL^{-1}).

Turbidimetric measurements were performed to investigate the interaction between the TP and the PLUR stabilizing agent in a pure aqueous solution and in PBS at 25 °C and 37 °C (pH = 7.4, 0.9% NaCl); the results are presented in Figure 5. In MQ water (Figure 5A), the turbidity of TP is systematically decreased till ca. 0.9 mg·mL^{-1} of PLUR concentration. Over time, more and more TP can dissolve in this medium. In contrast, in the PBS solution at 25 °C and at 37 °C, the titration curves exhibit steeper decreasing intensity, which may be due to the reduced critical micellization concentration (cmc) of PLUR in the presence of salt. In the case of the PBS solution, the turbidity remains constant from 0.7 mg·mL^{-1} at 25 °C, while an increase in the temperature to 37 °C 0.6 mg·mL^{-1} value is observed. It is important to mention that the solubility of the TP scarcely depends on time at 37 °C, which allows the possible use of the PLUR stabilizing agent for in vitro drug release measurements.

It is well known that the surfactant affects the solubility of the TP drug in the absence of a polymer carrier. Namely, above cmc, due to the micellization ability of the PLUR, the solubilization of the drug dominates forming TP-loaded individual micelles, while below cmc, only the solubility increases. Accordingly, the cmc of the PLUR was measured by surface tension measurements (Figure 6). In the literature, very different values can be found; the obtained range of cmc is 2–7 mg·mL^{-1} [30,31]. Similar values were measured, but we determined that at 25 °C, the obtained cmc is decreased from 4.92 mg·mL^{-1} to 1.99 mg·mL^{-1} in the presence of the phosphate buffer. If the temperature rises from 25 °C to 37 °C, these values are further decreased. We can conclude that the concentration of the PLUR in the composites is significantly lower than the cmc (4.92 mg·mL^{-1}) value, which excludes the presence of TP-loaded individual micelles.

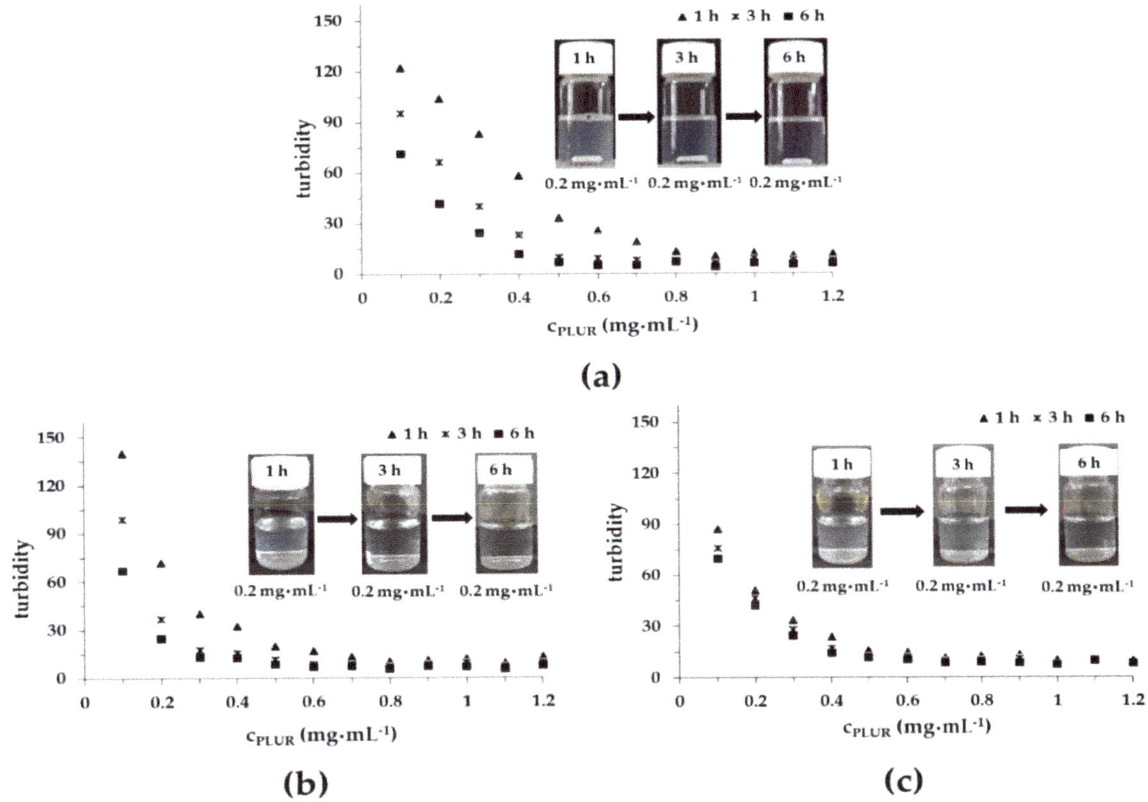

Figure 5. The turbidity of the TP in the PLUR solution at 25 °C in an aqueous medium (**a**), in a PBS buffer at 25 °C (**b**) and at 37 °C (**c**) (pH = 7.4, 0.9 *w/w*% NaCl) (c_{TP} = 0.05 mg·mL^{-1}).

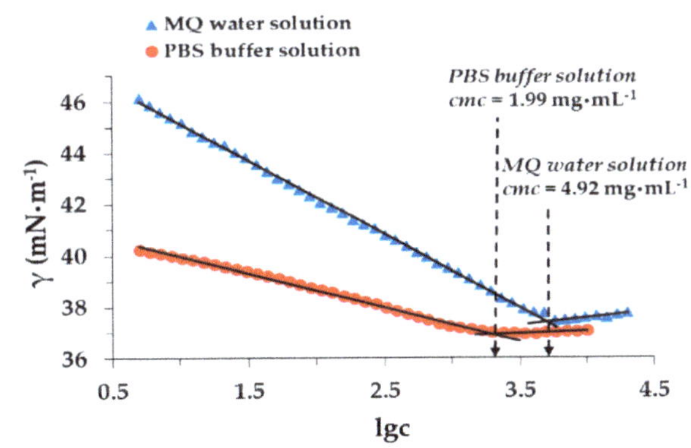

Figure 6. Determination of PLUR cmc at 25 °C in MQ water and in a PBS solution.

3.3. In Vitro Drug Release Experiments

The determination of the exact TP amount released from the different composites was carried out by the UV-Vis spectrophotometric method. The spectra of the TP and the calibration curve are presented in Figure 7. The absorption bands of the TP appear in the UV range.

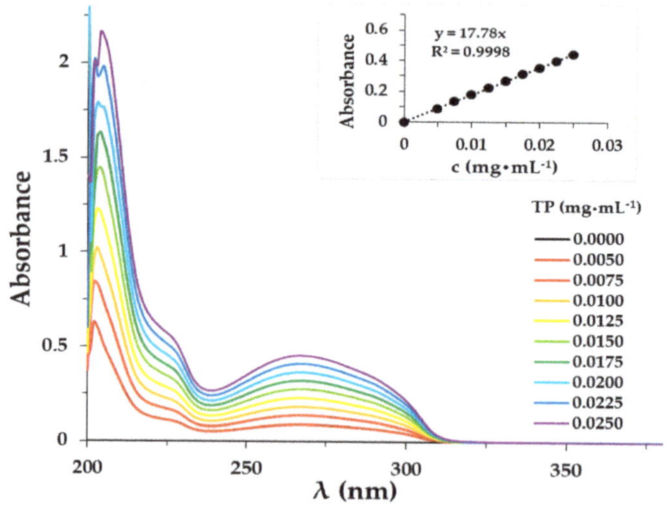

Figure 7. UV spectra of the TP in the PBS solution (c_{PLUR} = 1.0 mg·mL^{-1}, 0.9 *w*/*w*% NaCl).

After the characterization of the TP-loaded PLA and PLGA NPs, the mechanism of the drug release was investigated. The drug dissolution profiles and the fitting of these curves by different kinetic models are demonstrated in Figure 8 (Figure S5). The suitability of several models like Korsmeyer–Peppas, Peppas–Sahlin, the first-order and the Weibull models were investigated. The release curves clearly show that a high amount of TP is retained in the polymers after 7 h. It was also observed that in the first half an hour, the dissolution of the drug occurs relatively quickly, but after that, measurable slow dissolution is observed. Moreover, we found that the active substance is released slowly with a decrease of the lactide part (PLA, 35.0%, PLGA75, 28.3%, PLGA65, 19.8%) in 7 h. The slowest dissolution occurred in the carrier-free TP (15%). Because of the higher hydrophobicity, a higher amount of the non-encapsulated drug can be attached to the surface of the particles, which confirms the above-mentioned dissolution order [13]. Thanks to the application of the nanosized drug carrier systems (polymer NPs), the TP molecules can bind to the enhanced specific surface area of the NPs, which facilitates the dissolution of more TP, in contrast to the bulk TP.

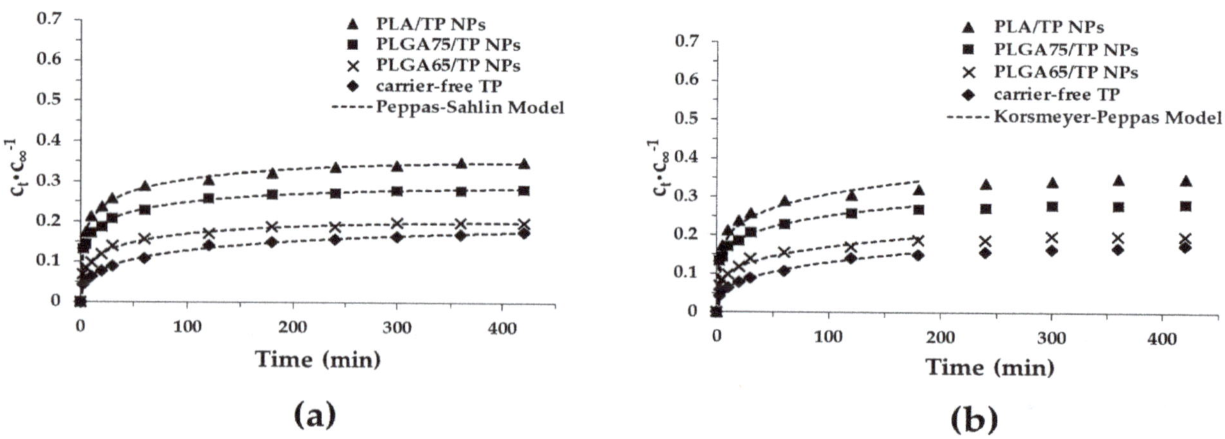

Figure 8. Release profiles and different kinetic models-predicted (Peppas-Sahlin model (**a**), Korsmeyer-Peppas model (**b**)) for the release curves of TP from PLA and PLGA NPs in the PBS buffer (pH = 7.4, 0.9 *w*/*w*% NaCl).

Taking into account the coefficient of the determination (R^2), the Peppas–Sahlin model was the best kinetic formula for our systems (Table 2). The values of the Case II relaxation contribution (k_2) were negative in all cases; therefore, this model does not provide complete information about the dissolution of the TP, but the low diffusion exponent (m) is referred to for the Fickian release.

Table 2. Determined parameters of the TP release by fitting several kinetic equations.

Peppas–Sahlin Formulation	k_1 (min^{-m})	k_2 (min^{-2m})	m	R^2
PLA/TP NPs	0.1371	−0.01346	0.260	0.9974
PLGA75/TP NPs	0.1165	−0.01189	0.248	0.9986
PLGA65/TP NPs	0.0572	−0.00412	0.317	0.9974
TP	0.0304	−0.00124	0.366	0.9978
Korsmeyer–Peppas Formulation	k_m (min^{-n})	n	R^2	
PLA/TP NPs	0.1339	0.182	0.9898	
PLGA75/TP NPs	0.1120	0.175	0.9982	
PLGA65/TP NPs	0.0592	0.223	0.9904	
TP	0.0310	0.311	0.9977	
Weibull Formulation	a	b	R^2	
PLA/TP NPs	6.52	0.178	0.9896	
PLGA75/TP NPs	7.85	0.166	0.9819	
PLGA65/TP NPs	15.45	0.220	0.9898	
TP	28.19	0.285	0.9945	
First Order Formulation	k (min^{-1})	R^2		
PLA/TP NPs	0.0094	0.9792		
PLGA75/TP NPs	0.0113	0.9532		
PLGA65/TP NPs	0.0130	0.9514		
TP	0.0079	0.9856		

The second-best kinetic model was the Korsmeyer–Peppas model where the diffusion dissolution index (n) gives the information about the diffusion and the erosion of the matrix. The values of the n are increased from $n = 0.182$ (PLA) to $n = 0.223$ (PLGA65), which is referred to for the diffusion-controlled quasi Fickian drug release. Furthermore, it is important to note that the value of the diffusion dissolution index is lower than 0.42. This is caused by the high polydispersity of the particles (because they are lyophilized) and the very low degradation of the polymers [32]. Presumably, the Case II relaxation contribution from the Peppas–Sahlin model will be low by these effects.

During the slow degradation of the PLA/PLGA carrier, the drug diffuses with difficulty from the core of the particles. The measured and calculated results clearly stated that the released drug originates from the surface region of the particles. Based on this, we could calculate the approximate quantity of the TP in the core of the particles after 7 h: 65.0% (PLA), 71.7% (PLGA75) and 80.2% (PLGA65) from the encapsulated mass of the TP; therefore, a significant amount of the active ingredient can be encapsulated inside the particles.

4. Conclusions

In the work presented here, the successful encapsulation of the hydrophobic α-Tocopherol, one of the determinative natural forms of vitamin E, was carried out using the PLA, PLGA75 and PLGA65 biocompatible polymer carriers by increasing hydrophilicity. To the best of our knowledge, we first proved the formation of well-defined nanosized TP-core PLA/PLGA-shell structured nanocomposites. Optimization of the experimental conditions, such as optimal concentration of drug, polymer carrier and stabilizing PLUR non-ionic surfactant, resulted in the formation of core-shell NPs within the diameter range of ~200–220 nm. For the PLA-based system 14.7% of drug loading was achieved, where most of the TP molecules are encapsulated in the core (65%), while the remaining part of the active ingredient is located on the surface of the polymer shell. By replacing the hydrophobic PLA to PLGA copolymers, both the drug loading (PLGA75: 16%, PLGA65: 18%) as well the EE% can be increased (PLA/TP: 69.1%; PLGA75/TP: 75.7%; PLGA65/TP: 87.7%). Furthermore, the PLGA-based composites contain 71.7% and 80.2% of the encapsulated TP in the core. Considering the slower precipitation ability of the PLGA copolymers in contrast to the PLA and the active ingredient, the higher encapsulation efficiency can be explored. Besides the preparation and the characterization of the composites, the drug release was also studied. The dissolution curves clearly show that depending on the polymer, more than 65–80% of the TP is contained in the composites after 7 h. In the first half an hour, the dissolution of the drug occurs relatively quickly, but after that, measurable slow dissolution was observed. Moreover, we found that the active substance is released slowly with decreasing lactide part (PLA, 35.0%; PLGA75, 28.3%; PLGA65, 19.8%) in 7 h. Thanks to the biocompatibility, cost-effectivity and tuneable hydrophilic properties, the PLA/PLGA polymers are potential candidates for controlled drug release and for the encapsulation of hydrophobic TP or similar sized and structured molecules in core-shell nanosized particles.

Supplementary Materials:
Figure S1: UV spectra of TP in 1,4-dioxane at different concentrations, Figure S2: The turbidity of TP (a) and PLA (b) in PLUR solution at 25°C in aqueous medium ($c_{TP} = 0.25$ mg·mL^{-1}, $c_{PLA} = 0.25$ mg·mL^{-1}), Figure S3: IR spectra of the TP- free (a) and TP- loaded (b) PLGA75 NPs ($c_{TP} = 2.5$ mg·mL^{-1}, $c_{PLA} = 10$ mg·mL^{-1}, $c_{PLUR} = 0.1$ mg·mL^{-1}), Figure S4: IR spectra of the TP- free (a) and TP- loaded (b) PLGA65 NPs ($c_{TP} = 2.5$ mg·mL^{-1}, $c_{PLA} = 10$ mg·mL^{-1}, $c_{PLUR} = 0.1$ mg·mL^{-1}), Figure S5: Release profiles and different kinetic models-predicted (First Order model (a), Weibull model (b)) release curves of TP from PLA and PLGA NPs in PBS solution (pH = 7.4, 0.9 *w/w*% NaCl).

Author Contributions: Conceptualization, E.C.; methodology, N.V.; investigation, N.V. and Á.T. and V.H.; data curation, Á.T.; writing—original draft preparation, E.C.; writing—review and editing, V.H.; supervision, E.C.

Acknowledgments: The research was supported by the National Research, Development and Innovation Office-NKFIH through the project GINOP-2.3.2-15-2016-00060. V.H. acknowledges the Premium Post Doctorate Research Program of the Hungarian Academy of Sciences for the financial support. This paper was supported by the János Bolyai Research Scholarship of the Hungarian Academy of Sciences (E. Csapó). The Ministry of Human Capacities, Hungary grant TUDFO/47138-1/2019-ITM is acknowledged.

References

1. Kumari, A.; Yadav, S.K.; Yadav, S.C. Biodegradable polymeric nanoparticles based drug delivery systems. *Colloids Surf. B Biointerfaces* **2010**, *75*, 1–18. [CrossRef] [PubMed]
2. Nair, L.S.; Laurencin, C.T. Biodegradable polymers as biomaterials. *Prog. Polym. Sci.* **2007**, *32*, 762–798. [CrossRef]
3. Rancan, F.; Papakostas, D.; Hadam, S.; Hackbarth, S.; Delair, T.; Primard, C.; Verrier, B.; Sterry, W.; Blume-Peytavi, U.; Vogt, A. Investigation of Polylactic Acid (PLA) Nanoparticles as Drug Delivery Systems for Local Dermatotherapy. *Pharm. Res.* **2009**, *26*, 2027–2036. [CrossRef] [PubMed]
4. Chanphai, P.; Vesper, A.R.; Bariyanga, J.; Bérubé, G.; Tajmir-Riahi, H.A. Review on the delivery of steroids by carrier proteins. *J. Photochem. Photobiol. B Biol.* **2016**, *161*, 184–191. [CrossRef] [PubMed]
5. Janovák, L.; Turcsányi, Á.; Bozó, É.; Deák, Á.; Mérai, L.; Sebők, D.; Juhász, Á.; Csapó, E.; Abdelghafour, M.M.; Farkas, E.; et al. Preparation of novel tissue acidosis-responsive chitosan drug nanoparticles: Characterization and in vitro release properties of Ca2+ channel blocker nimodipine drug molecules. *Eur. J. Pharm. Sci.* **2018**, *123*, 79–88. [CrossRef] [PubMed]
6. Sarmento, B.; Ferreira, D.; Veiga, F.; Ribeiro, A. Characterization of insulin-loaded alginate nanoparticles produced by ionotropic pre-gelation through DSC and FTIR studies. *Carbohydr. Polym.* **2006**, *66*, 1–7. [CrossRef]
7. Csapó, E.; Szokolai, H.; Juhász, Á.; Varga, N.; Janovák, L.; Dékány, I. Cross-linked and hydrophobized hyaluronic acid-based controlled drug release systems. *Carbohydr. Polym.* **2018**, *195*, 99–106. [CrossRef] [PubMed]
8. Lassalle, V.; Ferreira, M.L. PLA Nano- and Microparticles for Drug Delivery: An Overview of the Methods of Preparation. *Macromol. Biosci.* **2007**, *7*, 767–783. [CrossRef]
9. Jia, W.J.; Gu, Y.C.; Gou, M.L.; Dai, M.; Li, X.Y.; Kan, B.; Yang, J.L.; Song, Q.F.; Wei, Y.Q.; Qian, Z.Y. Preparation of Biodegradable Polycaprolactone/Poly(ethylene glycol)/Polycaprolactone (PCEC) Nanoparticles. *Drug Deliv.* **2008**, *15*, 409–416. [CrossRef]

10. Zhang, Y.; Zhuo, R. Synthesis and drug release behavior of poly(trimethylene carbonate)–poly(ethylene glycol)–poly(trimethylene carbonate) nanoparticles. *Biomaterials* **2005**, *26*, 2089–2094. [CrossRef]
11. Leach, J.B.; Schmidt, C.E. Characterization of protein release from photocrosslinkable hyaluronic acid-polyethylene glycol hydrogel tissue engineering scaffolds. *Biomaterials* **2005**, *26*, 125–135. [CrossRef] [PubMed]
12. Jiang, X.; Xin, H.; Ren, Q.; Gu, J.; Zhu, L.; Du, F.; Feng, C.; Xie, Y.; Sha, X.; Fang, X. Nanoparticles of 2-deoxy-d-glucose functionalized poly(ethylene glycol)-co-poly(trimethylene carbonate) for dual-targeted drug delivery in glioma treatment. *Biomaterials* **2014**, *35*, 518–529. [CrossRef] [PubMed]
13. Varga, N.; Hornok, V.; Janovák, L.; Dékány, I.; Csapó, E. The effect of synthesis conditions and tunable hydrophilicity on the drug encapsulation capability of PLA and PLGA nanoparticles. *Colloids Surf. B Biointerfaces* **2019**, *176*, 212–218. [CrossRef] [PubMed]
14. Kiss, É.; Gyulai, G.; Pénzes, C.B.; Idei, M.; Horváti, K.; Bacsa, B.; Bősze, S. Tuneable surface modification of PLGA nanoparticles carrying new antitubercular drug candidate. *Colloids Surf. A Physicochem. Eng. Asp.* **2014**, *458*, 178–186. [CrossRef]
15. Duse, L.; Agel, M.R.; Pinnapireddy, S.R.; Schäfer, J.; Selo, M.A.; Ehrhardt, C.; Bakowsky, U. Photodynamic Therapy of Ovarian Carcinoma Cells with Curcumin-Loaded Biodegradable Polymeric Nanoparticles. *Pharmaceutics* **2019**, *11*, 282. [CrossRef] [PubMed]
16. Molina, I.; Li, S.; Martinez, M.B.; Vert, M. Protein release from physically crosslinked hydrogels of the PLA/PEO/PLA triblock copolymer-type. *Biomaterials* **2001**, *22*, 363–369. [CrossRef]
17. Hu, Y.; Jiang, X.; Ding, Y.; Zhang, L.; Yang, C.; Zhang, J.; Chen, J.; Yang, Y. Preparation and drug release behaviors of nimodipine-loaded poly(caprolactone)–poly(ethylene oxide)–polylactide amphiphilic copolymer nanoparticles. *Biomaterials* **2003**, *24*, 2395–2404. [CrossRef]
18. Duhem, N.; Danhier, F.; Préat, V. Vitamin E-based nanomedicines for anti-cancer drug delivery. *J. Control. Release* **2014**, *182*, 33–44. [CrossRef]
19. Zigoneanu, I.G.; Astete, C.E.; Sabliov, C.M. Nanoparticles with entrapped α-tocopherol: Synthesis, characterization, and controlled release. *Nanotechnology* **2008**, *19*, 105606. [CrossRef]
20. Alqahtani, S.; Simon, L.; Astete, C.E.; Alayoubi, A.; Sylvester, P.W.; Nazzal, S.; Shen, Y.; Xu, Z.; Kaddoumi, A.; Sabliov, C.M. Cellular uptake, antioxidant and antiproliferative activity of entrapped α-tocopherol and γ-tocotrienol in poly(lactic-co-glycolic) acid (PLGA) and chitosan covered PLGA nanoparticles (PLGA-Chi). *J. Colloid Interface Sci.* **2015**, *445*, 243–251. [CrossRef]
21. Astete, C.E.; Dolliver, D.; Whaley, M.; Khachatryan, L.; Sabliov, C.M. Antioxidant Poly(lactic-*co*-glycolic) Acid Nanoparticles Made with α-Tocopherol–Ascorbic Acid Surfactant. *ACS Nano* **2011**, *5*, 9313–9325. [CrossRef] [PubMed]
22. Murugeshu, A.; Astete, C.; Leonardi, C.; Morgan, T.; Sabliov, C.M. Chitosan/PLGA particles for controlled release of α-tocopherol in the GI tract via oral administration. *Nanomedicine* **2011**, *6*, 1513–1528. [CrossRef] [PubMed]
23. Simon, L.C.; Stout, R.W.; Sabliov, C. Bioavailability of Orally Delivered Alpha-Tocopherol by Poly(Lactic-Co-Glycolic) Acid (PLGA) Nanoparticles and Chitosan Covered PLGA Nanoparticles in F344 Rats. *Nanobiomedicine* **2016**, *3*, 8. [CrossRef] [PubMed]
24. Benkő, M.; Varga, N.; Sebők, D.; Bohus, G.; Juhász, Á.; Dékány, I. Bovine serum albumin-sodium alkyl sulfates bioconjugates as drug delivery systems. *Colloids Surf. B Biointerfaces* **2015**, *130*, 126–132. [CrossRef] [PubMed]
25. Dash, S.; Murthy, P.N.; Nath, L.; Chowdhury, P. Kinetic modeling on drug release from controlled drug delivery systems. *Acta Pol. Pharm.* **2010**, *67*, 217–223.
26. Costa, P.; Sousa Lobo, J.M. Modeling and comparison of dissolution profiles. *Eur. J. Pharm. Sci.* **2001**, *13*, 123–133. [CrossRef]
27. Peppas, N.A.; Sahlin, J.J. A simple equation for the description of solute release. III. Coupling of diffusion and relaxation. *Int. J. Pharm.* **1989**, *57*, 169–172. [CrossRef]
28. Silva, M.E.S.R.; Freitas, R.F.S.; Sousa, R.G. Synthesis, Characterization, and Study of PLGA Copolymer in Vitro Degradation. *J. Biomater. Nanobiotechnol.* **2015**, *6*, 8–19. [CrossRef]
29. Che Man, Y.B.; Ammawath, W.; Mirghani, M.E.S. Determining α-tocopherol in refined bleached and deodorized palm olein by Fourier transform infrared spectroscopy. *Food Chem.* **2005**, *90*, 323–327. [CrossRef]

30. Gyulai, G.; Magyar, A.; Rohonczy, J.; Orosz, J.; Yamasaki, M.; Bosze, S.; Kiss, E. Preparation and characterization of cationic Pluronic for surface modification and functionalization of polymeric drug delivery nanoparticles. *Express Polym. Lett.* **2016**, *10*, 216–226. [CrossRef]
31. Bouchemal, K.; Agnely, F.; Koffi, A.; Ponchel, G. A concise analysis of the effect of temperature and propanediol-1, 2 on Pluronic F127 micellization using isothermal titration microcalorimetry. *J. Colloid Interface Sci.* **2009**, *338*, 169–176. [CrossRef] [PubMed]
32. Ritger, P.L.; Peppas, N.A. A simple equation for description of solute release I. Fickian and non-fickian release from non-swellable devices in the form of slabs, spheres, cylinders or discs. *J. Control. Release* **1987**, *5*, 23–36. [CrossRef]

9

Formulation, Colloidal Characterization and In Vitro Biological Effect of BMP-2 Loaded PLGA Nanoparticles for Bone Regeneration

Teresa del Castillo-Santaella [1], Inmaculada Ortega-Oller [2], Miguel Padial-Molina [2], Francisco O'Valle [3], Pablo Galindo-Moreno [2], Ana Belén Jódar-Reyes [1,4] and José Manuel Peula-García [1,5,*]

1. Biocolloid and Fluid Physics Group, Department of Applied Physics, University of Granada, 18071 Granada, Spain
2. Department of Oral Surgery and Implant Dentistry, University of Granada, 18071 Granada, Spain
3. Department of Pathology, School of Medicine & IBIMER, University of Granada, 18071 Granada, Spain
4. Excellence Research Unit "Modeling Nature" (MNat), University of Granada, 18071 Granada, Spain
5. Department of Applied Physics II, University of Malaga, 29071 Malaga, Spain

* Correspondence: jmpeula@uma.es

Abstract: Nanoparticles (NPs) based on the polymer poly (lactide-co-glycolide) acid (PLGA) have been widely studied in developing delivery systems for drugs and therapeutic biomolecules, due to the biocompatible and biodegradable properties of the PLGA. In this work, a synthesis method for bone morphogenetic protein (BMP-2)-loaded PLGA NPs was developed and optimized, in order to carry out and control the release of BMP-2, based on the double-emulsion (water/oil/water, W/O/W) solvent evaporation technique. The polymeric surfactant Pluronic F68 was used in the synthesis procedure, as it is known to have an effect on the reduction of the size of the NPs, the enhancement of their stability, and the protection of the encapsulated biomolecule. Spherical solid polymeric NPs were synthesized, showing a reproducible multimodal size distribution, with diameters between 100 and 500 nm. This size range appears to allow the protein to act on the cell surface and at the cytoplasm level. The effect of carrying BMP-2 co-adsorbed with bovine serum albumin on the NP surface was analyzed. The colloidal properties of these systems (morphology by SEM, hydrodynamic size, electrophoretic mobility, temporal stability, protein encapsulation, and short-term release profile) were studied. The effect of both BMP2-loaded NPs on the proliferation, migration, and osteogenic differentiation of mesenchymal stromal cells from human alveolar bone (ABSC) was also analyzed in vitro.

Keywords: BMP-2; PLGA nanoparticles; Pluronic F68

---

1. Introduction

In the context of nanomedicine, tissue regeneration using colloidal micro- and nano-structures having unique size and surface activity has received increasing attention over recent years. Many efforts have been made to improve the engineering of these nano-systems in order to reach a "smart" delivery of bioactive molecules in order to optimize their therapeutic advantages and minimize harmful side effects [1]. With this aim, a broad spectrum of biocompatible nanocarriers has been described, showing properties suitable for different biological and therapeutic applications [2]. Among these varied proposals, polymeric nanosystems represent a major group in which poly lactic-co-glycolic acid (PLGA) is one of the most widely used due to its biocompatibility, biodegradability, and low cytotoxicity, gaining the approval from different drug agencies for human use [3,4].

PLGA-based structures are described as micro- and nanocarriers to deliver a wide variety of active molecules and drugs, synthetic or natural molecules with hydrophilic or hydrophobic properties, and biomolecules from proteins to nucleic acids [5–7]. PLGA micro- and nanosystems can be set up using different formulation techniques, with the possibility of a systemic or local distribution. These systems can be applied not only in tissue regeneration but also in very diverse therapies: Anticancer drug delivery, infections, inflammatory diseases, or gene therapy [3]. Despite this great potential, certain applications, especially in protein encapsulation, are hindered by problems, such as an uncontrolled release profile and protein denaturation [8–11].

The water-in oil-in water (W/O/W) double emulsion method is an "emulsion solvent evaporation" technique frequently used to encapsulate hydrophilic molecules as proteins in PLGA NPs [6,12]. The appropriate choice of organic solvents, the use of polymer-surfactant blends, and the addition of stabilizer-protective agents have proved to be key aspects for optimizing the resulting systems [9,11]. Additionally, a surface specific functionalization can be used to improve their versatility, allowing the chemical surface immobilization of different molecules in order to confer targeting or adhesive properties to these nanocarriers [13].

Within tissue engineering, bone regeneration has a broad range of applications, mostly in the field of dentistry, where PLGA is suggested as a reference polymer to formulate NPs with bone-healing uses [14]. The literature describes the delivery of bioactive molecules, normally growth factors, using polymeric microparticles (MPs) and NPs with PLGA as the main component [13]. Among the bone morphogenetic growth factors, BMP-2 (bone morphogenetic protein 2) has been the most frequently cited, with many examples in which encapsulation or surface adsorption enables adequate entrapment efficiency and diverse release patterns [15–19]. For proteins with a very short half-life, such as BMPs, biodegradable PLGA nanosystems provide protection and optimal dosage for an adequate stimulation of cell differentiation [20,21].

Thus, within this scenario, in the present work, we seek to optimize a nano-particulate system in order to carry out and control the release of BMP-2 using as a starting point the synthesis procedure of a lysozyme-loaded NP system, previously described for the encapsulation of that model protein [11]. Also, to encapsulate BMP-2, we prepared a second system in which this protein was co-adsorbed with bovine serum albumin onto the surface of empty NPs. The size and morphology, the protein encapsulation efficiency, the surface characteristics, and the colloidal and temporal stability were studied to complete the physico-chemical characterization of both NP systems.

The release profile of BMP-2 indicates the potential of a PLGA nanocarrier for bone regeneration and depends heavily on the polymer degradation by hydrolysis [22]. However, over the short term, during which the release does not depend on this chemical degradation, proper control of release is necessary in order to modulate other physical processes. Thus, we focused our release experiments on the short-term using different techniques to compare the two NP samples and establish the corresponding BMP-2 release profiles. Finally, the biological activity (cell migration, proliferation, and osteogenic differentiation) was tested in vitro using mesenchymal stromal cells (MSCs) derived from alveolar bone [23].

2. Materials and Methods

2.1. Nanoparticle Synthesis

2.1.1. Formulation

Poly(lactide-co-glycolide) acid (PLGA 50:50) ($[C_2H_2O_2]_x[C_3H_4O_2]_y$), x = 50, y = 50 (Resomer® 503H, (Evonik, Essen, Germany), 32–44 kDa was used as the polymer, and polymeric surfactant Pluronic F68 (Poloxamer 188) (Sigma-Aldrich, St. Louis, MO, USA) as the emulsifier. Their structure, based on a poly(ethylene oxide)-block-poly(propylene oxide)-block-poly(ethylene oxide), is expressed as PEOa-PPOb-PEOa with a = 75 and b = 30. Human recombinant bone morphogenetic protein, rhBMP-2 (Sigma-H4791), was used as therapeutic biomolecule. Water was purified in a Milli-Q

Academic Millipore system. A double-emulsion synthesis method was used following a procedure previously described with slight modifications [11]. In this method, 100 mg of PLGA and 3 mg of deoxycholic acid (DC) were dissolved in a tube containing 1 mL of ethyl acetate (EA) and vortexed. In total, 40 μL of a buffered solution at pH 12.8, with or without rhBMP-2 (200 μg/mL), were added and immediately sonicated (Branson Ultrasonics 450 Analog Sonifier) for 1 min (Duty cycle dial: 20%, Output control dial: 4) with the tube surrounded by ice. This primary W/O emulsion was poured into a plastic tube containing 2 mL of a buffered solution (pH 12) of F68 at 1 mg/mL, and vortexing for 30 s. Then, the tube surrounded by ice was sonicated at the maximum amplitude for the micro tip for 1 min (Output control: 7). This second W/O/W emulsion was poured into a glass containing 10 mL of the buffered F68 solution and kept under magnetic stirring for 2 min. The organic solvent was then rapidly extracted by evaporation under vacuum to a final volume of 8 mL. The resulting empty and BMP-2 encapsulated NP systems were named NP and NP-BMP2, respectively. A detailed scheme of the synthesis procedure, with a yield based on the PLGA component always higher than 85%, is shown in Figure S1 of the Supplementary Materials.

2.1.2. Cleaning and Storage

After the organic solvent evaporation, the sample was centrifuged for 10 min at 20 °C at 12,000 rpm. The supernatant was filtered using Millipore nanofilters, 0.1 μm for measuring the free non-encapsulated protein. The pellet was then resuspended in phosphate buffer (1.15 mM NaH_2PO_4), PB, to a final volume of 4 mL and kept refrigerated at 4 °C. Under these conditions, the systems kept colloidal stability at least for one month.

2.1.3. Protein Loading and Encapsulation Efficiency

The initial protein loading was optimized for the nanoparticle formulation, preserving the final colloidal stability after the evaporation step and taking into account the amounts shown in the literature for this growth factor when encapsulated inside PLGA NPs [24,25]. Thus, we chose 2 μg as the initial total mass of rhBMP-2, which means a relation of $2 \times 10^{-5}\%$ *w/w* (rhBMP-2/PLGA). The amount of encapsulated rhBMP-2 was calculated by measuring the difference between the initial added amount, and the free non-encapsulated protein present in the supernatant after the cleaning step, which was tested by a specific enzyme-linked immuno-sorbent assay following the instructions of the manufacturer (ELISA, kit RAB0028 from Sigma-Aldrich, St. Louis, MO, USA). Then, protein-encapsulation efficiency (EE) was calculated as follows:

$$EE = \frac{M_I - M_F}{M_I} \times 100$$

where M_I is the initial total mass of rhBMP-2, and M_F is the total mass of rhBMP-2 in the aqueous supernatant.

2.1.4. Physical Protein Adsorption

Bovine serum albumin (BSA) and rhBMP-2 were coupled on the empty nanoparticle surface by a physical adsorption method. The appropriate volume of an aqueous protein solution containing 0.5 mg of BSA and 2 μg of rhBMP-2 was mixed with 5 mL of acetate buffer (pH 5) containing empty NPs with 12.5 mg of PLGA. This provided a starting amount of proteins corresponding to 0.04% *w/w* (protein/PLGA), while the mass relation between proteins was 0.4 *w/w* (rhBMP-2/BSA). This solution was incubated at room temperature for 2 h under mechanical stirring. The nanoparticles were separated from the buffer solution by centrifugation, and after the supernatants were filtered (Millipore nanofilters, 0.1 μm), they were qualitatively analyzed by gel electrophoresis while the protein quantification was made by a bicinchoninic acid protein assay (BCA) (Sigma-Aldrich, St. Louis, MO, USA) for BSA and the specific ELISA for rhBMP-2. The nanoparticle pellet was resuspended in phosphate buffer (pH 7.4) and stored at 4 °C. This system was named NP-BSA-BMP2.

2.1.5. Protein Separation by Gel Electrophoresis, SDS-PAGE

The protein-loaded NPs and different supernatants were treated at 90 °C for 10 min in the following buffer: 62.5 mM Tris-HCl (pH 6.8 at 25 °C), 2% (*w*/*v*) sodium dodecyl sulfate (SDS), 10% glycerol, 0.01% (*w*/*v*) bromophenol blue, 40 mM dithiothreitol (DTT). Samples were then separated by size in porous 12% polyacrylamide gel (1D SDS polyacrylamide gel electrophoresis), under the effect of an electric field. The electrophoresis was run under constant voltage (130 V, 45 min) and the gels were stained using a Coomassie Blue solution (0.1% Coomassie Brilliant Blue R-250, 50% methanol and 10% glacial acetic acid) and destained with the same solution lacking the dye.

2.2. Nanoparticle Characterization: Morphology, Size, Concentration, and Electrokinetic Mobility

NPs were imaged by scanning electron microscopy (SEM) with a Zeiss SUPRA 40VP field-emission scanning electron microscope from the Scientific Instrumentation Center of the University of Granada (CIC, UGR).

The hydrodynamic size distribution of the NPs was evaluated by nanoparticle tracking analysis (NTA) with a NanoSight LM10-HS (GB) FT14 (NanoSight, Amesbury, UK) and an sCMOS camera. The particle concentration according to the diameter (size distribution) was calculated as an average of at least three independent size distributions. The total concentration of NPs of each system was determined in order to control the number of particles used in cell experiments. The measurement conditions for all samples were 25 °C, a viscosity of 0.89 cP, a measurement time of 60 s, and a camera gain of 250. The camera shutter was 11 and 15 ms for the empty and BMP-loaded NPs, respectively. The detection threshold was fixed at 5.

The electrophoretic mobility of the NPs was determined using a Zetasizer® NanoZeta ZS device (Malvern Instrument Ltd., Malvern, UK) working at 25 °C with an He-Ne laser of 633 nm, and a 173° scattering angle. Each data point was taken as an average over three independent sample measurements. For each sample, the electrophoretic mobility distribution and the average electrophoretic mobility (μ-average) were determined by the technique of laser Doppler electrophoresis.

2.3. Colloidal and Temporal Stability in Biological Media

The average hydrodynamic diameter and the polydispersity index (PDI) by dynamic light scattering (DLS) of each NP system were measured in different media (phosphate buffer (PB) saline phosphate buffer (PBS), and cell culture medium: Dulbecco's modified Eagle's medium, DMEM (Sigma)). Also, data on temporal stability were gathered by repeating these analyses at different times after synthesis (0, 1, and 5 days) and after 1 month under storage conditions.

In vitro release experiments were conducted as follows: 1 mL of each sample for each incubation time was suspended in PBS at 37 °C. After the corresponding time (24, 48, 96, 168 h), NPs were separated from the supernatant of released proteins by centrifugation for 10 min at 14,000 rpm (10 °C). The NP pellet was suspended in 1 mL of 0.05 M NaOH and stirred for 2 h for a complete polymer degradation. The alkaline protein solution was assayed by BCA and ELISA to quantify the unreleased amount. The protein released was calculated taking into account the total encapsulated amount. All experiments were made in triplicate.

2.4. Cell Interactions

For all biological in vitro studies, a cell population cultured from the maxillary alveolar bone was used. This population was previously characterized and confirmed to present all characteristics of a mesenchymal stromal cell population (MSC) [23]. Cells were taken from healthy human donors after the approval from the Ethics Committee for Human Research from the University of Granada (424/CEIH/2018). Regular Dulbecco's modified Eagle's medium (DMEM) with 1 g/L glucose (DMEM-LG) (Gibco), 10% fetal bovine serum (FBS) (Sigma-Aldrich, St. Louis, MO, USA), 1:100 of non-essential amino acid solution (NEAA) (Gibco), 0.01 μg/mL of basic fibroblast growth factor (bFGF)

(PeproTech, London, UK), 100 U/mL of penicillin/streptomycin, and 0.25 μg/mL of amphotericin B was used as culture medium for all experiments. Cultures were maintained at 37 °C in a 5% CO_2 atmosphere (2000 cells/well). All biological experiments were repeated in triplicate at least 3 times per condition.

2.4.1. Cell Migration

A cell-migration assay was conducted as previously described [26,27]. Briefly, MSCs were distributed on to three wells for each condition and allowed to grow to a cell confluency close to 99%, in 24-wells/plate at 3000 cells/cm^2, and in each well three different scratches were made. Then, cells were starved for 24 h by adding culture medium without serum. A scratch was made using a pipette tip along the diameter of the well. A wash step with PBS was performed to remove the scratched cells. Fresh complete culture media was added and supplemented depending on the assigned group (BMP-2, NP- BMP2, and NP-BSA-BMP2 at 1.25, 2.5, and 5 ng/mL of BMP-2). Afterwards, nine images were taken from the same area in each condition until 48 h later. On these images, the scraped area was measured by ImageJ software (National Institute of Health, Bethesda, MD, USA; http://rsbweb.nih.gov/ij/). The reduction in the scratched area over time was measured considering the area at time 0 as 100% open.

2.4.2. Cell Proliferation

Proliferation was evaluated by a sulphorhodamine (SRB) assay [28]. The assay was conducted by seeding the cells at 1500 cells/cm^2 in a 96-well plate at a confluence not higher than 50%. After cell attachment, the different supplements were added (BMP-2, NP- BMP2, and NP-BSA-BMP2 at 1.25, 2.5, and 5 ng/mL of BMP-2) and the cells were maintained in culture for up to 7 days. At each time point, the cells were washed with 1X PBS and fixed by adding ice-cold 10% trichloroacetic acid for 20 min at 4 °C. Then, the cells were washed 3 times with dH_2O and dried until all time points were collected. Each well received 0.4% SRB in 1% acetic acid for 20 min at room temperature with gentle shaking. The staining was finished by washing each well 3 times with 1% acetic acid and drying it at room temperature for 24 h. The dye was retrieved from the cells by adding 10 mM Tris Base at pH 10.5 and gently shaking for 10 min. The solution recovered was then distributed in a 96-well plate and the optical absorbance was read at 492 nm.

2.4.3. Osteogenic Differentiation

Osteogenic differentiation was evaluated by adding osteogenic media to the cell culture in combination with free BMP-2, NP-BMP2, and NP-BSA-BMP2 at the highest dosages used in previous experiments. Cells were seeded at 3000 cells/cm^2 and cultured to reach an 85% to 90% confluency. This was followed by the addition of induction media containing 10 mM of β-glycerophosphate (Fluka, 50020), 0.1 μM of dexamethasone (Sigma-Aldrich, D2915) and 0.05 mM of L-ascorbic acid (Sigma-Aldrich, A8960). Cell cultures were maintained for 7 days to analyze early activity. At day 7, cells were collected in 1 mL of TRIzol®. Then, RNA was extracted and converted to cDNA. Alkaline phosphatase (ALP) was then evaluated, expression being calculated relative to glyceraldehyde-3-phosphate dehydrogenase protein (GAPDH) by the $2^{-\Delta\Delta Ct}$ method. These procedures were conducted as described elsewhere [23]. Forward and reverse primer sequences were AGCTCATTTCCTGGTATGACAAC and TTACTCCTTGGAGGCCATGTG for GAPDH, and TCCAGGGATAAAGCAGGTCTTG and CTTTCTCTTTCTCTGGCACTAAGG for ALP.

2.4.4. Statistical Evaluation

Cell migration and proliferation were evaluated by ANOVA followed by Tukey multiple comparisons test for pairwise analysis. Comparison between the levels of ALP at 4 vs. 7 days were analyzed by paired Student's t test. In all cases, a p value lower than 0.05 was established as statistical significance.

3. Results and Discussion

3.1. Nanoparticle Formulation

Double emulsion-solvent evaporation has been described as a robust and frequently used method to produce biomolecule-loaded PLGA NPs [6,12,13,29]. A formulation previously optimized by our group enabled the preservation of the biological activity of encapsulated biomolecules using a slightly aggressive organic solvent. Moreover, deoxycholic acid has been used in the first step of the formulation in order to improve the colloidal stability of NPs and, simultaneously, to obtain NP surfaces enriched with carboxylic groups, improving their versatility and allowing a subsequent chemical immobilization of different specific ligands [30]. By means of this improved formulation, in the present work, we developed empty nanoparticles (NPs) or nanoparticles encapsulating rhBMP-2 (NP-BMP2). A schematic description of the synthesis procedure is shown in Figure S1 of the Supplementary Data. For NP-BMP2, we achieved a protein-encapsulation efficiency (EE) of 97 ± 2%. This result is consistent with the literature in which several authors have reported similarly high values encapsulating this protein inside PLGA nano- and microparticles [31,32]. Our formulation has several factors leading to this very high EE value: The low protein/polymer relation in mass [33], the affinity of rhBMP-2 to an unspecific interaction with hydrophobic surfaces [31], or the addition of stabilizers (poloxamer) in the second step of the double-emulsion procedure [13]. The absence of rhBMP-2 in the supernatant resulting from the centrifugation step in the cleaning process was verified by ELISA and SDS-PAGE, in which a clear band corresponding to 14 kD of rhBMP-2 polypeptidic chains is shown for lane A in Figure 1, corresponding to NP-BMP2. The mass of protein encapsulated, around 2 μg, is similar to that of different PLGA micro- and nanosystems described in the literature [18,34,35]. Taking into account the storage conditions for our samples, this corresponds to 500 ng/mL, which represents a sufficient concentration for practical applications since this growth factor shows in vitro biological activities at very low dosages (5–20 ng/mL) [13].

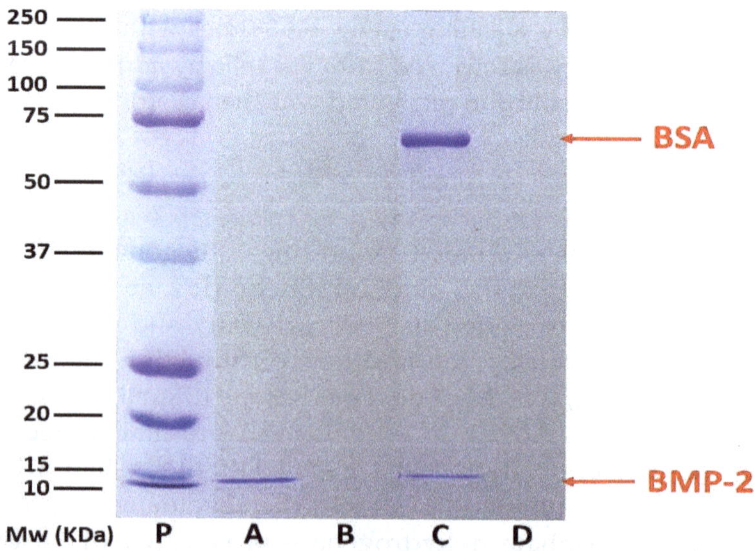

Figure 1. SDS polyacrylamide gel electrophoresis (SDS-PAGE) analysis under reducing conditions of solid PLGA Nanoparticles (PLGA NPs) and liquid (supernatant) fractions of different NP systems. Lane **P**: Protein standards; lane **A**: NP-BMP2 (bone morphogenetic protein); lane **B**: supernatant of NP-BMP2 after synthesis and encapsulation of rhBMP-2; lane **C**: NP after physical adsorption of BSA/rhBMP-2; lane **D**: supernatant after physical adsorption of BSA(bovine serum albumin)/rhBMP-2 on NP system.

On the other hand, a second nanosystem resulted, modifying the way in which rhBMP-2 is incorporated in the nanocarrier. There are several examples of surface adsorption of different growth factors in micro- and nanoparticles [35–37], and surface immobilization over the encapsulation has recently been proposed as a way to modulate the later release of biomolecules. This process, which depends on the slow diffusion of biomolecules through the polymeric matrix, is consequently highly influenced by the protein–polymer interaction [38,39] and polymer degradation [3,6]. Thus, this new focus on the use of PLGA NPs for biomolecule delivery was explored by immobilizing the protein rhBMP-2 on the surface of empty NPs by means of simple physical adsorption. This process is known to be governed by electrostatic and hydrophobic interactions between protein molecules and NP surfaces [40].

For this, the surface-charged groups, the hydrophilicity, the net charge of the protein molecules, and the characteristics of the adsorption medium are the reference parameters. Thus, we designed a co-adsorption experiment in which a mixture of rhBMP-2 and BSA (0.4% *w/w*, rhBMP-2/BSA) interact simultaneously with the PLGA NP surface. Albumins are routinely used as protective proteins when growth factors are incorporated in PLGA NPs [13,19]. Moreover, a surface distribution of BSA molecules can improve the colloidal stability of NPs at physiological pH due to their net negative charge under these conditions [41]. Figure S2 from Supplementary Materials shows a scheme of the co-adsorption process. The adsorption efficiency is higher than 95% and in SDS-PAGE from Figure 1, two bands characteristic of both proteins can be seen in lane C, corresponding to the NP-BSA-BMP2 nanosystem. However, lane D, corresponding to the run of the supernatant from the centrifugation of the nanosystem after adsorption processes, shows the absence of any protein. This result is fully explained by taking into account the pH of the medium (pH 5.0), near the isoelectric point of BSA, where the adsorption of this protein onto negatively charged nanoparticles presents a maximum [40,42]. The immobilization of rhBMP-2 on the negatively charged surface of NPs proves they are electrostatically favored due to the positive net charge of this protein at acid and neutral pH.

3.2. Nanoparticle Characterization

3.2.1. Nanoparticle Size

SEM and STEM micrographs (Figure 2) show that the samples consist of spherical particles of different diameters (between 150 and 450 nm), a range similar to that found in a previous work in which NPs were loaded with lysozyme following a similar synthesis protocol [11]. In that work, the DLS technique failed to provide a reliable size distribution. Therefore, the NTA technique was directly used to determine the hydrodynamic size of the BMP2-loaded NPs (see NTA video in the Supplementary Material).

The size distributions for empty (NP) and BMP-loaded NPs (NP-BMP2) from NTA (Figure 3 and videos S1, S2) were consistent with the SEM images. Particles with diameters between 100 and 500 nm were found to have the highest particle concentration at around 200 nm. The loading with BMP had an effect on the size distribution, leading to more defined peaks. These measurements enabled us to determine the concentration of particles in the measured sample: $6.88 \pm 0.09 \times 10^8$ pp/mL and $5.19 \pm 0.12 \times 10^8$ pp/mL for NP and NP-BMP2 nanosystems, respectively. These values were used (by taking into account the corresponding dilution) to control the number of particles added in the cell experiments.

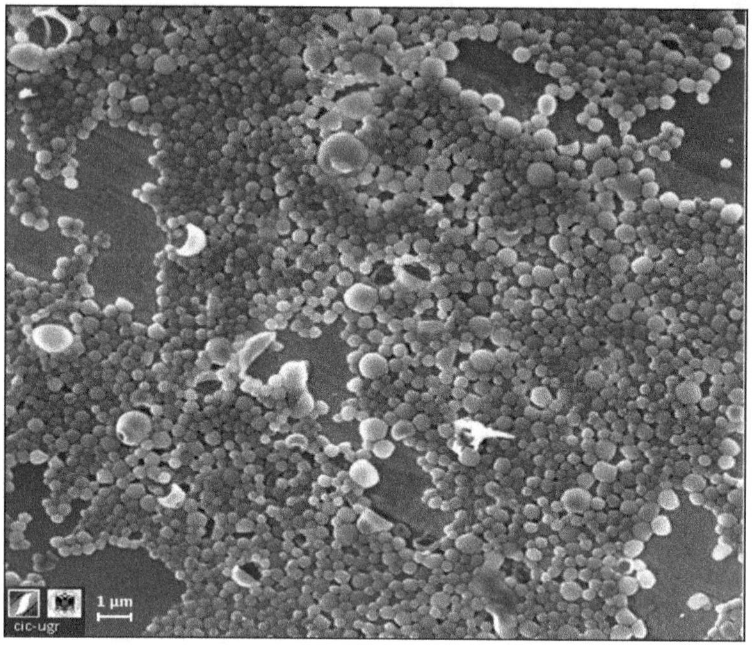

Figure 2. Scanning electron microscopy (SEM) micrograph of rhBMP-2-loaded nanoparticles (NP-BMP2).

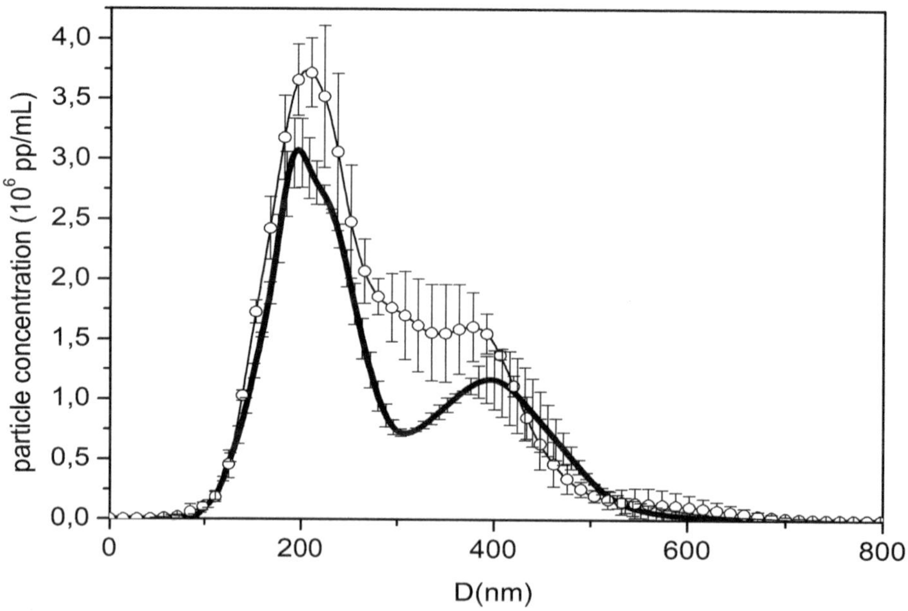

Figure 3. Hydrodynamic diameter distribution of NP (circles) and NP-BMP2 (thick black line) measured at pH 7.0 (phosphate buffer) by nanoparticle tracking analysis (NTA).

3.2.2. Electrokinetic Mobility and Colloidal Stability

The surface charge of nanoparticles can be analyzed using an electrokinetic study by measuring the electrophoretic mobility (μ_e) under different conditions. Figure 4 shows the μ_e and zeta potential values for the three nanosystems: NP, NP-BMP2, and NP-BSA-BMP2, at low ionic strength and different pH values. The electric surface charge of NPs resides in the carboxylic groups of the uncapped PLGA and deoxycholic acid molecules. These functionalized groups are additionally useful due to the possibility of a chemical surface vectorization in order to develop directed delivery nanocarriers [43]. It was previously confirmed that protonation of these acidic surface groups at pH values under their pKa value was tightly correlated with a loss of surface charge and consequently a reduction (in absolute value) of the electrophoretic mobility of the colloidal system [44,45]. Usually, when colloidal particles are coated by protein molecules, the μ_e values change markedly compared with the same bare surfaces and are influenced by the electrical charge of the adsorbed protein molecules [46,47]. The electrokinetic behavior of the NP-BMP2 system remains similar to that of NP, and encapsulation of rhBMP-2 does not affect the surface charge distribution. A similar result was reported by d'Angelo et al. on encapsulating different growth factors in PLGA-poloxamer blend nanoparticles in the same proportion *w/w* of protein/polymer [24]. This may be due to the low amount of encapsulated protein and its distribution in the inner part of the NPs (far from the surface). In our system, this internal distribution may be favored by the encapsulating conditions where the basic pH (pH 12.0) of the water phase containing rhBMP-2 allows a negative charge of these protein molecules, thereby preventing their electrostatic specific interaction with acidic groups of the NPs.

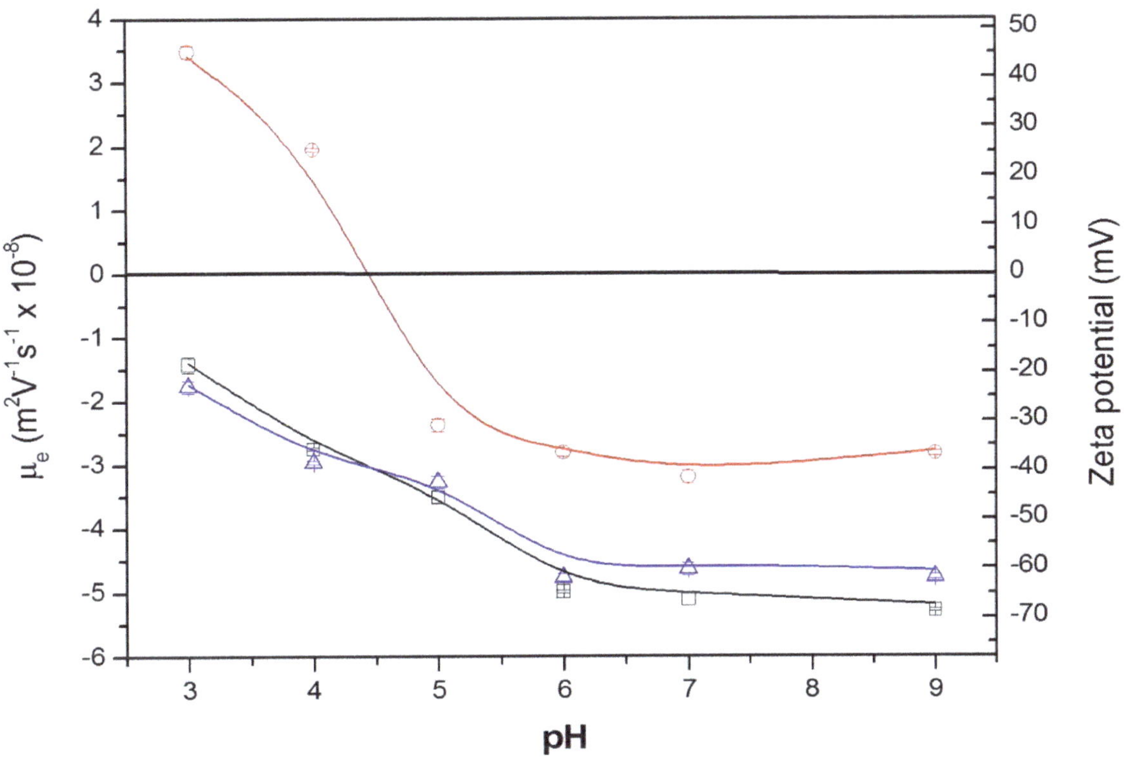

Figure 4. Electrophoretic mobility and zeta potential vs. pH in buffered media of low salinity (ionic strength equal to 0.002 M) for the different nanosystems: (black square) NP; (blue triangle) NP-BMP2; (red circle) NP-BSA-BMP2.

The electrokinetic distribution for the NP-BSA-BMP2 system radically changes. As previously shown, the very high adsorption efficiency leads to NPs with both proteins adsorbed around their surface. This situation is closely correlated with the μ_e values from Figure 4. Taking into account the *w/w* relation between adsorbed proteins (250 times higher for BSA), albumin molecules modulate the behavior at pH values below their isoelectric point (pI 4.7), where the positive net charge of BSA masks the original surface charge of NPs and even changes their original values to positive ones. This is a typical result found for this protein-covering colloidal particles [42,48]. At neutral and basic pH values, BSA molecules have a negative net charge, and the slight decrease in the absolute μ_e values could be due to the reduction of the negative net surface charge of NPs, which may be shielded, at least in a small part, by the positive charge of rhBMP-2 molecules under their basic isoelectric point (pI 9.0).

The colloidal stability for the different nanosystems (NP, NP-BMP2, and NP-BSA-BMP2) was determined by analyzing the size distributions in various media (PB, PBS, and DMEM) at different times after synthesis (0, 1, and 5 days). Size distributions similar to the original ones were found for the two formulations, NP and NP-BMP2, in all the media analyzed. This result was similar to that previously found for these types of NPs encapsulating lysozyme [11], in which the combination of electrostatic and steric interactions generated by surface chemical groups of NPs confer the stability mechanism that prevents colloidal aggregation [33]. The decrease of the absolute value of the zeta potential for the NP-BSA-BMP2 system as a consequence of surface protein distribution does not affect its colloidal stability. This system also maintains the same size distribution in the different media. It is commonly accepted that a zeta potential higher than +30 or −30 mV will give rise to a stable colloidal system [49] and the zeta potential value for NP-BSA-BMP2 is above −30 mV. Colloidal stability in PBS and DMEM, typically used media for the development of scaffold or cell interactions, respectively, assures the potential use of these nanosystems for in vitro or in vivo living environments. Additionally, these systems maintained their size under storage in PB, at 4 °C for at least 1 month (data not shown), showing this to be an adequate medium for sample storage.

3.2.3. Protein Release

One of the main problems for micro- or nanosystems of PLGA drug delivery is to find the appropriate release pattern for encapsulated/attached protein molecules. A wide spectrum of formulations modulates this property by the use of different types of synthesis processes, PLGA polymers, co-polymers, and stabilizers [3,13]. An adequate limitation and control in the burst release is critical for BMPs in order to ensure long-term continuous release that, favored by the polymer degradation, provides better in vivo action in driving bone and cartilage regeneration [20]. Therefore, we previously developed a dual PLGA nanosystem for controlled short-term release, where protein diffusion and protein–polymer interaction are the main factors governing this process [11].

In the present work, NP-BMP2 and NP-BSA-BMP2 nanosystems represent two different ways in which rhBMP-2 was incorporated into the nanocarrier. Figure 5A shows the cumulative release of both proteins, rhBMP-2 and BSA, for different systems as a function of time in a short-term period (7 days). The encapsulated rhBMP-2 protein reaches an amount released of around 30% of the initial encapsulated one while adsorbed rhBMP-2, despite its surface distribution, is three times lower. However, BSA shows released amounts up to 80% of the initial adsorbed ones. In all cases, error bars correspond to the standard deviations from three independent experiments. Under these conditions, the growth factor encapsulated in NP-BMP2 presents a release pattern similar to that previously found with the same formulation but using lysozyme as the protein [11]. Poloxamer in the water phase of the synthesis process can be key in modulating both specific and unspecific interfacial protein interactions [50]. Thus, the relation between protein–polymer interaction and protein diffusion appears to be well balanced, preventing an excessive initial burst and simultaneously maintaining the needed protein flux to release around a third of the encapsulated rhBMP-2 in 7 days. Although an excessive initial burst has been widely reported for PLGA NPs related with protein molecules close to the surface [6], this situation did not appear for the NP-BMP2 system, this being consistent with the electrokinetic behavior that did not show the presence of protein near surface. The literature offers some examples with reduced short-term release of BMP-2 using more hydrophilic PLGA-PEG co-polymers [16] or a different synthesis process [25].

The release performance for the NP-BSA-BMP2 system, also shown in Figure 5A, presents notable differences. The electrokinetic profile has previously justified the surface location of BSA and rhBMP-2 on the surface, which could lead to a fast release of both proteins. However, results from Figure 5A,B show this trend only for the BSA protein that is released from NPs, with about 20% of the initial amount remaining after seven days. However, up to 90% of the initial load of rhBMP-2 protein, unlike BSA, remains attached to the surface. The NP surface with hydrophilic groups form poloxamer molecules and a negative charge due to the abundant presence of carboxylic groups (end-groups of PLGA and deoxycholic acid molecules) favor a desorption process for BSA, whose molecules have a negative charge under release conditions (physiological pH). This agrees with the results of other authors who, even after encapsulating BSA in PLGA-poloxamer blend NPs, achieved a fast burst release of above

40% to 50% of the initial protein amount [33]. Moreover, the co-encapsulation of albumins with growth factors could strongly affect its release profile, causing an initial burst [21,24]. Otherwise, the specific electrostatic attraction between positive rhBMP-2 molecules and negative surface groups slows down the short time release of this protein. This result is in agreement with the low release of adsorbed BMP previously found using PLGA micro- and nanoparticles with uncapped acid end groups [38,51]. Thus, the combination of different methods for trapping BMP-2 into and around NPs shows up the possibility of attaining a properly controlled release, balancing the interactions between polymers, stabilizers, and protein.

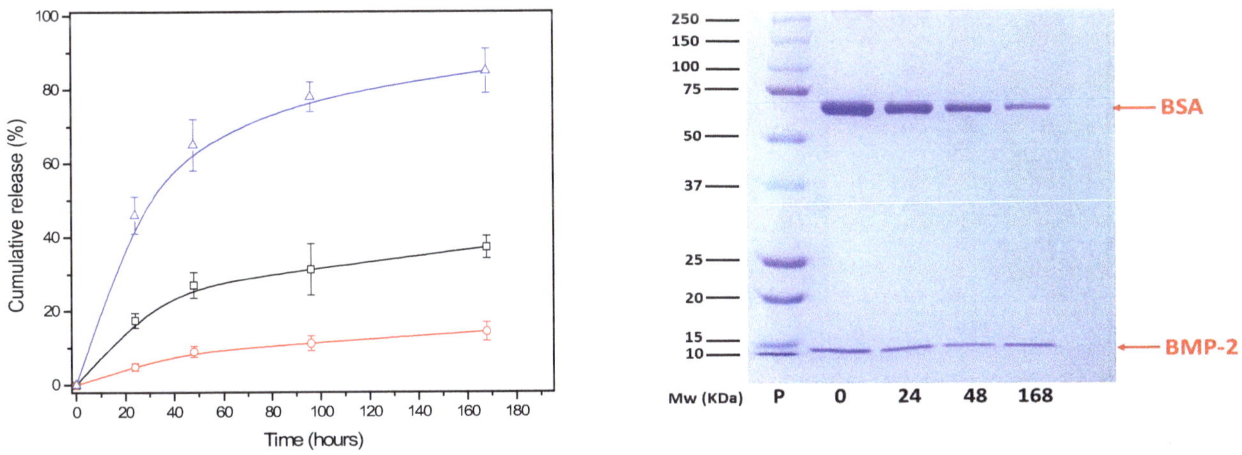

(A) (B)

Figure 5. (**A**) Cumulative release of rhBMP-2 for NP-BMP2 (black square) and NP-BSA-BMP2 (red circle) systems; and cumulative release of BSA for NP-BSA-BMP2 (blue triangle) system, incubated for different times at 37 °C in saline phosphate buffer (pH 7.4). (**B**) SDS-PAGE analysis under reducing conditions of solid fraction of NP-BSA-BMP2 after release at different times where the number of each lane corresponds to the time in hours.

3.3. Biological Activity and Interactions

3.3.1. Cell Migration

Cell migration is the first and necessary step in tissue regeneration [52]. Thus, a regenerative agent must accelerate cell migration or, at least, not interfere with it. In the present study, we found no differences between the groups, doses, and control in terms of closure of a scratched area (ANOVA with Tukey multiple comparisons test) (Figure 6). In contrast to our findings, previously published data suggests a positive effect of BMP-2 on cell migration [53,54]. However, in those studies, the doses applied, and the cell types were different than in the current experiments. We used lower doses of BMP-2 in order to test whether, even at low dosages, BMP-2 could still provide benefits if protected in a nanoparticle system. As mentioned, we demonstrated no negative effect of the system on cell migration. Our results nonetheless support the idea that BMP-2 activity is mediated by the activation of the phosphoinositide 3-kinase (PI3K) pathway, a common group of signaling molecules that participate in several process with BMP-2 and other molecules [26,54]. It should also be mentioned that the timeframe of a migration assay is short. Thus, the potential advantages of a controlled-release system as the one under study might be limited. That is, the release of BMP-2 from the nanoparticles, as demonstrated in Figure 5, is limited to the first 48 h. Thus, a sustained positive effect on migration activity over time could be hypothesized.

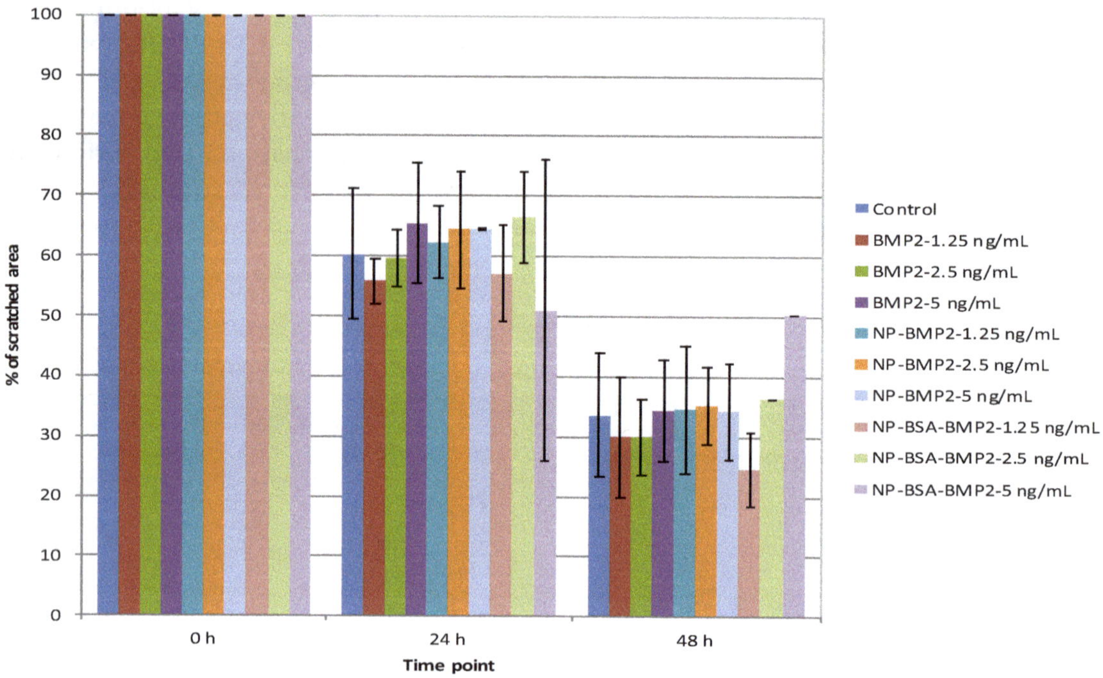

Figure 6. Migration assay. Percentage of scratched area closure at 24 and 48 h on different groups and doses.

3.3.2. Cell Proliferation

Proliferation is another of the cell activities required for tissue regeneration. However, this property must be balanced with both migration and differentiation, and not all three characteristics increase at the same time and with the same ratios [55]. In fact, reportedly, when a dose of BMP-2 induces higher proliferation, it decreases differentiation [56]. This property has been extensively analyzed but discrepancies can still be detected in the literature. Therefore, Kim et al. analyzed different doses of BMP-2 and its effect on cell proliferation and apoptosis. It was confirmed in vitro that high doses, but still lower than those used clinically, reduce cell proliferation and increase apoptosis [57]. This should be avoided. We have found that although free BMP-2 does not induce higher proliferation than the control at any of the doses applied nor time points (ANOVA with Tukey multiple comparisons test), the same amount of BMP-2 encapsulated or adsorbed onto PLGA nanoparticles boosts proliferation, this being statistically significant when using a dose of 2.5 ng/mL or higher (ANOVA with Tukey multiple comparisons test) (Figure 7). These dosages are still lower than those suggested in previous studies. Apart from that difference, a positive effect on proliferation was still achieved. Moreover, following the release pattern from Figure 5, more BMP-2 is expected to be released over time beyond the 7-day time frame. Thus, a sustained induction effect could be expected as well until full confluency of the cell culture.

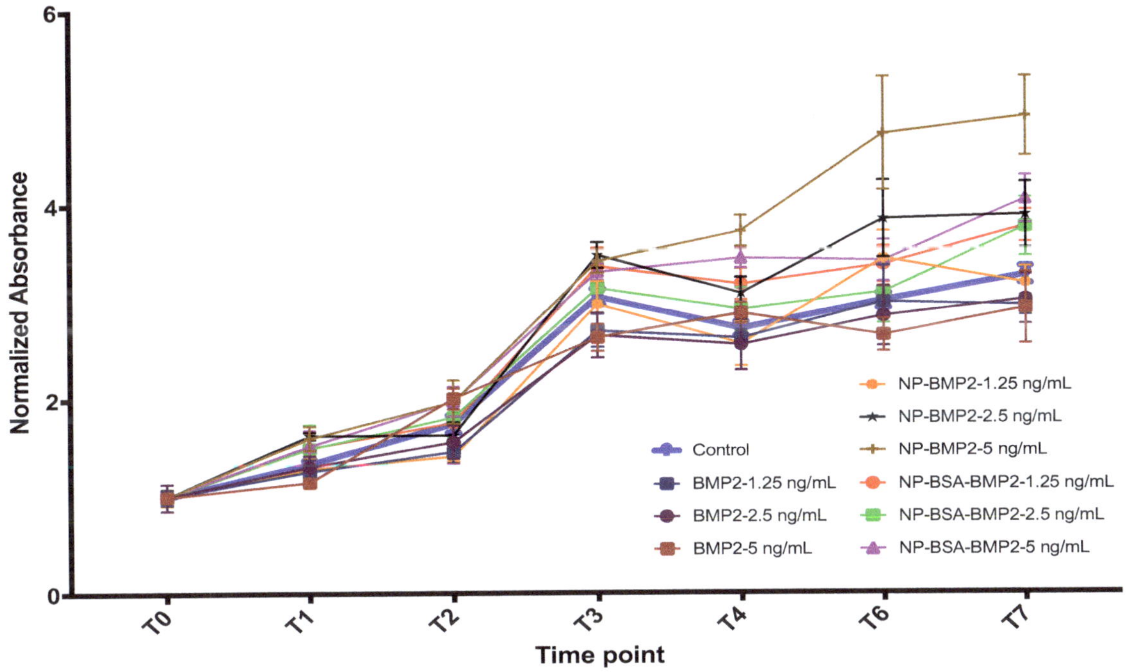

Figure 7. Proliferation of human mesenchymal stromal cells (MSCs) as measured by sulphorhodamine (SRB) absorbance. Results were normalized to T0 in each group.

3.3.3. Osteogenic Differentiation

It has been confirmed that cell differentiation induced by BMP-2 needs the presence of permissive osteoinductive components. Particularly, β-glycerophosphate has been shown to exert a synergistic effect with BMP-2 in inducing cell differentiation [56]. Thus, to test for osteogenic differentiation, we analyzed the expression of ALP mRNA. Maximum ALP activity was found to occur 10 days after stimulation with PLGA-based microparticles containing BMP-2 in co-encapsulation with human serum albumin [16]. Although other tests could have been used to reinforce our findings, ALP is known to modulate the deposition of mineralized nodules, thus indicating osteoblastic activity. For all of this, we supplemented the differentiation media with β-glycerophosphate and either free BMP-2, NP-BMP2, or NP-BSA-BMP2 for 4 and 7 days so that we could capture the early dynamics of the expression of the gene. In our study, we identified an increase in the expression of ALP in all groups from day 4 to day 7 (Figure 8). Although ALP at day 7 in the BMP-2 group appears to be higher than for the other two groups, the change did not prove significant. In fact, differences between groups were not statistically significant within any time period. Noteworthy though, the increase was not significant within the BMP-2 group ($p = 0.141$, Student's t test), but it was significant within the other two groups ($p = 0.025$ and $p = 0.003$; NP-BMP2 and NP-BSA-BMP2 groups, respectively). This, again, could be taken as a confirmation of the sustained release of the protein from the nanoparticle system beyond the earlier time points.

This and both the migration and proliferation studies described below lead us to confirm that the system proposed can maintain a proper release of BMP-2 over time, sustaining a positive effect on cell migration and proliferation with initial reduced doses of BMP-2. The fact that the excessive initial burst is prevented is important for the application of this nanotechnology in bone regeneration, as in dentistry. In this way, the negative effects of initial high doses of BMP-2 are avoided at the same time as the molecule is protected from denaturalization inside the NP. Thus, the regenerator effects are maintained over time.

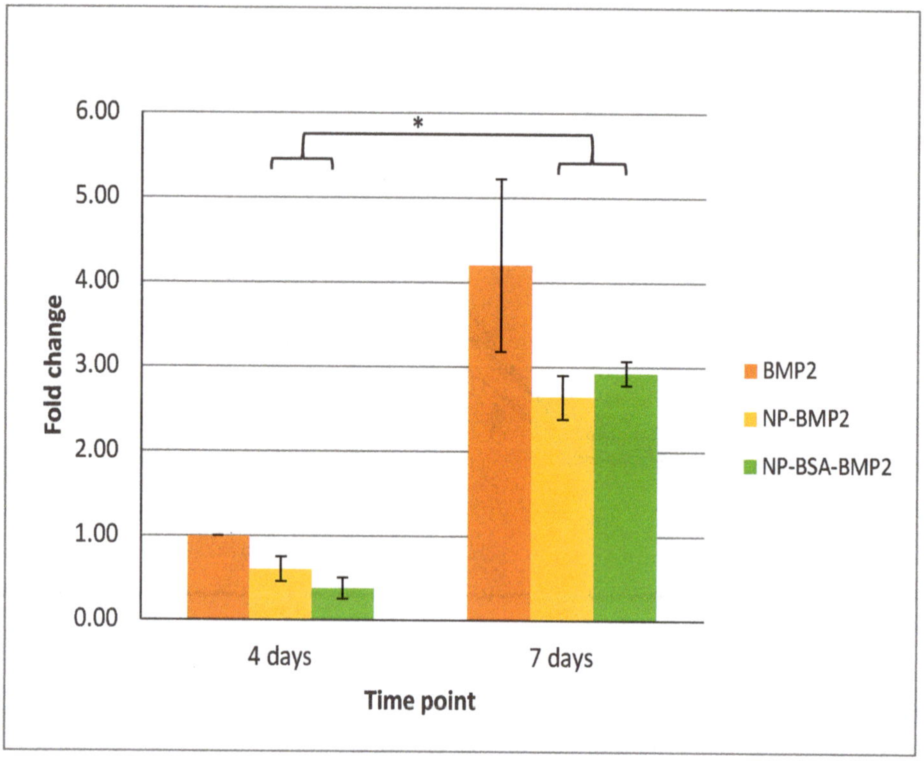

Figure 8. Relative fold change in the expression of ALP mRNA (control group: BMP2 at 4 days). * = Statistical significance of the comparison over time ($p = 0.025$ and $p = 0.003$, Student's t test; NP-BMP2 and NP-BSA-BMP2 groups).

4. Conclusions

In this work, a delivery PLGA-nanosystem previously developed for model proteins was chosen as the reference system to carry and deliver the growth factor BMP-2. This NP system, with a dual size distribution, was developed following a double-emulsion formulation in which the process and the components used were optimized to reach the appropriate colloidal and biological behavior. Encapsulation and adsorption are two different processes to load BMP-2 in PLGA NPs. Both were tested to elucidate the factors controlling them and their influence in the physico-chemical and biological properties of nanosystems. We verified that protein–polymer specific interactions have a major role in the way that protein molecules are carried and delivered from NPs. In vitro experiments showed that BMP-2-loaded PLGA NPs are the nanocarriers with the best release profile over the short-term without an initial burst and with moderate and sustained release of active protein before the onset of polymer degradation. Therefore, the biological activity is positive with no negative interaction with migration or proliferation but rather the induction of cell differentiation through the expression of ALP.

Author Contributions: Conceptualization, J.M.P.-G. and P.G.-M.; methodology, J.M.P.-G., A.B.J.-R. and M.P.-M.; investigation, T.d.C.-S., I.O.-O., J.M.P.-G., A.B.J.-R. and M.P.-M.; resources, A.B.J.-R., P.G.-M., F.O.-R.; writing—original draft preparation, J.M.P.-G. and M.P.-M.; writing—review and editing, J.M.P.-G., M.P.-M., A.B.J.-R., T.d.C.-S.; supervision, J.M.P.-G., P.G.-M. and F.O.-R.; funding acquisition, A.B.J.-R. and P.G.-M.

Acknowledgments: The authors wish to express their appreciation for the technical support to D. Darío Abril-García.

References

1. Van Rijt, S.; Habibovic, P. Enhancing regenerative approaches with nanoparticles. *J. R. Soc. Interface* **2017**, *14*. [CrossRef]
2. Kumar, B.; Jalodia, K.; Kumar, P.; Gautam, H.K. Recent advances in nanoparticle-mediated drug delivery. *J. Drug Deliv. Sci. Technol.* **2017**, *41*, 260–268. [CrossRef]

3. Mir, M.; Ahmed, N.; Rehman, A.U.R. Recent applications of PLGA based nanostructures in drug delivery. *Colloids Surf. B Biointerfaces* **2017**, *159*, 217–231. [CrossRef] [PubMed]
4. Jana, S.; Jana, S. Natural polymeric biodegradable nanoblend for macromolecules delivery. In *Recent Developments in Polymer Macro, Micro and Nano Blends*; Woodhead Publishing: Cambridge, UK, 2017; pp. 289–312. ISBN 9780081004081.
5. Danhier, F.; Ansorena, E.; Silva, J.M.; Coco, R.; Le Breton, A.; Préat, V. PLGA-based nanoparticles: An overview of biomedical applications. *J. Control. Release* **2012**, *161*, 505–522. [CrossRef] [PubMed]
6. Ding, D.; Zhu, Q. Recent advances of PLGA micro/nanoparticles for the delivery of biomacromolecular therapeutics. *Mater. Sci. Eng. C* **2018**, *92*, 1041–1060. [CrossRef] [PubMed]
7. Arias, J.L.; Unciti-Broceta, J.D.; Maceira, J.; del Castillo, T.; Hernández-Quero, J.; Magez, S.; Soriano, M.; García-Salcedo, J.A. Nanobody conjugated PLGA nanoparticles for active targeting of African Trypanosomiasis. *J. Control. Release* **2015**, *197*, 190–198. [CrossRef]
8. Giteau, A.; Venier-Julienne, M.C.; Aubert-Pouëssel, A.; Benoit, J.P. How to achieve sustained and complete protein release from PLGA-based microparticles? *Int. J. Pharm.* **2008**, *350*, 14–26. [CrossRef]
9. Fredenberg, S.; Wahlgren, M.; Reslow, M.; Axelsson, A. The mechanisms of drug release in poly(lactic-co-glycolic acid)-based drug delivery systems—A review. *Int. J. Pharm.* **2011**, *415*, 34–52. [CrossRef]
10. White, L.J.; Kirby, G.T.S.; Cox, H.C.; Qodratnama, R.; Qutachi, O.; Rose, F.R.A.J.; Shakesheff, K.M. Accelerating protein release from microparticles for regenerative medicine applications. *Mater. Sci. Eng. C* **2013**, *33*, 2578–2583. [CrossRef]
11. Ortega-Oller, I.; del Castillo-Santaella, T.; Padial-Molina, M.; Galindo-Moreno, P.; Jódar-Reyes, A.B.; Peula-García, J.M. Dual delivery nanosystem for biomolecules. Formulation, characterization, and in vitro release. *Colloids Surf. B Biointerfaces* **2017**, *159*, 586–595. [CrossRef]
12. McClements, D.J. Encapsulation, protection, and delivery of bioactive proteins and peptides using nanoparticle and microparticle systems: A review. *Adv. Colloid Interface Sci.* **2018**, *253*, 1–22. [CrossRef]
13. Ortega-Oller, I.; Padial-Molina, M.; Galindo-Moreno, P.; O'Valle, F.; Jódar-Reyes, A.B.; Peula-García, J.M. Bone Regeneration from PLGA Micro-Nanoparticles. *BioMed Res. Int.* **2015**, *2015*, 1–18. [CrossRef] [PubMed]
14. Bapat, R.A.; Joshi, C.P.; Bapat, P.; Chaubal, T.V.; Pandurangappa, R.; Jnanendrappa, N.; Gorain, B.; Khurana, S.; Kesharwani, P. The use of nanoparticles as biomaterials in dentistry. *Drug Discov. Today* **2019**, *24*, 85–98. [CrossRef]
15. Ji, Y.; Xu, G.P.; Zhang, Z.P.; Xia, J.J.; Yan, J.L.; Pan, S.H. BMP-2/PLGA delayed-release microspheres composite graft, selection of bone particulate diameters, and prevention of aseptic inflammation for bone tissue engineering. *Ann. BioMed. Eng.* **2010**, *38*, 632–639. [CrossRef] [PubMed]
16. Kirby, G.T.S.; White, L.J.; Rahman, C.V.; Cox, H.C.; Qutachi, O.; Rose, F.R.A.J.; Hutmacher, D.W.; Shakesheff, K.M.; Woodruff, M.A. PLGA-Based Microparticles for the Sustained Release of BMP-2. *Polymers* **2011**, *3*, 571–586. [CrossRef]
17. Qutachi, O.; Shakesheff, K.M.; Buttery, L.D.K. Delivery of definable number of drug or growth factor loaded poly(dl-lactic acid-co-glycolic acid) microparticles within human embryonic stem cell derived aggregates. *J. Control. Release* **2013**, *168*, 18–27. [CrossRef] [PubMed]
18. Wang, Y.; Wei, Y.; Zhang, X.; Xu, M.; Liu, F.; Ma, Q.; Cai, Q.; Deng, X. PLGA/PDLLA core-shell submicron spheres sequential release system: Preparation, characterization and promotion of bone regeneration in vitro and in vivo. *Chem. Eng. J.* **2015**, *273*, 490–501. [CrossRef]
19. Zhang, H.-X.; Zhang, X.-P.; Xiao, G.-Y.; Hou, -Y.; Cheng, L.; Si, M.; Wang, S.-S.; Li, Y.-H.; Nie, L. In vitro and in vivo evaluation of calcium phosphate composite scaffolds containing BMP-VEGF loaded PLGA microspheres for the treatment of avascular necrosis of the femoral head. *Mater. Sci. Eng. C* **2016**, *60*, 298–307. [CrossRef]
20. Begam, H.; Nandi, S.K.; Kundu, B.; Chanda, A. Strategies for delivering bone morphogenetic protein for bone healing. *Mater. Sci. Eng. C* **2017**, *70*, 856–869. [CrossRef]
21. Balmayor, E.R.; Feichtinger, G.A.; Azevedo, H.S.; Van Griensven, M.; Reis, R.L. Starch-poly-ε-caprolactone microparticles reduce the needed amount of BMP-2. *Clin. Orthop. Relat. Res.* **2009**, *467*, 3138–3148. [CrossRef]
22. Xu, Y.; Kim, C.S.; Saylor, D.M.; Koo, D. Polymer degradation and drug delivery in PLGA-based drug–polymer applications: A review of experiments and theories. *J. BioMed. Mater. Res. Part B Appl. Biomater.* **2017**, *105*, 1692–1716. [CrossRef] [PubMed]

23. Padial-Molina, M.; de Buitrago, J.G.; Sainz-Urruela, R.; Abril-Garcia, D.; Anderson, P.; O'Valle, F.; Galindo-Moreno, P. Expression of Musashi-1 during osteogenic differentiation of oral MSC: An in vitro study. *Int. J. Mol. Sci.* **2019**, *20*, 2171. [CrossRef] [PubMed]
24. D'Angelo, I.; Garcia-Fuentes, M.; Parajó, Y.; Welle, A.; Vántus, T.; Horváth, A.; Bökönyi, G.; Kéri, G.; Alonso, M.J. Nanoparticles based on PLGA:poloxamer blends for the delivery of proangiogenic growth factors. *Mol. Pharm.* **2010**, *7*, 1724–1733. [CrossRef] [PubMed]
25. Chang, H.-C.; Yang, C.; Feng, F.; Lin, F.-H.; Wang, C.-H.; Chang, P.-C. Bone morphogenetic protein-2 loaded poly(D,L-lactide-co-glycolide) microspheres enhance osteogenic potential of gelatin/hydroxyapatite/β-tricalcium phosphate cryogel composite for alveolar ridge augmentation. *J. Formos. Med. Assoc.* **2017**, *116*, 973–981. [CrossRef] [PubMed]
26. Padial-Molina, M.; Volk, S.L.; Rios, H.F. Periostin increases migration and proliferation of human periodontal ligament fibroblasts challenged by tumor necrosis factor -α and Porphyromonas gingivalis lipopolysaccharides. *J. Periodontal Res.* **2014**, *49*, 405–414. [CrossRef] [PubMed]
27. Liang, C.-C.; Park, A.Y.; Guan, J.-L. In vitro scratch assay: A convenient and inexpensive method for analysis of cell migration in vitro. *Nat. Protoc.* **2007**, *2*, 329–333. [CrossRef]
28. Houghton, P.; Fang, R.; Techatanawat, I.; Steventon, G.; Hylands, P.J.; Lee, C.C. The sulphorhodamine (SRB) assay and other approaches to testing plant extracts and derived compounds for activities related to reputed anticancer activity. *Methods* **2007**, *42*, 377–387. [CrossRef]
29. Iqbal, M.; Zafar, N.; Fessi, H.; Elaissari, A. Double emulsion solvent evaporation techniques used for drug encapsulation. *Int. J. Pharm.* **2015**, *496*, 173–190. [CrossRef]
30. Sánchez-Moreno, P.; Ortega-Vinuesa, J.L.; Boulaiz, H.; Marchal, J.A.; Peula-García, J.M. Synthesis and characterization of lipid immuno-nanocapsules for directed drug delivery: Selective antitumor activity against HER2 positive breast-cancer cells. *Biomacromolecules* **2013**, *14*, 4248–4259. [CrossRef]
31. Lochmann, A.; Nitzsche, H.; von Einem, S.; Schwarz, E.; Mäder, K. The influence of covalently linked and free polyethylene glycol on the structural and release properties of rhBMP-2 loaded microspheres. *J. Control. Release* **2010**, *147*, 92–100. [CrossRef]
32. Kempen, D.H.R.; Lu, L.; Hefferan, T.E.; Creemers, L.B.; Maran, A.; Classic, K.L.; Dhert, W.J.A.; Yaszemski, M.J. Retention of in vitro and in vivo BMP-2 bioactivities in sustained delivery vehicles for bone tissue engineering. *Biomaterials* **2008**, *29*, 3245–3252. [CrossRef]
33. Santander-Ortega, M.J.; Csaba, N.; González, L.; Bastos-González, D.; Ortega-Vinuesa, J.L.; Alonso, M.J. Protein-loaded PLGA–PEO blend nanoparticles: Encapsulation, release and degradation characteristics. *Colloid Polym. Sci.* **2010**, *288*, 141–150. [CrossRef]
34. Chung, Y.I.; Ahn, K.M.; Jeon, S.H.; Lee, S.Y.; Lee, J.H.; Tae, G. Enhanced bone regeneration with BMP-2 loaded functional nanoparticle-hydrogel complex. *J. Control. Release* **2007**, *121*, 91–99. [CrossRef]
35. La, W.-G.; Kang, S.-W.; Yang, H.S.; Bhang, S.H.; Lee, S.H.; Park, J.-H.; Kim, B.-S. The Efficacy of Bone Morphogenetic Protein-2 Depends on Its Mode of Delivery. *Artif. Organs* **2010**, *34*, 1150–1153. [CrossRef]
36. Fu, Y.; Du, L.; Wang, Q.; Liao, W.; Jin, Y.; Dong, A.; Chen, C.; Li, Z. In vitro sustained release of recombinant human bone morphogenetic protein-2 microspheres embedded in thermosensitive hydrogels. *Die Pharm.* **2012**, *67*, 299–303. [CrossRef]
37. Rahman, C.V.; Ben-David, D.; Dhillon, A.; Kuhn, G.; Gould, T.W.A.; Müller, R.; Rose, F.R.A.J.; Shakesheff, K.M.; Livne, E. Controlled release of BMP-2 from a sintered polymer scaffold enhances bone repair in a mouse calvarial defect model. *J. Tissue Eng. Regen. Med.* **2014**, *8*, 59–66. [CrossRef]
38. Pakulska, M.M.; Elliott Donaghue, I.; Obermeyer, J.M.; Tuladhar, a.; McLaughlin, C.K.; Shendruk, T.N.; Shoichet, M.S. Encapsulation-free controlled release: Electrostatic adsorption eliminates the need for protein encapsulation in PLGA nanoparticles. *Sci. Adv.* **2016**, *2*, e1600519. [CrossRef]
39. Fu, C.; Yang, X.; Tan, S.; Song, L. Enhancing Cell Proliferation and Osteogenic Differentiation of MC3T3-E1 Pre-osteoblasts by BMP-2 Delivery in Graphene Oxide-Incorporated PLGA/HA Biodegradable Microcarriers. *Sci. Rep.* **2017**, *7*, 12549. [CrossRef]
40. Peula, J.M.; de las Nieves, F.J. Adsorption of monomeric bovine serum albumin on sulfonated polystyrene model colloids 1. Adsorption isotherms and effect of the surface charge density. *Colloids Surf. A Physicochem. Eng. Asp.* **1993**, *77*, 199–208. [CrossRef]
41. Peula, J.M.; de las Nieves, F.J. Adsorption of monomeric bovine serum albumin on sulfonated polystyrene

model colloids 3. Colloidal stability of latex—Protein complexes. *Colloids Surf. A Physicochem. Eng. Asp.* **1994**, *90*, 55–62. [CrossRef]

42. Peula, J.M.; Hidalgo-Alvarez, R.; De Las Nieves, F.J. Coadsorption of IgG and BSA onto sulfonated polystyrene latex: I. Sequential and competitive coadsorption isotherms. *J. Biomater. Sci. Polym. Ed.* **1996**, *7*, 231–240. [CrossRef]
43. Siafaka, P.I.; Üstündağ Okur, N.; Karavas, E.; Bikiaris, D.N. Surface modified multifunctional and stimuli responsive nanoparticles for drug targeting: Current status and uses. *Int. J. Mol. Sci.* **2016**, *17*, 1440. [CrossRef]
44. Peula-García, J.M.; Hidalgo-Alvarez, R.; De Las Nieves, F.J. Colloid stability and electrokinetic characterization of polymer colloids prepared by different methods. *Colloids Surf. A Physicochem. Eng. Asp.* **1997**, *127*, 19–24. [CrossRef]
45. Santander-Ortega, M.J.; Lozano-López, M.V.; Bastos-González, D.; Peula-García, J.M.; Ortega-Vinuesa, J.L. Novel core-shell lipid-chitosan and lipid-poloxamer nanocapsules: Stability by hydration forces. *Colloid Polym. Sci.* **2010**, *288*, 159–172. [CrossRef]
46. Peula-Garcia, J.M.; Hidaldo-Alvarez, R.; De las Nieves, F.J. Protein co-adsorption on different polystyrene latexes: Electrokinetic characterization and colloidal stability. *Colloid Polym. Sci.* **1997**, *275*, 198–202. [CrossRef]
47. Santander-Ortega, M.J.; Bastos-González, D.; Ortega-Vinuesa, J.L. Electrophoretic mobility and colloidal stability of PLGA particles coated with IgG. *Colloids Surf. B Biointerfaces* **2007**, *60*, 80–88. [CrossRef]
48. Peula, J.M.; Callejas, J.; de las NIeves, F.J. Adsorption of Monomeric Bovine Serum Albumin on Sulfonated Polystyrene Model Colloids. II. Electrokinetic Characterization of Latex-Protein Complexes. In *Surface Properties of Biomaterials*; Butterworth and Heinemann: Oxford, UK, 1994; pp. 61–69.
49. Sun, D. Effect of Zeta Potential and Particle Size on the Stability of SiO_2 Nanospheres as Carrier for Ultrasound Imaging Contrast Agents. *Int. J. Electrochem. Sci.* **2016**, 8520–8529. [CrossRef]
50. del Castillo-Santaella, T.; Peula-García, J.M.; Maldonado-Valderrama, J.; Jódar-Reyes, A.B. Interaction of surfactant and protein at the O/W interface and its effect on colloidal and biological properties of polymeric nanocarriers. *Colloids Surf. B Biointerfaces* **2019**, *173*, 295–302. [CrossRef]
51. Schrier, J.A.; DeLuca, P.P. Porous bone morphogenetic protein-2 microspheres: Polymer binding and in vitro release. *AAPS PharmSciTech* **2001**, *2*, 66–72. [CrossRef]
52. Padial-Molina, M.; O'Valle, F.; Lanis, A.; Mesa, F.; Dohan Ehrenfest, D.M.; Wang, H.-L.; Galindo-Moreno, P. Clinical application of mesenchymal stem cells and novel supportive therapies for oral bone regeneration. *BioMed Res. Int.* **2015**, *2015*. [CrossRef]
53. Inai, K.; Norris, R.A.; Hoffman, S.; Markwald, R.R.; Sugi, Y. BMP-2 induces cell migration and periostin expression during atrioventricular valvulogenesis. *Dev. Biol.* **2008**, *315*, 383–396. [CrossRef]
54. Gamell, C.; Osses, N.; Bartrons, R.; Rückle, T.; Camps, M.; Rosa, J.L.; Ventura, F.; Imamura, T. BMP2 induction of actin cytoskeleton reorganization and cell migration requires PI3-kinase and Cdc42 activity. *J. Cell Sci.* **2008**, *121*, 3960–3970. [CrossRef]
55. Friedrichs, M.; Wirsdöerfer, F.; Flohé, S.B.; Schneider, S.; Wuelling, M.; Vortkamp, A. BMP signaling balances proliferation and differentiation of muscle satellite cell descendants. *BMC Cell Biol.* **2011**, *12*, 26. [CrossRef]
56. Hrubi, E.; Imre, L.; Robaszkiewicz, A.; Virág, L.; Kerényi, F.; Nagy, K.; Varga, G.; Jenei, A.; Hegedüs, C. Diverse effect of BMP-2 homodimer on mesenchymal progenitors of different origin. *Hum. Cell* **2018**, *31*, 139–148. [CrossRef]
57. Kim, H.K.W.; Oxendine, I.; Kamiya, N. High-concentration of BMP2 reduces cell proliferation and increases apoptosis via DKK1 and SOST in human primary periosteal cells. *Bone* **2013**, *54*, 141–150. [CrossRef]

10

Risperidone-Loaded PLGA–Lipid Particles with Improved Release Kinetics: Manufacturing and Detailed Characterization by Electron Microscopy and Nano-CT

Christopher Janich [1], Andrea Friedmann [2], Juliana Martins de Souza e Silva [3], Cristine Santos de Oliveira [3], Ligia E. de Souza [1], Dan Rujescu [4], Christian Hildebrandt [5], Moritz Beck-Broichsitter [5], Christian E. H. Schmelzer [2] and Karsten Mäder [1,*]

1. Institute of Pharmacy, Faculty of Biosciences, Martin Luther University Halle-Wittenberg, 06120 Halle (Saale), Germany; christopher.janich@pharmazie.uni-halle.de (C.J.); ligia.souza@pharmazie.uni-halle.de (L.E.d.S.)
2. Department of Biological and Macromolecular Materials, Fraunhofer Institute for Microstructure of Materials and Systems IMWS, 06120 Halle (Saale), Germany; andrea.friedmann@imws.fraunhofer.de (A.F.); christian.schmelzer@imws.fraunhofer.de (C.E.H.S.)
3. Institute of Physics, Martin Luther University Halle-Wittenberg, 06120 Halle (Saale), Germany; juliana.martins@physik.uni-halle.de (J.M.d.S.eS.); cristine.santos-de-oliveira@physik.uni-halle.de (C.S.d.O.)
4. Department of Psychiatry, Psychotherapy and Psychosomatics, Martin Luther University Halle-Wittenberg, 06120 Halle (Saale), Germany; dan.rujescu@uk-halle.de
5. MilliporeSigma a Business of Merck KGaA, 64293 Darmstadt, Germany; christian.hildebrandt@merckgroup.com (C.H.); moritz.beck-broichsitter@merckgroup.com (M.B.-B.)

* Correspondence: karsten.maeder@pharmazie.uni-halle.de

Abstract: For parenteral controlled drug release, the desired zero order release profile with no lag time is often difficult to achieve. To overcome the undesired lag time of the current commercial risperidone controlled release formulation, we developed PLGA–lipid microcapsules (MCs) and PLGA–lipid microgels (MGs). The lipid phase was composed of middle chain triglycerides (MCT) or isopropylmyristate (IPM). Hydroxystearic acid was used as an oleogelator. The three-dimensional inner structure of Risperidone-loaded MCs and MGs was assessed by using the invasive method of electron microscopy with focused ion beam cutting (FIB-SEM) and the noninvasive method of high-resolution nanoscale X-ray computed tomography (nano-CT). FIB-SEM and nano-CT measurements revealed the presence of highly dispersed spherical structures around two micrometres in size. Drug release kinetics did strongly depend on the used lipid phase and the presence or absence of hydroxystearic acid. We achieved a nearly zero order release without a lag time over 60 days with the MC-MCT formulation. In conclusion, the developed lipid-PLGA microparticles are attractive alternatives to pure PLGA-based particles. The advantages include improved release profiles, which can be easily tuned by the lipid composition.

Keywords: controlled release; PLGA; risperidone; microparticles; microcapsules; oleogels; electron microscopy; three-dimensional X-ray imaging; nano-CT; biodegradable polymers; hydroxy-stearic acid

---

1. Introduction

The use of parenteral controlled release drug delivery systems (CR-DDS) is a highly attractive and rational way to improve drug therapy. Potential benefits include decrease of administration frequency, increase of bioavailability and less side effects. Polylactic acid (PLA) and poly(lactic-*co*-glycolic acid

(PLGA) products have existed for several decades and are, by far, the most widely used polymers for CR-DDS [1,2]. The major clinical use is the peptide-based treatment of GnrH-dependent diseases such as breast and prostate cancer. Other important and increasingly used applications include the local delivery of drugs to the eye [3], the brain [4], or the inner ear [5,6]. An important application of CR-DDS is also the controlled release of antipsychotic compounds to treat schizophrenia. Long-acting parenteral controlled release of antipsychotic drugs overcomes the poor compliance of patients with oral administration [7,8]. Risperidone is an important drug in the treatment of schizophrenia. Several oral and one parenteral controlled release formulations are available and a PLGA based CR-DDS formulation is marketed (Risperdal® Consta®). According to the treatment schedule [9], patients initially have to take tablets, although the CR-DDS has already been injected. This situation is not a favorable scenario of pharmacotherapy, because schizophrenia patients do frequently not comply and double medication should be avoided. The release mechanisms of Risperdal® Consta® have been studied in detail by the group of Burgess and good in vitro and in vivo correlations have been observed by means of scaling factors [10,11]. Initially, a lag phase with almost no release is observed, followed by a faster release. The group clearly showed that the release onset is related to the water penetration and polymer degradation-induced drop of the polymer glass transition temperature T_g to 37 °C.

Several publications describe alternative PLGA formulations for the controlled release of risperidone. However, commonly, the presence of lag times, sigmoidal release curves, and rather short release times (<1 month) have been observed [10–15]. Souza et al. tested different formulations with single or repeated doses in vivo [16]. For single dose injections, peak maxima were observed after around one week. Unfortunately, no in vitro release data were published in the paper [16]. Therefore, it is clearly still desirable to develop biodegradable DDS with better risperidone release kinetics. The CR-DDS should provide a constant release over the 1–2 months without a lag time and the need for initial oral comedication. It should also be cost effective. Unfortunately, the selection possibility for biodegradable materials for parenteral controlled release is rather limited. In addition to PLA and PLGA, there are few other polymers and lipids. Liquid lipids are used clinically, but they provide only release control for a short period of few days. Solid lipids are also attractive as parenteral depot systems [17], but their use is often linked with problems of polymorphic transitions and limited enzymatic degradability due to the crystalline structure of the lipid. The use of polymer–lipid hybrid structures—compared to pure polymer or pure lipid-based DDS—offers additional opportunities. For example, increased drug loads may be achieved by the lipid component and the release rate might be controlled by the polymer shell. The incorporation of liquid oil into a microparticle might compromise the mechanical stability of the particle and could potentially lead to oily leakage and loss of release control. The incorporation of solid lipids will overcome this problem, but this advantage is at the cost of drug solubility in the crystalline lipid matrix and the problem of polymorphic transitions. It is desirable to combine the advantages of a liquid lipid phase with high mechanical stability. Therefore, we decided to investigate oleogels as possible alternatives. A suitable oleogelator for parenteral applications is 12-hydroxystearic acid (HS). Hydroxystearic acid induces gel formation in lipids due to its precipitation as a HS-fiber network [18,19]. Preclinical studies on injectable oleogels demonstrate the good biocompatibility and degradability of HS-oleogels in vivo [20,21].

We selected PLGA Expansorb® 75-7E from Merck KGaA (Darmstadt, Germany), which has the following properties: lactide/glycolide (L/G) ratio of 75/25, a molecular weight (MW) 80–115 kDa, and the end groups are esterified. The physical chemical properties of Expansorb®75-7E were similar to the PLGA in the market product Risperdal Consta® which contains a lactide/glycolide (L/G) ratio of 78/22, a molecular weight (MW) ~111 kDa and the end groups are esterified [22]. As the oil phase, we incorporated isopropyl myristate (IPM) or middle chain triglycerides (MCT) to form a microcapsule (MC) structure. Oily components with saturated fatty acids were used to avoid the danger of oxidation problems connected with unsaturated fatty acids.

The properties and the release kinetics of the micro-DDS will depend on the general structure and the physicochemical state of the drug and the excipients. Possible structures of (drug-free) micro-DDS are shown in Figure 1.

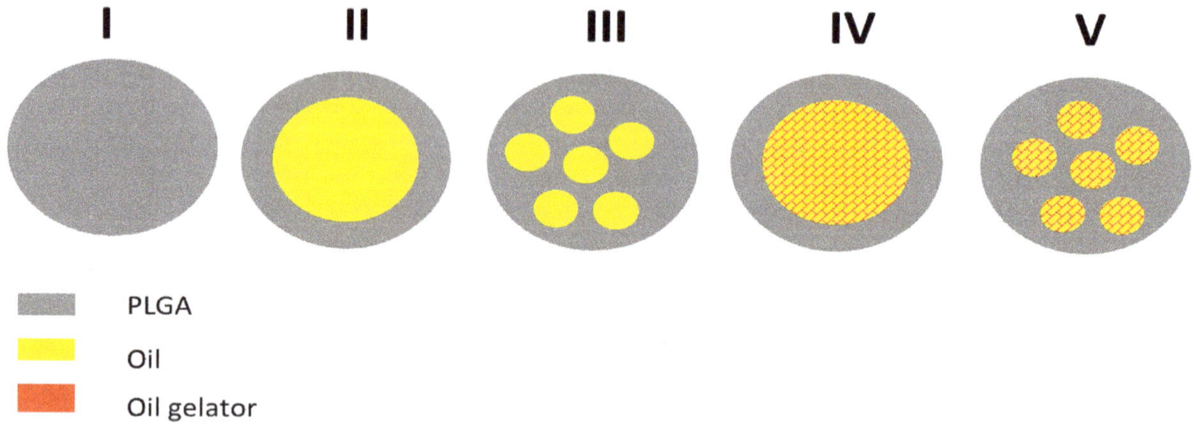

Figure 1. Possible structures of poly(lactic-*co*-glycolic acid (PLGA) and PLGA/lipid microparticles: I: PLGA microparticle; II: microcapsule with core–shell structure; III: microcapsule with multiple oily droplets; IV: microgel with core–shell structure; microgel with multiple gelled lipid domains.

PLGA microparticles are expected to form a homogeneous polymer matrix (structure I). Microcapsules composed of PLGA and oil could show structures with a single oily core and a PLGA shell (structure II) or multiple oily droplets encapsulated in PLGA (structure III). The addition of the oil gelator will increase the viscosity, but again, the oily phase could exist as a single core (structure IV) or as multiple cores (structure V). The drug could be dissolved in the polymer and the oil and/or exist as an own solid (crystalline or amorphous) phase. A rational development of the DDS requires an appropriate characterization. For particle sizing of micro-DDS, static light scattering is the standard method. We decided to use X-ray diffraction for the detection of crystalline structures in our DDS. In addition, we wanted to explore the microstructure inside the DDS. For this purpose, we used two complementary imaging techniques, which were focus ion beam scanning electron microscopy (FIB-SEM) and Zernike phase-contrast X-ray nano-computed tomography (nano-CT). By means of focused ion-beam preparation, we could cut the particles in situ and we were able to visualize the morphology of the microstructure at the location of the cut. In addition, we performed nano-CT experiments. Due to the high penetration depth of X-rays, nano-CT provided high-resolution three-dimensional images of the DDS and we were able to visualize their internal structures at any virtual slice without the need for cutting or slicing them.

In summary, the main goals of this work were:

(i) development of risperidone loaded PLGA–lipid microcapsules (MCs) and PLGA–lipid microgels (MGs) with an optimized release profile (no lag time, constant release rate)
(ii) characterization of the three-dimensional inner structure of risperidone-loaded MCs and MGs by using focused ion beam (FIB) preparation and three-dimensional X-ray imaging (nano-CT).

2. Materials and Methods

2.1. Materials

Expansorb DLG 75-7E, batch number C100010962, (Merck, Darmstadt, Germany) PVA 4-88 (Merck, Darmstadt, Germany) Risperidone 95+% (Activate Scientific, Shanghai, China), Pioneer MCT (middle chain triglycerides) batch number: 1132229 (Hansen & Rosenthal, Hamburg, Germany); isopropylmyristate Ph-Eur. batch number: 1407015-01, (Euro OTC Pharma GmbH, Bönen, Germany); dichloromethane 99.9% (Carl-Roth, Karlsruhe, Germany); hydroxystearic acid was a gift from Alberdingk Boley GmbH, (Krefeld, Germany). Risperdal Consta® 50 mg batch number: GCSK002,

(Janssen-Cilag GmbH, Neuss, Germany); 2.5 mL GASTIGHT® syringe (Hamilton Germany GmbH, Planegg, Martinsried, Germany), syringe pump (Pump 11 Elite, Harvard Apparatus, Holliston, MA, USA).

2.2. Methods

2.2.1. Preparation of PLGA Microcapsules (MC) and PLGA Microgels (MG)

Risperidone-loaded microcapsules were prepared using an oil-in-water (o/w) emulsion solvent extraction/evaporation technique.

For this purpose, 100 mg PLGA 75-7E, 100 mg of the oil phase (MCT or IPM), and 50 mg of Risperidone were weighted into a 4 mL glass vial and dissolved into the final volume of 2 mL dichloromethane by vortexing. The organic solutions were drawn up into a 2.5 mL GASTIGHT® syringe (Hamilton Germany GmbH, Planegg, Martinsried, Germany) and injected with a flow rate 5.2 μL/min by a syringe pump (Pump 11 Elite, Harvard Apparatus, Holliston, MA, USA) directly into 300 mL of aqueous PVA 4-88 (Merck, Darmstadt, Germany) solution 0.25% (*w/v*) stirred with a Rotating Paddle, USP at 240 rpm at room temperature. The aqueous phase contains double distilled and filtrated water with 0.25% polyvinyl alcohol PVA 4-88 (Merck, Darmstadt, Germany). When particle formation was completed, the suspensions were transferred into a 500 mL round bottom flask and the remaining DCM were removed under vacuum 40 mbar for 20 min. Thereafter, sedimented microcapsules were transferred by a glass pipette into a 15 mL tube and the supernatants were removed carefully. Then, the microcapsules were washed thrice with sterile filtrated double distilled water, filled up to the final volume of 1 mL and lyophilized.

2.2.2. Lyophilization

For freeze-drying, the samples were frozen rapidly with liquid nitrogen at −196 °C and lyophilised on a Christ Alpha 2–4 freeze dryer (Martin Christ Gefriertrocknungsanlagen GmbH, Osterode am Harz, Germany) in combination with a Vacuubrand RC 6 vacuum pump (Vacuubrand GmbH, Wertheim, Germany) for 24 h. The chamber was evacuated to 0.05 mbar, corresponding to −48 °C on the sublimation curve of ice. The prepared microcapsules were stored at −20 °C until further use.

2.2.3. Static Light Scattering Measurements

Routine measurements of the size distribution were carried out by laser diffractometry on a Mastersizer 2000 (Malvern Instruments, Malvern, United Kingdom) combined with a Hydro 2000 S wet dispersion unit. The samples were measured at a laser obscuration of 5%, corresponding to 11%–15% obscuration of the blue laser, in purified water. A series of five runs was evaluated by the Mastersizer 2000 software version 5.60, using the Mie theory, assuming spherical particles with a refractive index of 1.44, absorption of 0.001, and a refractive index of 1.33 for the dispersant as optical properties.

2.2.4. Powder XRD

XRD analysis was performed on a Bruker D8-Advance diffractometer, equipped with a one-dimensional silicon strip detector (LynxEye) operating with Cu Kα radiation. Diffraction was measured from $2\theta = 5°$ to $70°$ with a step size of $0.01°$ and a counting time of 1 s.

2.2.5. High-Performance Liquid Chromatography (HPLC)

A HPLC Agilent 1100 Series (Agilent, Santa Clara, CA, USA) was used. Separations were carried out using a BDS-Hypersil® C18 5 μm 250 × 4.6 column (Thermo Fisher Scientific, Waltham, MA, USA) and a mobile phase of 75% (*v/v*) methanol/25% (*v/v*) water, 1% (*v/v*) tetramethylammoniumhydroxid pentahydrate solution 25% *w/v*. Runs were carried out at 0.5 mL/min over 16 min and the absorption at 280 nm was recorded. The retention time of risperidone was 7.5 min. Injection volumes of 20 μL were used for determination of drug loading.

2.2.6. Drug Loading and Encapsulation Efficiency (EE)

Risperidone-loaded microcapsules were weighed and diluted in methanol to get a final concentration of 0.5mg/mL. All the samples were sonicated for 10 min to accelerate the dissolving of MC. Thereafter all samples were diluted 0.05 mg/mL and filtered (Minisart SRP 4, 0.45 μm syringe filter, Sartorius Stedim Biotech GmbH, Göttingen, Deutschland). The concentration of risperidone was determined via HPLC. Drug loading and EE were calculated as following equations from literature: Drug loading = (weight of drug entrapped/weight of MC used) × 100%; EE = (experimental drug loading/theoretically drug) × 100% [23].

2.2.7. In Vitro Drug Release Assay

The in vitro release of risperidone from MCs was carried out in a heated bath shaker (Memmert GmbH + Co. KG, Schwabach, Germany) at 37 °C and constant shaking at 50 rpm. A total of 6 mg of formulation I-IV and 3 mg of Risperdal Consta® were suspended in 1 mL of 10 mmol phosphate buffer saline (PBS) at pH 7.4 and transferred into a Spectra Por Float-A_Lyzer ® G2 1000kD. The float-A Lyzer was placed into a 100 mL measuring cylinder and filled up with PBS to the final volume of 60 mL so that the float-A Lyzer is submerged in PBS. To maintain sink conditions, the buffer solution was drawn off half (half change) when the risperidone concentration reaches 7%–8% of the solubility in PBS. Drug quantity was determined by UV-1800 spectrophotometer (Shimadzu, Kyoto, Japan). All measurements were performed in triplicate and the measurement points were represented as the mean ± SD.

2.2.8. Scanning Electron Microscopy and Focused Ion Beam Preparation

High resolution investigations of the microparticle morphology were done by scanning electron microscopy (SEM) using a Quanta 3D FEG (field emission gun) instrument from FEI Company, (Hillsboro, OH, USA). The microparticles were carefully placed on SEM sample holders using carbon tape and subsequently coated with a thin layer of platinum using a magnetron sputtering system (HVD, Dresden, Germany) to achieve a conducting surface. The SEM images were obtained under high vacuum conditions using an acceleration voltage of 5 keV, a working distance of 6–10 mm and electron beam currents of 12 pA determined with an Everhart–Thornley detector.

The microscope is designed as a dual beam (electron and ion beam) which gives the possibility to perform FIB preparations in the same device. Here, the gallium ion beam and the electron beam operate independently of each other. The point of coincidence of the two beams is located at a working distance of 10 mm. The angle between both beams is 52°. To allow vertical cutting with the FIB, the sample was tilted by this angle. Thus observation of the cross-sections with the electron beam was also done at an angle of 52°. After screening the samples by conventional SEM, the particle of interest was selected for cross-sectional preparation (target preparation). As the first step in cross-section preparation at predefined areas of interest coarse material was ablated with gallium ions accelerated at 30 kV with ion currents of 15 nA. After this coarse milling step lower beam currents of Afterwards, 1–0.5 nA were used to polish the cross sections. The samples were not cooled during FIB milling. The patterning conditions used conform to the standard patterning conditions for silicon materials. The SEM observation can be done during ion milling or after subsequent milling steps.

2.2.9. Nano-CT

X-ray imaging experiments were performed at the Institute of Physics, Martin Luther University Halle-Wittenberg, in a Carl Zeiss Xradia 810 Ultra (Cr source, 5.4 keV, for instrument details see [24]). Phase-contrast imaging mode was used with a phase-ring positioned near the back focal plane of the zone plate. In each experiment, a total of 901 projections with a field-of-view (FOV) of 65 μm were obtained over 180°, with an exposure time of 15 s per projection, a detector binning of 2, and voxel size of 128 nm. Image reconstruction was performed by filtered back-projection algorithm using the software integrated into the Xradia 810 Ultra. For each sample, two or three imaging experiments were performed, moving the sample vertically to enable the visualization of one entire microsphere in one single direction (from now on named Z-direction). For each sample's datasets, the brightness and contrast were adjusted in ImageJ® and the datasets were then stitched together using the Merge module of the Thermo Fisher Scientific Avizo® software (version 9.2, Thermo Fisher Scientific, Hillsboro, OR, USA). Median denoising and nonlocal mean filter were applied to the datasets. The 3D renderings presented here were created using either the commercial software arivis Vision4D® (version 2.12.6, arivis AG, Rostock, Germany) or Avizo®. For the dispersed internal spherical structures (ISS) evaluation, a volume located in the center of the 3D image was extracted consisting of 325 × 325 × Z voxels. Z varies among the samples, as it is almost equal to the number of pixels of the microsphere diameter, but is smaller than it to prevent voxels that do not consist of sample to be added to the calculation. The results obtained here represent the ratio of ISS compared to the total extracted volume of the sample (PLGA+ISS). For binarization of the datasets into PLGA and ISS, automatic thresholding with IsoData criterion was used, followed by island removal for the removal of small clusters of voxels (<15). A surface was generated from the segmented dataset in order to smooth sharp voxel edges and the specific surface area (SSA) values obtained represent the ratio of the constructed surface area (SA) to the volume (V) for each sample.

3. Results and Discussion

3.1. *Preparation of MCs and MGs*

For the preparation of MCs and MGs, the conventional oil-in-water (o/w) emulsion solvent evaporation method was used [2,25]. All components were dissolved in dichloromethane. The components of the four different formulations are listed in the Table 1. In general, the composition followed a 2:2:1 mass ratio of PLGA/Lipid/Risperidone. Therefore, the theoretical drug load was 20% [m/m]. High encapsulation efficiencies (>92%) were achieved, as seen in Table 1.

Table 1. Composition and encapsulation efficiency of Risperidone-loaded PLGA microcapsules (MC) and microgels (MG).

Sample	PLGA (mg)	Risperidone [mg]	MCT (mg)	IPM (mg)	HS (mg)	% Encapsul. Efficiency [+/−% SD]
MC-IPM	100	50	0	100	0	92.62 [0.94]
MG-IPM	100	50	0	90	10	100.82 [5.50]
MG-MCT	100	50	90	0	10	96.05 [3.98]
MC-MCT	100	50	100	0	0	92.79 [3.23]

MC = microcapsule, MG = microgel, PLGA = poly(lactide-*co*-glycolide), MCT = middle chain triglycerides, IPM = isopropylmyristate, HS = hydroxystearic acid.

To get reproducible particle sizes, it was important to keep all size-influencing parameters constant, e.g., the o-phase volume and solvent, the concentration and type of polymer, the volume of the continuous phase and the type and concentration of stabilizer, the temperature, and the stirring speed [26]. After lyophilization the MCs did not agglomerate and were resuspendable in water.

3.2. *Characterization*

3.2.1. Particle Size Measurements

The particle size and morphology of MC are key factors which potentially affect EE, drug release rate, and the biodistribution [27,28]. The optimal size range for microparticles with controlled release characteristics is considered to be 10–200 μm. Particles in the lower micron range will show a faster drug release, and they are also more easily phagocytosed by immune cells [29]. Sizes larger than

200 μm are difficult to inject and will show more inhomogeneous degradation [30]. The particle size distribution is shown in Figure 2.

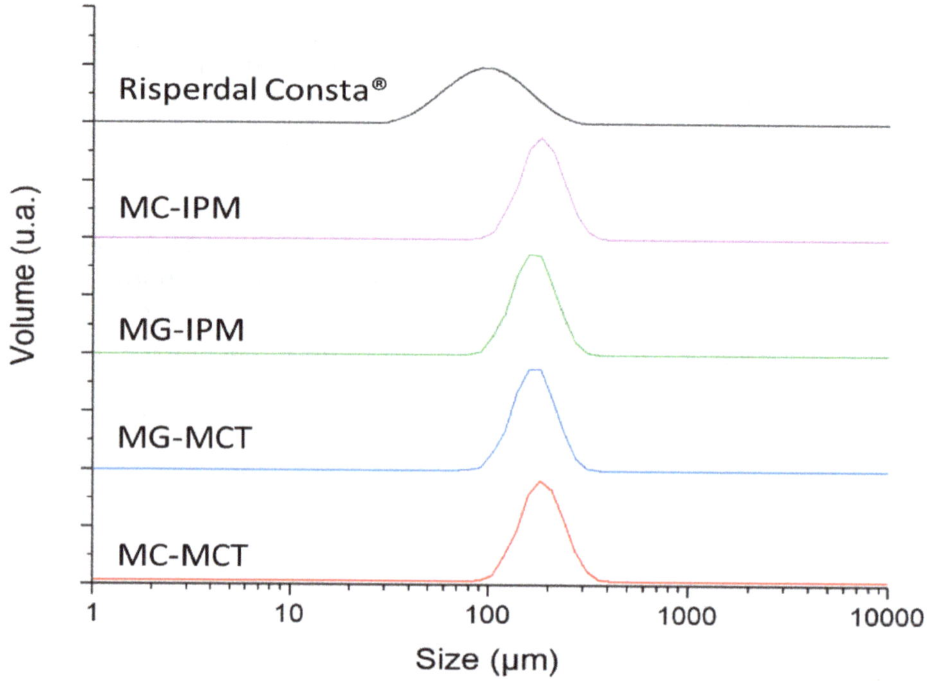

Figure 2. Volume-averaged particle sizes of microcapsules, microgels, and the reference product.

The particle size of the microcapsule formulations MC-IPM and MC-MCT are very similar ($D_{(0.5)}$ = 172.8 μm and 169.5 μm). The particle sizes for the corresponding microgels MG-IPM and MG-MCT were smaller compared to the microcapsules, but again very similar between IPM and MCT ($D_{(0.5)}$ = MG-IPM 157.2 μm; MG-MCT 155.9 μm), as seen Figure 2 and Table 2. It can be concluded, therefore, that the incorporation of hydroxystearic acid leads to slightly smaller particles, probably due to the impact on the surface tension during particle formation. The determined $D_{(0.5)}$ of the market product is 89.1 μm, which is in line with a size range between 25 and 150 μm reported in the literature [31]. The particle size distribution of the commercial product is considerably broader compared to our formulations (Span Risperdal Consta® 1.165 vs. span values between 0.612 and 0.637), as seen in Table 2.

Table 2. Particle size distributions determined by static light scattering.

Sample	D(0.1) (μm)	D(0.5) (μm)	D(0.9) (μm)	Mean $D_{(4,3)}$ (μm)	Span	Uniformity
Risperdal Consta®	50.7	89.1	154.5	96.9	1.165	0.36
MC-IPM	126.1	172.8	236.3	178.1	0.637	0.202
MG-IPM	116.4	157.2	212.6	161.2	0.612	0.193
MG-MCT	115.3	155.9	211.8	160.2	0.620	0.196
MC-MCT	123.7	169.5	230.8	174.4	0.631	0.197

3.2.2. Scanning Electron Microscopy and Focused Ion Beam Investigations

SEM images of Risperdal Consta® are shown in Figure 3. The market product Risperdal Consta® shows a high heterogeneity of particle size, shape, and surface structures. Surprisingly, structures showing partial engulfment, as seen in Figure 3d, and collapsed structures are visible, as seen in Figure 3c. Larger magnification of the surface indicated the presence of anisotropic material, which are most likely drug crystals, as seen in Figure 3e,f.

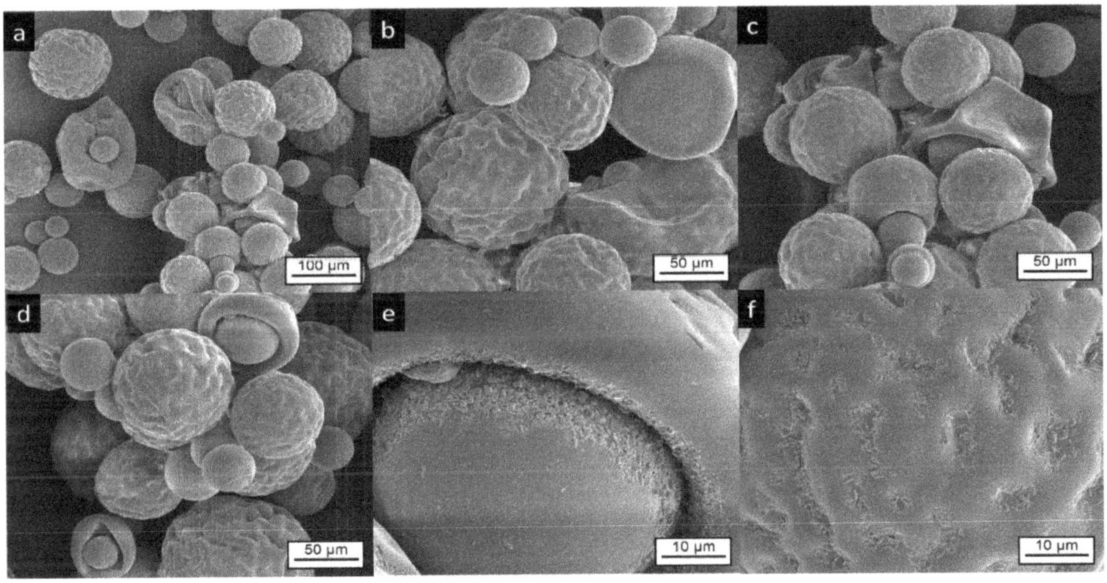

Figure 3. Electron microscopic pictures of Risperdal Consta®. The pictures at lower magnifications (**a**–**d**) show the presence of different particle sizes and shapes. Most particles show wrinkled surfaces; some have a smooth surface. High magnification shows the presence of small anisotropic material on the surface (**e**,**f**).

The microcapsules and microgels do not show the irregular structures of the commercial product. Most of MCT microcapsules are spherical, some show an elongated shape, which probably results from the coalescence of two particles, as seen in Figure 4a, white stars. The surface of the MC-MCT microcapsules shows a pattern similar to golf balls, as seen in Figure 4b,c. Very rarely, small anisotropic structures are found on the particle surface, as seen in Figure 4c, top middle, which most likely represent risperidone crystals. Cutting of the particles by focused ion beam (FIB) provides insights into the internal structure, as seen in Figure 4b,d. A multicore structure with dimensions in the lower micron range becomes visible. Within the internal structures, anisotropic shapes are visible which most likely present precipitated drug crystals, as seen in Figure 4d.

The electron microscopic pictures of the corresponding microgel MG-MCT shows spherical particles with a structured surface that appears smoother compared to the MC-MCT surface (Figure 5). In contrast to the MC-MCT microcapsules, we could not detect elongated shapes, as indicated by white stars in Figure 4a, which emerge from the coalescence of two particles. The pictures obtained by FIB cutting of the particles show internal multicore structures with dimensions in the lower micron range, as seen in Figure 5b,d.

IPM loaded microcapsules (MC-IPM) have a spherical shape, as seen in Figure 6a. The surface appears similar to the MC-MCT capsules. Very rarely, small crystals can be detected on the particle surface, as seen in Figure 6c. After FIB cutting, multicore structures in the lower micron range become visible, as seen in Figure 6b,d.

The electron microscopy investigation on MG-IPM microgels shows the presence of spherical particles, as seen in Figure 7a. Higher magnifications of the particle surface show surface dips ("golf ball structure") similar to the MG-MCT microgels. In addition, elongated "hair-like" structures are visible, as seen in Figure 7c,d, which are not detectable in the other samples. Most likely, they are mainly composed of hydroxystearic acid, which is known to induce gel formation by elongated structures. Again, FIB cutting was used to explore the interior of the particles. Multicore microdomains became visible, as seen in Figure 7b, similar to the MG-MCT microgel particles with dimensions in the lower micron range.

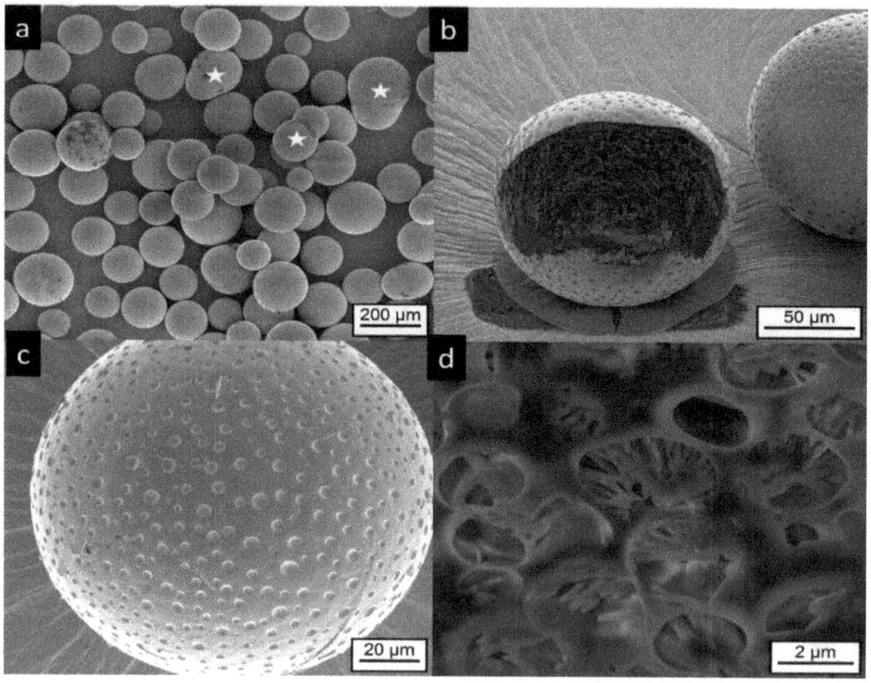

Figure 4. Electron microscopic pictures of MC-MCT microcapsules, (for composition details see Table 1). Intact particles are presented at lower (**a**,**c**) higher magnification. Focused ion beam (FIB) cut particles are shown at lower magnification in (**b**) and after deeper FIB milling and higher magnification in (**d**). The white stars in (**a**) indicate anisotropic particles, which were most likely formed by coalescence of two particles.

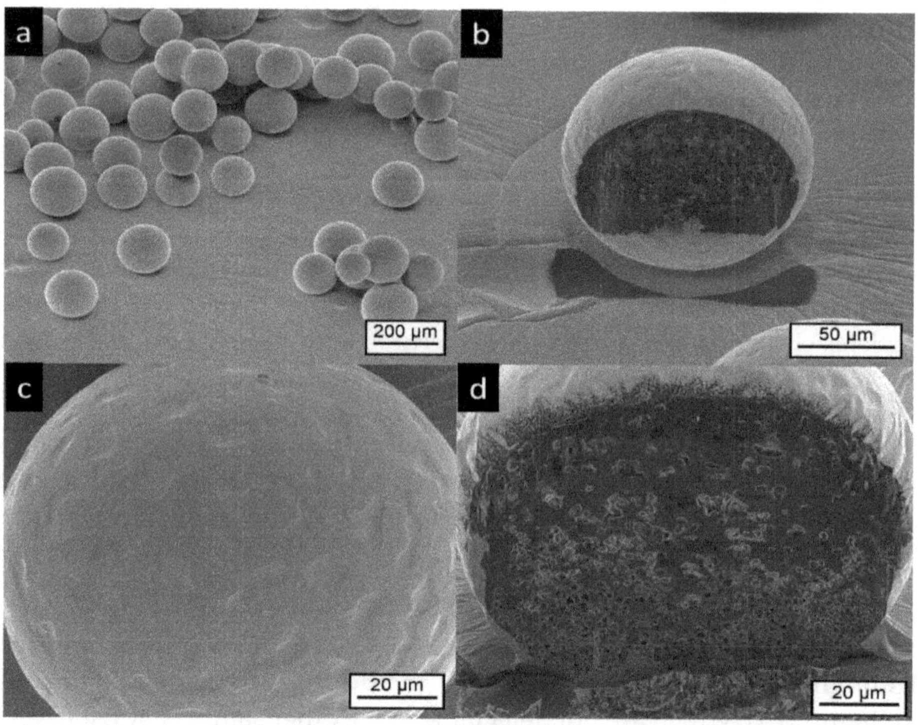

Figure 5. Electron microscopic pictures of MG-MCT microgels (for composition see Table 1). Intact particles are presented at lower (**a**,**c**) higher magnification. FIB cut particles are shown at lower magnification in (**b**) and at higher magnification at (**d**).

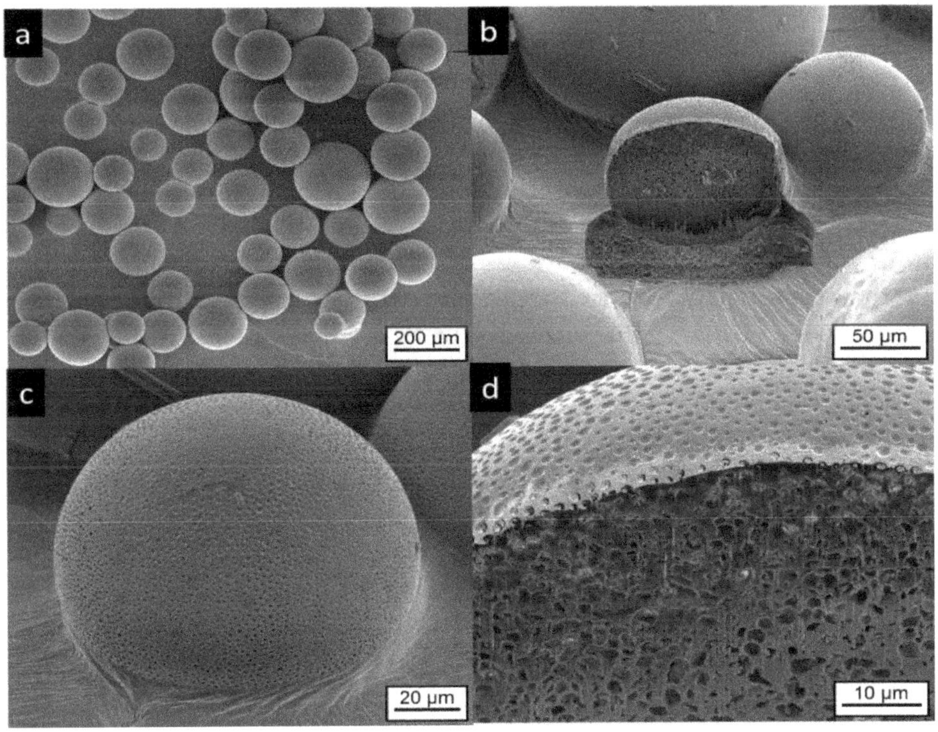

Figure 6. Electron microscopic pictures of MC-IPM microcapsules (composition details are given in Table 1). Intact particles are presented at lower (**a**,**c**) higher magnification. FIB cut particles are shown at lower magnification in (**b**) and at higher magnification at (**d**).

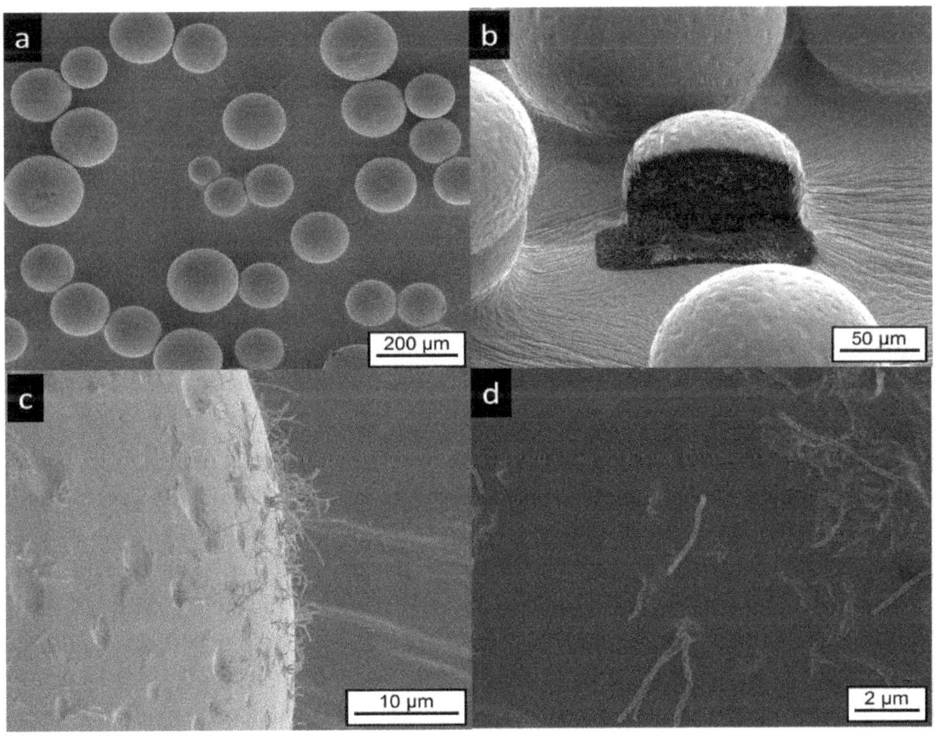

Figure 7. Electron microscopic pictures of MG-IPM microgels (sample composition is given in Table 1). Intact particles are presented at lower (**a**,**b**) and higher (**c**,**d**) magnifications. A FIB cut particle is shown in (**b**). Elongated, "worm like" structures (most likely precipitated hydroxyl-stearic acid) are visible in (**c**,**d**).

The crystallinity of the formulations was evaluated by X-ray diffraction. The diffractograms of PLGA, the pure drug risperidone, the commercial product, and the developed microcapsules and microgels are shown in Figure 8. It is known that the drug can exist in different polymorphs [32–34]. As expected, the polymer PLGA does not show sharp peaks, but only broad lines, indicating an amorphous state. The pure drug shows multiple sharp peaks. The X-ray diffractograms of the commercial product Risperdal Consta® and the developed formulations show a similar pattern, but they are different from the pure drug. From the measurements, it can be concluded that risperidone exists in all formulations at least partially in the crystalline state. The crystalline state in the formulation is different from the crystal structure of the parent drug, but very similar to the crystal form of risperidone, which has been observed after micronization with supercritical fluids [33].

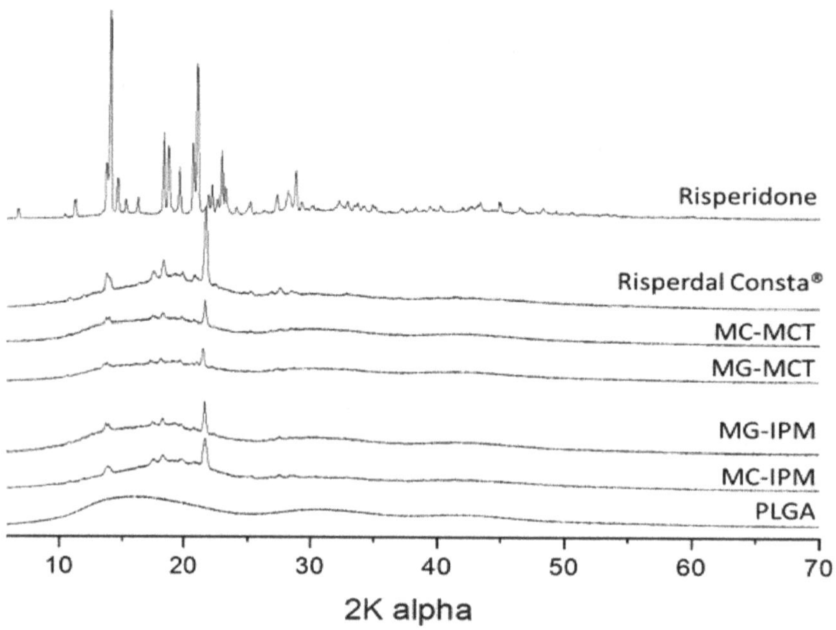

Figure 8. Wide angle X-ray diffractograms of microcapsules, microgels, Risperdal Consta®, and the pure drug risperidone.

4. X-Ray Nano-Imaging (Nano-CT)

X-ray imaging comprises a class of nondestructive techniques that are used to visualize the internal structure of different materials. In conventional X-ray imaging, differences in the X-ray absorption cross-section of different materials results in the image contrast [35,36]. Therefore, if the different parts composing one sample show only small differences in the X-ray attenuation, a poor image contrast will be obtained in conventional absorption-based X-ray imaging. This is specially the case for samples composed of elements with low electron density, making the characterization of the structures and visualization of the sample features a very hard task. Alternatively, phase-contrast imaging methods enable the visualization of features of weakly absorbing objects [35,37,38]. X-ray phase-contrast imaging is based on a different physical principle, and the contrast of the image is generated by the detection of the changes in the phase of the wavefront [36,39]. In this work, we imaged the different microspheres using Zernike phase-contrast imaging in a benchtop nano-CT scanner (Xradia Ultra 810). Phase-contrast nano-CT was used to characterize the inner structure of the commercial product Risperdal Consta® (Figure 9) and the developed microcapsules and microgels (Figure 10). Videos Supplementary Videos S1–S5 show the inner 3D structure of the microparticles. The diameter and volume distributions of the internal structures are presented in Supplementary Figures S1 and S2.

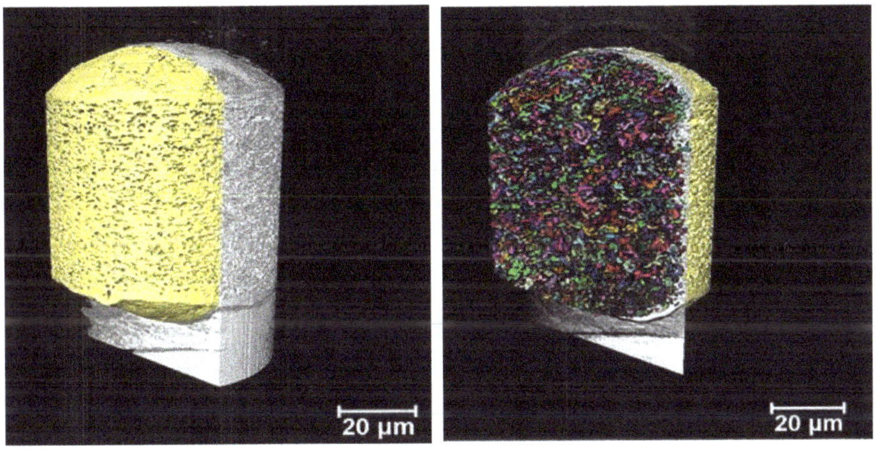

Figure 9. Volumetric representation the inner part of one reconstructed microsphere of Risperdal Consta® imaged with nano-CT. The left picture shows the X-ray signal in gray and the microsphere PLGA matrix pseudocolored in yellow. On the right, the small colored structures represent the dispersed internal spherical structures (ISS), which can be attributed to the dispersed drug particles. The volume of the ISS is about 13% of the total volume of the particle.

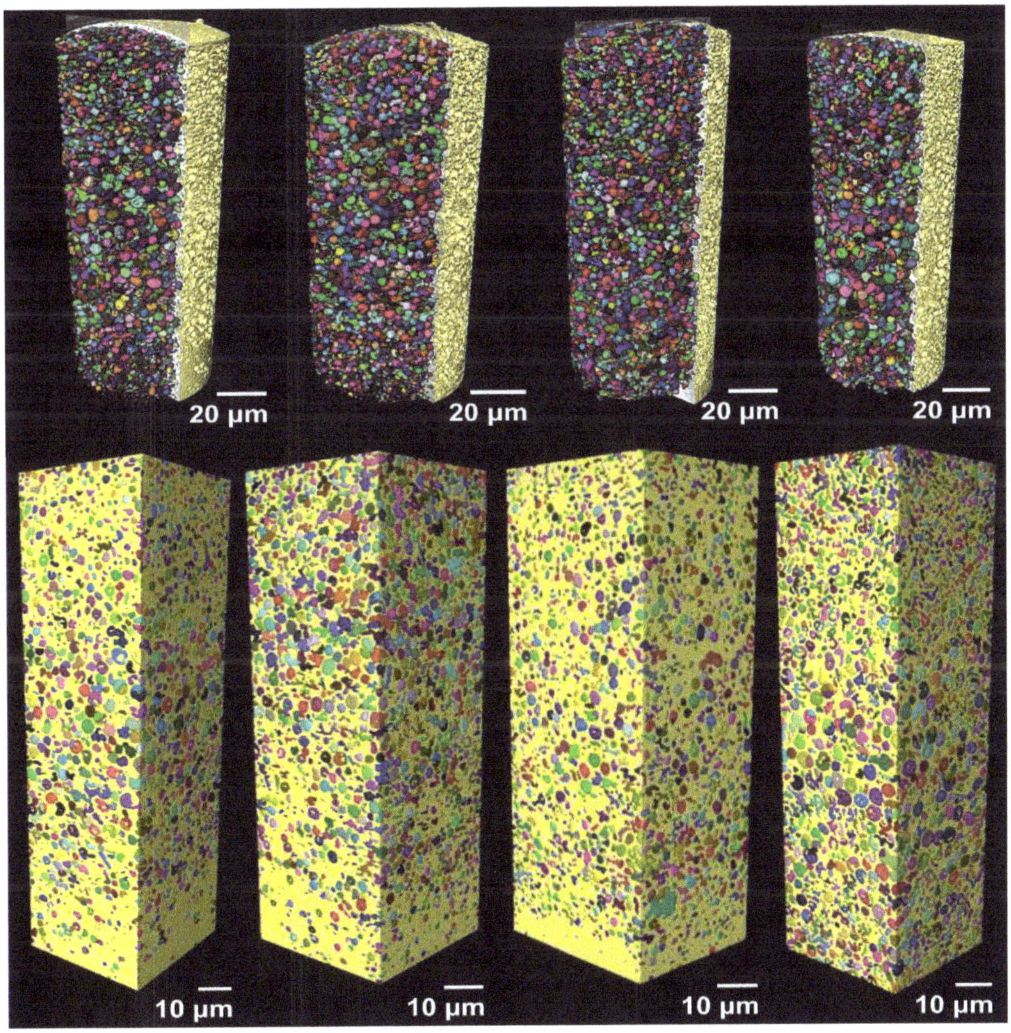

Figure 10. Volumetric representation of the inner part of the microspheres imaged with nano-CT. On the top from left to right, the MC-IPM, MG-IPM, MG-MCT, and MC-MCT microspheres pseudocolored in yellow are shown, with the dispersed internal spherical structures (ISS) represented in different colors. On the bottom, the volume used for the estimations done with nano-CT are shown for all samples.

All microgels and microcapsules show internal spherical structures (ISS) in the submicrometer range, with sphericity values close to unit. However, the volume percentage of the ISS in the microcapsules is between 35% and 46% and is, therefore, much higher than the volume percentage of the ISS phase in the Risperdal Consta® particles. The ISS phase can be attributed to the dispersed lipid phase for the microgels and microcapsules. In contrast, the ISS consists of risperidone only for the Risperdal Consta® system. A quantitative treatment of the 3D images indicates that the ISS have diameter around 2 μm for lipid-based systems and around 800 nm for the Risperdal Consta® product, as seen in Table 3. The ISS diameter and volume distributions are shown in Figures S1 and S2.

Table 3. Volume, diameter and sphericity of the internal dispersed phase (ISS), assessed by nano-CT.

Sample	Volume ISS	ISS Diameter	ISS Sphericity
Risperdal Consta®	13%	0.8 ± 0.2 μm	0.95 ± 0.02
MG-MCT	35%	2.0 ± 0.9 μm	0.8 ± 0.2
MC-MCT	46%	2.2 ± 0.8 μm	0.7 ± 0.1
MC-IPM	39%	1.9 ± 1.3 μm	0.8 ± 0.2
MG-IPM	43%	2.3 ± 1.0 μm	0.8 ± 0.3

Compared to other imaging techniques, Zernike phase-contrast nano-CT has the advantage of producing high-resolution three-dimensional images of low-absorbing samples, which enables the estimation of the values shown here. As with most high-resolution imaging techniques, nano-CT has the disadvantage of producing images limited to a small field of view, thus, to obtain the images of one single microparticle, it was necessary to image the sample two or three times and stitch the datasets. One of the benefits of phase-contrast nano-CT for imaging low-absorbing samples is that it does not require any special sample preparation procedure or induce any sample damage within the imaged area, in contrast with FIB-SEM. Overall, the results obtained by FIB-SEM correlate well with those obtained by nano-CT, and the same structures were observed. Both methods indicate the presence of a high percentage of internal structures (ISS) with sizes around two micrometers. Therefore, the microcapsules and microgels represent structures III and V of Figure 1, respectively.

5. Drug Release

The in vitro release of risperidone from the commercial product in the developed formulations is shown in Figure 11. For all formulations, a low percentage of the drug (<10%) is initially released. Most likely, drug molecules on the surface (which were observed by electron microscopy) are released very quickly. After the initial release, there is almost no release detectable for two weeks for Risperdal Consta®. Thereafter, the release accelerates. The developed formulations show different release profiles. The fastest release was observed for the MG-IPM microgel. The slowest release rate observed for the lipid formulations was for the MC-IPM microcapsules system. Therefore, it can be concluded that the oleogelator hydroxystearic acid had a strong impact on the release kinetics. The impact of the oleogelator hydroxystearic acid is also visible for the MCT systems, but to a smaller extent. Again, the microparticles with the incorporated oleogel (MG-MCT) release faster compared to the HS-free microcapsules (MC-MCT). The desired release profile was obtained with the MC-MCT microparticles: an almost linear release profile over two months with no lag time has been achieved.

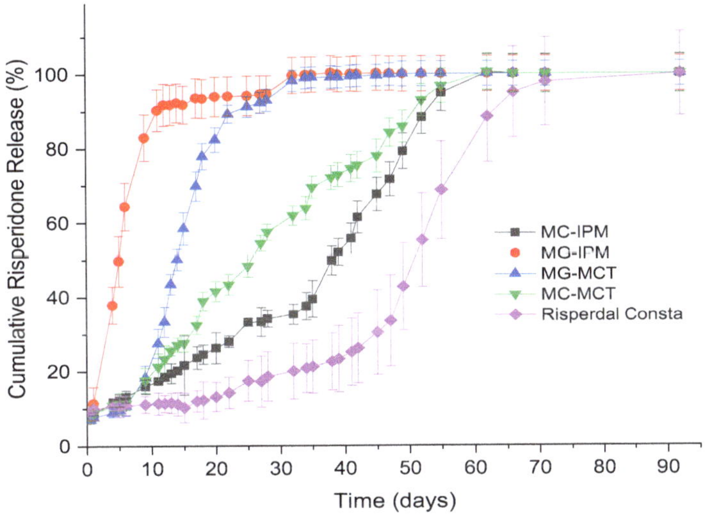

Figure 11. In vitro release profiles of Risperidone microcapsules (MC), microgels (MG), and Risperdal Consta®.

6. Conclusions

The results of our study show that lipid–PLGA hybrid systems are interesting alternatives to pure PLGA microparticles. The saturated liquid lipids MCT and IPM were incorporated in the form of microcapsules and microgels. Hydroxystearic acid (HS) was used as an oleogelator. The particle structure was investigated by FIB-SEM and nano-CT imaging. Both methods support the existence of a highly dispersed internal phase with spherical particle sizes of around 2 micrometers. The noninvasive nano-CT imaging enabled the production of 3D representations of the microparticles' structures in high-resolution images. After image processing and segmentation, it was possible to estimate the amount, size distribution, and sphericity of the internal structures. The presence of hydroxystearic acid accelerated the drug release. The drug release kinetics can be tuned by the lipid composition. An almost ideal release profile for risperidone was achieved with PLGA–MCT microcapsules (MC-MCT). In contrast to Risperdal Consta®, no lag time and an almost linear release over 60 days was observed. Therefore, the developed systems are suitable candidates to overcome the need for double medication (injected microparticles and tablets), which is currently needed due to the release lag time of Risperdal Consta®.

Supplementary Materials:
Figure S1: Diameter distribution of the internal spherical structures (ISS) determined by nano-CT. Figure S2: Volume distribution of the internal structures (ISS) determined by nano-CT. Video S1: Video of the internal structure obtained by nano-CT for Risperdal Consta. Video S2: Video of the internal structure obtained by nano-CT for MC-IPM. Video S3: Video of the internal structure obtained by nano-CT for MG-IPM. Video S4: Video of the internal structure obtained by nano-CT for MG-MCT. Video S5: Video of the internal structure obtained by nano-CT for MC-MCT.

Author Contributions: Conceptualization, K.M., C.J., L.E.d.S., D.R., C.H., M.B.-B.; Particle manufacturing and drug release studies: C.J., L.E.d.S., K.M. Nano-CT measurements and data evaluation: J.M.d.S.eS. and C.S.d.O. F.I.B.-SEM: A.F., C.S.d.O. writing—original draft preparation, C.J., K.M.; writing—review and editing, C.J., A.F., J.M.d.S.eS., C.S.d.O., D.R., C.H., M.B.-B., C.H., C.E.H.S., supervision: K.M.

Acknowledgments: The authors gratefully acknowledge Toni Buttler (Institute of Chemistry, Martin Luther University Halle-Wittenberg, Germany) for carrying out the powder-XRD measurements and Carl Zeiss for the loan of the phase-ring.

References

1. Jain, A.; Kunduru, K.R.; Basu, A.; Mizrahi, B.; Domb, A.J.; Khan, W. Injectable formulations of poly(lactic acid) and its copolymers in clinical use. *Adv. Drug Deliv. Rev.* **2016**, *107*, 213–227. [CrossRef] [PubMed]
2. Makadia, H.K.; Siegel, S.J. Poly Lactic-*co*-Glycolic Acid (PLGA) as biodegradable controlled drug delivery carrier. *Polymers* **2011**, *3*, 1377–1397. [CrossRef] [PubMed]

3. Bhat, P.V.; Goldstein, D.A. Dexamethasone intravitreal implant (allergan) for the treatment of noninfectious uveitis. *Expert Opin. Orphan Drugs* **2014**, *2*, 301–310. [CrossRef]
4. Hänggi, D.; Etminan, N.; Macdonald, R.L.L.; Steiger, H.J.H.J.; Mayer, S.A.S.A.; Aldrich, F.; Diringer, M.N.M.N.; Hoh, B.L.B.L.; Mocco, J.; Strange, P.; et al. NEWTON: Nimodipine microparticles to enhance recovery while reducing toxicity after subarachnoid hemorrhage. *Neurocrit. Care* **2015**, *23*, 274–284. [CrossRef]
5. Plontke, S.K.; Glien, A.; Rahne, T.; Mäder, K.; Salt, A.N. Controlled release dexamethasone implants in the round window niche for salvage treatment of idiopathic sudden sensorineural hearing loss. *Otol. Neurotol.* **2014**, *35*, 1168–1171. [CrossRef]
6. Mäder, K.; Lehner, E.; Liebau, A.; Plontke, S.K.S.K. Controlled drug release to the inner ear: Concepts, materials, mechanisms, and performance. *Hear. Res.* **2018**, *368*, 49–66. [CrossRef]
7. Citrome, L. Long-acting injectable antipsychotics update: Lengthening the dosing interval and expanding the diagnostic indications. *Expert Rev. Neurother.* **2017**, *17*, 1029–1043. [CrossRef]
8. Chou, Y.H.; Chu, P.C.; Wu, S.W.; Lee, J.C.; Lee, Y.H.; Sun, I.W.; Chang, C.L.; Huang, C.L.; Liu, I.C.; Tsai, C.F.; et al. A systemic review and experts' consensus for long-acting injectable antipsychot. *Clin. Psychopharmacol. Neurosci.* **2015**, *13*, 121–128. [CrossRef]
9. Available online: https://www.accessdata.fda.gov/drugsatfda_docs/label/2007/021346s015lbl.pdf (accessed on 4 December 2019).
10. Rawat, A.; Bhardwaj, U.; Burgess, D.J. Comparison of in vitro-in vivo release of Risperdal® Consta® microspheres. *Int. J. Pharm.* **2012**, *434*, 115–121. [CrossRef]
11. Shen, J.; Choi, S.; Qu, W.; Wang, Y.; Burgess, D.J. In vitro-in vivo correlation of parenteral risperidone polymeric microspheres. *J. Control. Release* **2015**, *218*, 2–12. [CrossRef]
12. Andhariya, J.V.; Shen, J.; Wang, Y.; Choi, S.; Burgess, D.J. Effect of minor manufacturing changes on stability of compositionally equivalent PLGA microspheres. *Int. J. Pharm.* **2019**, *566*, 532–540. [CrossRef] [PubMed]
13. Wu, Z.; Zhao, M.; Zhang, W.; Yang, Z.; Xu, S.; Shang, Q. Influence of drying processes on the structures, morphology and in vitro release profiles of risperidone-loaded PLGA microspheres. *J. Microencapsul.* **2019**, *36*, 21–31. [CrossRef] [PubMed]
14. Turek, A.; Borecka, A.; Janeczek, H.; Sobota, M.; Kasperczyk, J. Formulation of delivery systems with risperidone based on biodegradable terpolymers. *Int. J. Pharm.* **2018**, *548*, 159–172. [CrossRef] [PubMed]
15. Zhao, J.; Wang, L.; Fan, C.; Yu, K.; Liu, X.; Zhao, X.; Wang, D.; Liu, W.; Su, Z.; Sun, F.; et al. Development of near zero-order release PLGA-based microspheres of a novel antipsychotic. *Int. J. Pharm.* **2017**, *516*, 32–38. [CrossRef] [PubMed]
16. D'Souza, S.; Faraj, J.; Deluca, P.; D'Souza, S.; Faraj, J.; Deluca, P. Microsphere delivery of Risperidone as an alternative to combination therapy. *Eur. J. Pharm. Biopharm.* **2013**, *85*, 631–639. [CrossRef] [PubMed]
17. Vollrath, M.; Engert, J.; Winter, G. Long-term release and stability of pharmaceutical proteins delivered from solid lipid implants. *Eur. J. Pharm. Biopharm.* **2017**, *117*, 244–255. [CrossRef] [PubMed]
18. Fameau, A.-L.; Houinsou-Houssou, B.; Novales, B.; Navailles, L.; Nallet, F.; Douliez, J.-P. 12-Hydroxystearic acid lipid tubes under various experimental conditions. *J. Colloid Interface Sci.* **2010**, *341*, 38–47. [CrossRef]
19. Co, E.; Marangoni, A.G. The formation of a 12-hydroxystearic acid/vegetable oil organogel under shear and thermal fields. *J. Am. Oil Chem. Soc.* **2013**, *90*, 529–544. [CrossRef]
20. Mäder, K.; Windorf, M.; Kutza, J. Injizierbare Depotformulierungen zur Kontrollierten Wirkstofffreisetzung. WO2015062571, 29 October 2014.
21. Lampp, L.; Rogozhnikova, O.Y.; Trukhin, D.V.; Tormyshev, V.M.; Bowman, M.K.; Devasahayam, N.; Krishna, M.C.; Mäder, K.; Imming, P. A radical containing injectable in-situ-oleogel and emulgel for prolonged in-vivo oxygen measurements with CW EPR. *Free Radic. Biol. Med.* **2019**, *130*, 120–127. [CrossRef]
22. Garner, J.; Skidmore, S.; Park, H.; Park, K.; Choi, S.; Wang, Y. A protocol for assay of poly(lactide-*co*-glycolide) in clinical products. *Int. J. Pharm.* **2015**, *495*, 87–92. [CrossRef]
23. Hu, Z.; Liu, Y.; Yuan, W.; Wu, F.; Su, J.; Jin, T. Effect of bases with different solubility on the release behavior of risperidone loaded PLGA microspheres. *Colloids Surf. B Biointerfaces* **2011**, *86*, 206–211. [CrossRef] [PubMed]
24. Available online: https://www.zeiss.com/content/dam/Microscopy/us/download/pdf/technical-notes/x-ray-microscopy/en_44_013_027_tech-note_ultra-nanotomography.pdf (accessed on 4 October 2019).
25. O'Donnell, P.B.; McGinity, J.W. Preparation of microspheres by the solvent evaporation technique. *Adv. Drug Deliv. Rev.* **1997**, *28*, 25–42. [CrossRef]
26. Wischke, C.; Schwendeman, S.P. Principles of encapsulating hydrophobic drugs in PLA/PLGA microparticles. *Int. J. Pharm.* **2008**, *364*, 298–327. [CrossRef] [PubMed]

27. Han, F.Y.; Thurecht, K.J.; Whittaker, A.K.; Smith, M.T. Bioerodable PLGA-based microparticles for producing sustained-release drug formulations and strategies for improving drug loading. *Front. Pharmacol.* **2016**, *7*, 185. [CrossRef] [PubMed]
28. Barrow, W.W. Microsphere technology for chemotherapy of mycobacterial infections. *Curr. Pharm. Des.* **2004**, *10*, 3275–3284. [CrossRef] [PubMed]
29. Dawes, G.J.S.; Fratila-Apachitei, L.E.; Mulia, K.; Apachitei, I.; Witkamp, G.J.; Duszczyk, J. Size effect of PLGA spheres on drug loading efficiency and release profiles. *J. Mater. Sci. Mater. Med.* **2009**, *20*, 1089–1094. [CrossRef]
30. Anderson, J.M.; Shive, M.S. Biodegradation and biocompatibility of PLA and PLGA microspheres. *Adv. Drug Deliv. Rev.* **2012**, *64*, 72–82. [CrossRef]
31. D'Souza, S.; Faraj, J.A.; Giovagnoli, S.; DeLuca, P.P. Development of risperidone PLGA microspheres. *J. Drug Deliv.* **2014**, 620464. [CrossRef]
32. Krochmal, B.; Diller, D.; Dolitzky, B.-Z.; Aronhime, J. Preparation of Risperidone. WO2002012200A9, 8 August 2001.
33. Bagratashvili, V.N.; Bogorodskiy, S.E.; Egorov, A.M.; Krotova, L.I.; Mironov, A.V.; Parenago, O.O.; Pokrovskiy, O.I.; Ustinovich, K.B.; Chizhov, P.S.; Prokopchuk, D.I.; et al. Polymorphism of risperidone in supercritical fluid processes of micronization and encapsulation into aliphatic polyesters. *Russ. J. Phys. Chem. B* **2017**, *11*, 1163–1172. [CrossRef]
34. Karabas, I.; Orkoula, M.G.; Kontoyannis, C.G. Analysis and stability of polymorphs in tablets: The case of Risperidone. *Talanta* **2007**, *71*, 1382–1386. [CrossRef]
35. Pfeiffer, F.; Weitkamp, T.; Bunk, O.; David, C. Phase retrieval and differential phase-contrast imaging with low-brilliance X-ray sources. *Nat. Phys.* **2006**, *2*, 258–261. [CrossRef]
36. Kaulich, B.; Thibault, P.; Gianoncelli, A.; Kiskinova, M. Transmission and emission x-ray microscopy: Operation modes, contrast mechanisms and applications. *J. Phys. Condens. Matter* **2011**, *23*, 083002. [CrossRef] [PubMed]
37. Davis, T.J.; Gao, D.; Gureyev, T.E.; Stevenson, A.W.; Wilkins, S.W. Phase-contrast imaging of weakly absorbing materials using hard X-rays. *Nature* **1995**, *373*, 595–598. [CrossRef]
38. Núñez, J.A.; Goring, A.; Hesse, E.; Thurner, P.J.; Schneider, P.; Clarkin, C.E. Simultaneous visualisation of calcified bone microstructure and intracortical vasculature using synchrotron X-ray phase contrast-enhanced tomography. *Sci. Rep.* **2017**, *7*, 13289. [CrossRef] [PubMed]
39. Olivo, A.; Castelli, E. X-ray phase contrast imaging: From synchrotrons to conventional sources. *Riv. Nuovo Cim.* **2014**, *37*, 467–508.

11

Pharmacokinetic Profile and Anti-Adhesive Effect of Oxaliplatin-PLGA Microparticle-Loaded Hydrogels in Rats for Colorectal Cancer Treatment

Sharif Md Abuzar [1,2], Jun-Hyun Ahn [1,2], Kyung Su Park [3], Eun Jung Park [4,*], Seung Hyuk Baik [4,*] and Sung-Joo Hwang [1,2,*]

1 College of Pharmacy, Yonsei University, 85 Songdogwahak-ro, Yeonsu-gu, Incheon 21983, Korea
2 Yonsei Institute of Pharmaceutical Sciences, Yonsei University, 85 Songdogwahak-ro, Yeonsu-gu, Incheon 21983, Korea
3 Advanced Analysis Center, Korea Institute of Science and Technology, Hwarang-ro, Seongbuk-gu, Seoul 02792, Korea
4 Division of Colon and Rectal Surgery, Department of Surgery, Gangnam Severance Hospital, Yonsei University College of Medicine, Seoul 06273, Korea
* Correspondence: camp79@yuhs.ac (E.J.P.); whitenoja@yuhs.ac (S.H.B.); sjh11@yonsei.ac.kr (S.-J.H.)

Abstract: Colorectal cancer (CRC) is one of the most malignant and fatal cancers worldwide. Although cytoreductive surgery combined with chemotherapy is considered a promising therapy, peritoneal adhesion causes further complications after surgery. In this study, oxaliplatin-loaded Poly-(D,L-lactide-co-glycolide) (PLGA) microparticles were prepared using a double emulsion method and loaded into hyaluronic acid (HA)- and carboxymethyl cellulose sodium (CMCNa)-based cross-linked (HC) hydrogels. From characterization and evaluation study PLGA microparticles showed smaller particle size with higher entrapment efficiency, approximately 1100.4 ± 257.7 nm and 77.9 ± 2.8%, respectively. In addition, microparticle-loaded hydrogels showed more sustained drug release compared to the unloaded microparticles. Moreover, in an in vivo pharmacokinetic study after intraperitoneal administration in rats, a significant improvement in the bioavailability and the mean residence time of the microparticle-loaded hydrogels was observed. In HC21 hydrogels, $AUC_{0\text{–}48h}$, C_{max}, and T_{max} were 16012.12 ± 188.75 ng·h/mL, 528.75 ± 144.50 ng/mL, and 1.5 h, respectively. Furthermore, experimental observation revealed that the hydrogel samples effectively protected injured tissues from peritoneal adhesion. Therefore, the results of the current pharmacokinetic study together with our previous report of the in vivo anti-adhesion efficacy of HC hydrogels demonstrated that the PLGA microparticle-loaded hydrogels offer novel therapeutic strategy for CRC treatment.

Keywords: oxaliplatin; PLGA; hydrogel; intra-abdominal anti-adhesion barrier; colorectal cancer

---

1. Introduction

Colorectal cancer (CRC) is one of the most malignant cancers worldwide. Although the incidence of CRC is low, the number of new cases that are malignant and fatal is still the highest among both men and women. In addition, peritoneal carcinomatosis is one of the numerous manifestations of CRC identified at the first diagnosis in more than 10% of CRC patients, and it is extremely fatal, with median survival of approximately 6 months [1,2]. The treatment strategies for both CRC and peritoneal carcinomatosis patients depend on the type and stage, and optimal therapy comprises cytoreductive surgery combined with chemotherapy [3].

Peritoneal adhesion is one of the most common postoperative complications associated with cytoreductive surgery. Previous studies indicated their occurrence in more than 50% cases, and they have even higher recurrence rates (85–93%) [4,5]. As cytoreductive surgery and intraperitoneal chemotherapy are closely related to the completeness of cytoreduction, problems associated with cytoreductive surgery are still a big challenge in medical science. Therefore, hydrogel-based anti-adhesion barriers came into the spotlight to reduce adhesion by mechanical separation of injured tissue surfaces during peritoneal repair after surgery [6].

Oxaliplatin (Figure 1) is a third-generation, platinum-based, systemic chemotherapeutic agent for CRC [7], and it is expected to be similarly effective in peritoneal carcinomatosis. Therefore, it is currently being used as a part of the standard chemotherapy regimen, FOLFOX (oxaliplatin with 5-fluorouracil and leucovorin) [8], for the clinical treatment of metastatic CRC [9]. However, a recent study conducted in a murine model confirmed that intraperitoneally administered oxaliplatin enhanced peritoneal tissue concentration while reducing its systemic absorption, suggesting a possible decrease in toxicity associated with systemic chemotherapy [10]. Therefore, the new approach comprising cytoreductive surgery followed by intraperitoneal oxaliplatin delivery has resulted in significant improvement in the disease states of CRC and peritoneal carcinomatosis [11].

Biodegradable microparticles have been widely investigated for the controlled delivery of chemotherapeutic agents [12,13]. In addition, neither an initial burst release, nor the presence of a lag phase are desirable for the chemotherapeutic agents as it can be associated with adverse effects. Poly-(D,L-lactide-*co*-glycolide) (PLGA) is an unique copolymer approved by the regulatory agencies for the manufacturing of bioresorbable surgical sutures. Owing to its biodegradability and biocompatibility, PLGA become the first line materials for the production of injectable microparticle based controlled release system [14]. A recent report of metformin/irinotecan-loaded nanoparticles have shown an initial 2 h burst release, however, increase the drug retention time in tumor and increase drug circulation [15]. Moreover, alternative reports of paclitaxel-loaded PLGA microparticles have been evaluated for cancer therapy. These models revealed protection of the therapeutic payload from premature burst release, and enable the sustained release of paclitaxel [16,17].

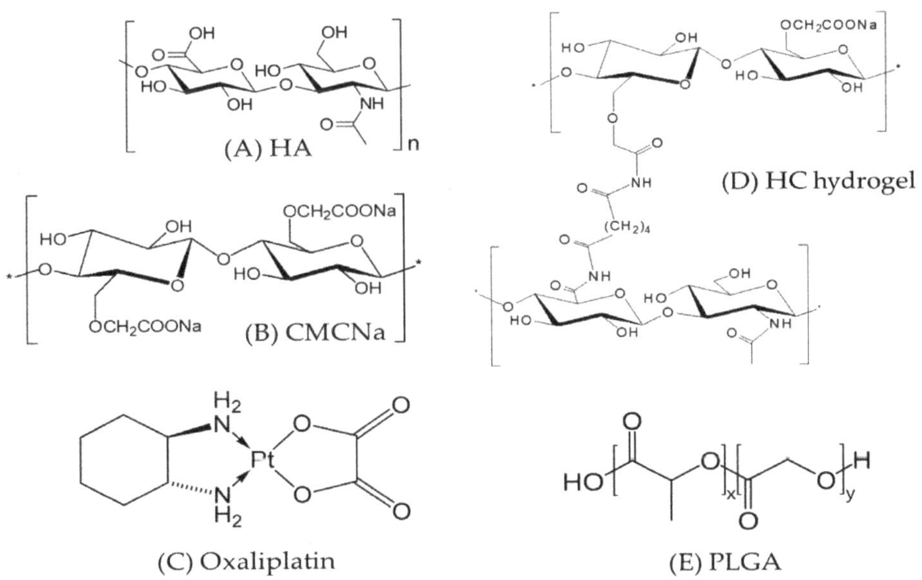

Figure 1. Chemical structures of Poly-(D,L-lactide-*co*-glycolide) (PLGA) microparticles and hyaluronic acid (HA) and carboxymethyl cellulose sodium (CMCNa)-based cross-linked (HC) hydrogel components (**A**) HA; (**B**) CMCNa; (**C**) HC hydrogel; (**D**) Oxaliplatin; and (**E**) PLGA.

Recently we succeeded in synthesizing novel hyaluronic acid (HA) and carboxymethyl cellulose sodium (CMCNa)-based cross-linked (HC) hydrogels loaded with oxaliplatin [18]. These novel HC hydrogels significantly prevented intraperitoneal adhesion and offered the highest anti-adhesion barrier in an in vivo rat model. However, pharmacokinetic evaluation of oxaliplatin-loaded HC hydrogels was not carried out. Several reports of microparticles-loaded hydrogels in various drug delivery system showed controlled drug release for over a prolonged period [19,20]. Therefore, to provide an adequate anti-adhesion barrier effect after cytoreductive surgery and deliver intraperitoneal chemotherapy, oxaliplatin-loaded PLGA microparticles were prepared, characterized, and loaded into HC hydrogels. In addition, an in vitro oxaliplatin release study of PLGA microparticle-loaded HC hydrogels in comparison with that of commercially available Guardix-Sol® hydrogel was carried out. Furthermore, in vivo pharmacokinetic analysis was carried out to demonstrate the efficacy of intraperitoneal chemotherapy with oxaliplatin-PLGA microparticles loaded into HC hydrogels.

2. Materials and Methods

2.1. Materials and Animals

Oxaliplatin was a gift from Boryung Pharm (Ansan, Korea). Resomer® RG 502 H (Poly-(D,L-lactide-*co*-glycolide)) PLGA, molecular weight (MW) approximately 7000–17,000, was purchased from Evonic Ind., (Darmstadt, Germany). Hyaluronic acid (HA, MW 1000 kDa) was a gift from Huons (Seongnam, Korea). Poly-(vinyl alcohol) (PVA, MW approximately 89,000–98,000), carboxymethyl cellulose sodium (CMCNa, MW approximately 700 kDa), and adipic acid dihydrazide (ADH) were obtained from Sigma Aldrich (St. Louis, MO, USA). 1-Ethyl-3-(3-(dimethylaminopropyl) carbodiimide (EDC) was purchased from Tokyo Chemical (Tokyo, Japan). All other chemicals were of reagent grade, and Milli-Q® water (Millipore1, Molsheim, France) was used throughout the study.

Male Sprague-Dawley (SD) rats were purchased from YoungBio (Seongnam, Republic of Korea). The animals were housed in a semi-specific pathogen free facility using standard cages at 19 ± 1 °C and 50 ± 5% relative humidity, with a 12-h light-dark cycle. The rats were fed a standard diet, provided with purified water, and allowed to move freely. All experiments were approved by the Institutional Animal Care and Use Committee (IACUC-201809-788-01) at Yonsei University, Seoul, Korea, and were performed according to IACUC guidelines.

2.2. Preparation of Oxaliplatin-PLGA Microparticles

Oxaliplatin-PLGA microparticles were prepared using a double emulsion method [21]. Briefly, oxaliplatin (20 mg) was dissolved in 5 mL of deionized water (first aqueous solution, W_1) containing 0.5% (*w/v*) PVA. The resulting oxaliplatin containing W_1 was added dropwise to 12.5 mL DCM, containing 1 g of PLGA 502 H, using a homogenizer ULTRA-TURRAX® (IKA-WERKE GMBH & Co. KG, Staufen, Germany) at 12,000 rpm for 2 min. This primary emulsion (W_1/O) was slowly added to 100 mL of 1% (*w/v*) PVA solution (second aqueous solution, W_2) and emulsified at 400 rpm using magnetic stirrer for 3 h while the DCM was allowed to evaporate completely under vacuum. The resultant microparticles were collected, washed using distilled water, centrifuged, and freeze-dried using an ilShinBioBase (Seoul, Korea) freeze-drier under vacuum (5 mTorr). Samples were pre-frozen for 2 h at −60 ± 1.0 °C prior to final drying at −88 ± 1.0 °C for 2 days. The collected freeze-dried microparticles were stored at 4 °C and further evaluated by scanning electronic microscopy (SEM) to characterize the morphological features.

2.3. Synthesis of HA-CMCNa Cross-Linked Hydrogels

Hydrogels were synthesized using variable ratios of HA and CMCNa (Figure 1) by chemical cross-linking, as described by our previous study [18]. Briefly, HA and CMCNa at ratios of 1:2 and 2:1 (*w/w*) were dissolved in deionized water with continuous stirring. After complete dissolution, 2 mM/L of ADH was added to the mixture, and the pH was adjusted to 4.75 ± 0.05 using 0.1 M HCl. After vortex mixing for 1 min, 2 mM/L EDC was added, and the resulting mixture was stirred thoroughly at room temperature (25 ± 1.0 °C) for at least 12 h to allow for complete cross-linking. The reaction was maintained at pH 4.75 ± 0.05 by the addition of 0.1 M HCl. Finally, the cross-linking reaction was terminated by elevating the pH of the mixture to 7.0 ± 0.05 via the slow addition of 0.1 M NaOH. The hydrogel samples were purified as previously described by Luo et al. [22]. Briefly, the hydrogel samples were dispensed into a dialysis bag (Mw cut-off 18,000 Da) previously treated with a 70% ethanol (EtOH) solution and dried. The bag was submerged and dialyzed for 12 h in 0.1 M NaCl followed by alternating solutions of 25% EtOH for 6 h and DW for 6 h. The remaining hydrogels in the dialysis bag were rinsed using EtOH, and then centrifuged at 2000 rpm for 10 min to remove the remaining ADH. Finally, the precipitated hydrogels (HC12 and HC21) were collected and stored until further experiments.

2.4. *Preparation of Oxaliplatin-PLGA Microparticle-Loaded Hydrogel*

Guardix-Sol® is a commercial anti-adhesive hydrogel used for the prevention of post-operative adhesion. Above, we synthesized HC12 and HC21 hydrogel composites with variable weight ratios of HA and CMCNa. Next, oxaliplatin-PLGA microparticles were dispersed gently in the hydrogel (HC12, HC21, and Guardix-Sol®). Briefly, precisely weighed oxaliplatin-PLGA microparticles were mixed with 10 mL of hydrogels at room temperature (25 ± 1.0 °C) with continuous stirring for 30 min. The final concentration of oxaliplatin was 2 mg/ mL of hydrogel. After complete dissolution was visually observed, samples were evaluated for in vitro and in vivo release of oxaliplatin.

2.5. *Characterization of Oxaliplatin-PLGA Microparticles*

2.5.1. Morphology

The morphology of oxaliplatin-PLGA microparticles was evaluated using SEM (JSM-6700F, JEOL, Tokyo, Japan). Briefly, a small amount of powder was sprinkled onto double-sided adhesive tape attached to an aluminum stub and was sputter-coated with gold under vacuum. Photographs were taken at 5× magnification with an accelerating voltage of 1–5 kV to reveal the surface characteristics of the particles.

2.5.2. Particle Size Analysis

The mean particle size and distribution of oxaliplatin-PLGA microparticles were analyzed by dynamic light scattering (DLS) using an electrophoretic light scattering spectrophotometer (ELS-Z, Otsuka Electronics, Hirakata, Japan).

2.5.3. Rheological Measurements

The rheological measurements for HC12, HC21, and Guardix-Sol® hydrogels were performed using a Brookfield rheometer (Brookfield Digital Rheometer Model DV-III, DV3T™ Rheometer, Middleboro, MA, USA) equipped with a Peltier system for temperature control. Precisely, about 0.5 g of sample was applied to the plate and allowed to equilibrate. Measurements were performed at 37 ± 0.5 °C with shear rates ranging from 200–500 s^{-1}. Before each measurement, the samples were allowed to rest for 5 min at 37 ± 0.5 °C. Results were analyzed with Brookfield software (Firmware version 1.2.2-9).

2.5.4. Encapsulation Efficiency

Freeze-dried oxaliplatin-PLGA microparticles (eq. 2 mg of oxaliplatin) were dissolved in 5 mL of DCM. After 5 min of vortexing, particles were allowed to dissolve properly, and the tube was gently swung in incubator at 37 ± 0.5 °C for 1 h. Then, 5 mL of DW was added to the tube and vortexed vigorously for 1 h. The suspension was centrifuged at 12,000 rpm for 5 min to precipitate PLGA. The upper aqueous phase was collected, and the concentration of oxaliplatin was determined by HPLC. Encapsulation efficiency (EE %) was calculated using the following Equation (1):

$$EE\ \% = M_{\text{actual oxaliplatin}}/M_{\text{theoretical oxaliplatin}} \times 100 \quad (1)$$

2.6. *In Vitro Oxaliplatin Release from PLGA Microparticles Loaded into Hydrogels*

To evaluate the in vitro oxaliplatin release rate from oxaliplatin-PLGA microparticles, an amount equivalent to 2 mg of oxaliplatin was weighed and suspended in 1 mL of HPLC grade water. The suspension was transferred into dialysis bags (MWCO 14,000) and then submerged in 20 mL of double distilled water in capped 50 mL Falcon® tube. Samples were shaken at 30 rpm at the predetermined time points (1, 2, 3, 4, 6, 8, and 12 h); 1 mL of sample was collected from the medium and 1 mL of pre-warmed medium was immediately added to the tubes. Experiments were performed in triplicate (n = 3), and the collected samples were analyzed with HPLC after necessary dilution. The release profile was expressed as the ratio of cumulative oxaliplatin release to initial oxaliplatin loading versus time, using the following Equation (2):

$$\text{Percent of oxaliplatin release} = M_t/M_0 \times 100 \quad (2)$$

For the in vitro oxaliplatin release from the PLGA microparticle-loaded hydrogels (from Section 2.4.), a similar method was used. Briefly, 1 mL PLGA microparticle-loaded hydrogel (HC12, HC21, or Guardix-Sol®) was transferred to one end-closed dialysis bags (MWCO 14,000). The other end of the bag was closed properly, and the samples were submerged in 20 mL of double distilled water in capped 50 mL Falcon® tube. Samples were shaken at 30 rpm at similar time points (1, 2, 3, 4, 6, 8, and 12 h). Subsequently, 1 mL of sample was collected from the medium and 1 mL of pre-warmed medium was immediately added to the tubes. Experiments were performed in triplicate (n = 3), and the collected samples were analyzed with HPLC after necessary dilution with the mobile phase. The release profile was expressed as cumulative oxaliplatin release calculated using Equation (2).

2.7. *In Vivo Oxaliplatin Release in SD Rat's Intraperitoneal Cavity*

In vivo oxaliplatin release from the prepared hydrogels was evaluated in the intraperitoneal cavity of SD rats, and oxaliplatin solution was also evaluated for comparison. Briefly, a total of fifteen male SD rats, aged 4–6 weeks, were randomly divided into three groups (n = 5, per group) and were anesthetized with isoflurane. Intra-abdominal adhesions were induced to mimic the postoperative surgical conditions, as described previously [23]. The peritoneum was exposed by a 5-cm ventral midline incision. The left abdominal sidewall was scraped with a 1 cm^2 piece of 100-grit sandpaper 200 times. In group 1, oxaliplatin solution was introduced, whereas, group 2 and 3 were exposed to oxaliplatin powder and oxaliplatin-PLGA microparticles, loaded into HC21 hydrogel, respectively. All the rats from each group were administered oxaliplatin in the form of a solution or loaded into hydrogel at a dose level of 5 mg/kg body weight [24]. The abdominal layers and skin incision were then completely closed, and each rat was kept separately in single cases. All surgeries were performed by the same individual. At predetermined time interval (0.5, 1, 1.5, 2, 3, 5, 8, 14, 24, and 48 h), approximately 1-mL blood samples were collected from the conjunctiva using a capillary tube and kept in an ice bath.

Blood samples collected from the rat's conjunctiva were centrifuged at 10,000 rpm (9425× *g*) for 10 min at 4 °C. The supernatant plasma was obtained and stored at −80 °C until analyzed. The frozen plasma samples were thawed, and approximately 200 ± 5 mg was weighed. The samples were oxidized into metals and organic materials by treating with 6 mL nitric acid using a microwave sample pre-treatment machine equipped with platinum (Pt) sensor (Microwave Reaction System, Multi-wave PRO, Anton Paar, Graz, Austria). Samples were heated at predefined temperature and pressure (200 ± 0.5 °C and 4.0 MPa) for 1 h and diluted up to 30 mL with deionized water, and the concentrations of Pt were analyzed using ICP-MS (NexION 300 D, PerkinElmer, Waltham, MA, USA). Pharmacokinetic parameters AUC_{0-48h} (area under curve), C_{max} (peak concentration), and T_{max} (time to peak concentration) were calculated using noncompartmental analysis.

After the last blood sample collection at 48 h, rats were housed individually in standard case with a 12-h light-dark cycle. The rats were fed a standard diet, provided with purified water, and were allowed to move freely. After 10 days, they were sacrificed, and the peritoneum was opened. For all rats, adhesion type and extent were assessed, and photographs were taken.

2.8. *High-Performance Liquid Chromatography (HPLC) Analysis*

In vitro oxaliplatin release and % EE were determined by using HPLC Agilent 1200 Infinity Series HPLC system (Agilent Technologies, Waldbronn, Germany). Briefly, XTerra™ RPC_{18} column (particle size 5 µm, inside diameter 4.6 mm, and length 250 mm; Waters Corporation, Milford, MA, USA) at 210 nm using an HPLC-UV spectrometer (Agilent 1290 infinity). The mobile phase was a 20:80 mixture of ACN and deionized water and was set to a flow rate of 0.8 mL/min (Model 1260 Quat Pump VL). The samples were diluted as necessary, and 20 µL of each sample was injected using an autosampler (Model 1260 ALS).2.9. Statistical Analysis

In vitro percent (%) cumulative oxaliplatin release and in vivo pharmacokinetic study data are expressed as the means ± standard deviations. The *t*-test or two-sided RM ANOVA and Bonferroni test were applied to the analyses of the differences between the groups. A p value < 0.05 was considered as a statistically significant difference.

3. Results and Discussion

3.1. *Characterization of PLGA Microparticles*

PLGA-based microparticles were prepared using the double emulsion method. The microparticles were characterized for size, morphology, and encapsulation efficiency. As shown in Table 1, oxaliplatin-loaded PLGA microparticles had a particle size of more than 1 µm diameter, with a small standard deviation. Encapsulation efficiency was 77.9 ± 2.8%, which is excellent for a hydrophilic drug like oxaliplatin. Although the encapsulation of hydrophilic drugs in PLGA microparticles is challenging due to the partitioning of weakly associated drugs from the oil phases to the external water phase, the double emulsion technique is the most commonly used method for encapsulating hydrophilic drugs. In addition, the SEM image shown in Figure 2A reveals the morphology of the microparticles. Uniform size and spherical particles were observed, which is in agreement with the particle size results. To fulfill the aims of this study, PLGA microparticles were further loaded into HC hydrogels and the in vitro release and in vivo pharmacokinetic studies were conducted.

Table 1. Compositions and characterizations of Poly-(D,L-lactide-*co*-glycolide) (PLGA) microparticles and hyaluronic acid (HA) and carboxymethyl cellulose sodium (CMCNa)-based cross-linked (HC) hydrogels.

Particles	Method	Weight Ratio				Particle Size (nm) (Mean ± SD)	Encapsulation Efficiency (%) (Mean ± SD)
		Oxaliplatin	PLGA 502 H	HA	CMCNa		
Oxaliplatin-PLGA Microparticles	Double Emulsion	1	50	-	-	1100.4 ± 257.7	77.9 ± 2.8
HC12 Hydrogel	Synthesis by cross-linking reaction	-	-	1	2	-	-
HC21 Hydrogel		-	-	2	1	-	-

3.2. *Preparation and Characterization of HC Hydrogels*

Cross-linked HC hydrogels were prepared using variable weight ratios of HA and CMCNa. HC hydrogel synthesis was carried out based on our previous description [18]. In the presence of ADH (as a nucleophile), EDC (a water-soluble carbodiimide) linked both HA and CMCNa molecules with its amine group. EDC is not incorporated into the final product, but converts into a non-toxic water-soluble urea derivative, which is removed by dialysis. Moreover, CH_2COO^-anions provided by CMCNa react with H^+ ions, leading to carboxyl group formation and facilitation of cross-linking. Therefore, the reaction in the presence of EDC is pH-dependent and was performed at pH 4.75 ± 0.05.

To evaluate the rheology of the HC hydrogel along with the commercial product Guardix-Sol®, a Brookfield Digital Rheometer was used. All measurements were performed at 37 ± 0.5 °C, with shear rates ranging from 200 to 500 s^{-1}. All hydrogels followed non-Newtonian shear thinning (pseudo) plastic flow behavior (Figure 2B). Decreasing viscosity with increasing shear rates was observed, which demonstrated viscosity-dependent shear rates [25].

In addition, variable ratios of the composition (HA and CMCNa) alter the viscosity of the HC hydrogels. The order could be written as follows: HC21 > HC12, as markedly increased viscosity was observed with HA. The highest viscosity was observed with the HC21 formulation, whereas the lowest viscosity was observed with HC12. The viscosity of Guardix-Sol® was measured for comparison with those of the synthesized HC hydrogels, and it showed moderate viscosity. The rheology results correlated with the mechanical characteristics of the polymer, in which viscosity scaled linearly with molecular weight. The mechanical properties (entanglement phenomenon) of the polymers increased with increasing molecular weight. Finally, the hydrogels were loaded with oxaliplatin-PLGA microparticles and their in vitro and in vivo characteristics were evaluated.

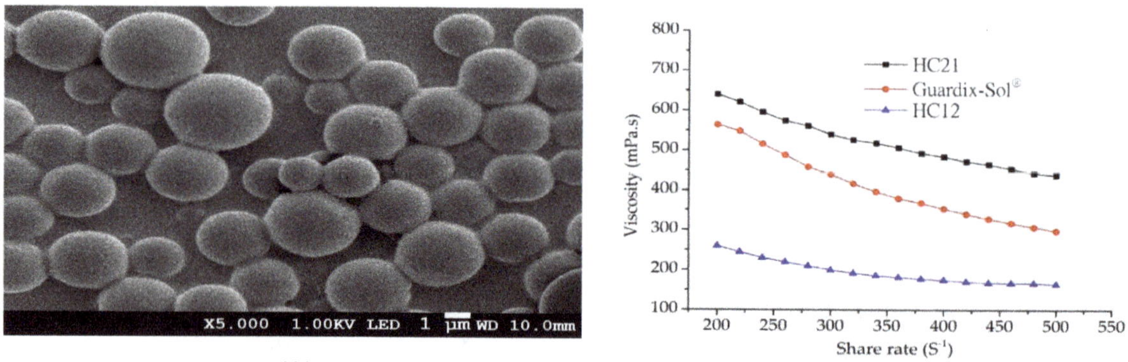

(A) (B)

Figure 2. (**A**) SEM image of oxaliplatin-PLGA microparticles (at X5.000 magnification); (B) rheology properties of hydrogel samples (■) HC21, (●) Guardix-Sol®, and (▲) HC12 (measurements were performed at 37 ± 0.5 °C).

3.3. *In Vitro Oxaliplatin Release Study*

An in vitro oxaliplatin release study was conducted on oxaliplatin-PLGA microparticles generated using the double emulsion method. In addition, oxaliplatin-PLGA microparticles and oxaliplatin powder were dispersed into hydrogels (HC12, HC21, and Guardix-Sol®), and an in vitro oxaliplatin release study was conducted. Plots of cumulative oxaliplatin release (%) versus time (h) are shown in Figure 3A–C. In vitro release profile for oxaliplatin-PLGA microparticles (red closed circle; (●) showed immediate release. With an initial burst release, about 63.2% oxaliplatin was released at 4 h. Oxaliplatin release from PLGA microparticles is a combination of diffusion and bioerosion mechanism [26]. During the diffusion stage, oxaliplatin release occurs by diffusion through aqueous channels. The release could also be triggered by the external pores on the surface or through leaching of the oxaliplatin at or near the surface, leading to an initial burst release. Besides, the standard deviation values of the results of the in vitro release study for the hydrogels were low, which indicate excellent reproducibility of the release behavior. However, when oxaliplatin-PLGA microparticles were loaded into three different hydrogel systems, HC12, HC21, and Guardix-Sol®, slight initial burst release was observed. Although the rate of burst release was almost the same for the three systems, HC12, with the lowest viscosity, showed the maximum release. In contrast, the higher the viscosity of the hydrogel system, the lower the burst and sustained release observed. This may be due to low leaching of the drugs and high protection of the microparticles by the hydrogels.

Table 2 demonstrated the kinetic models adopted for evaluation. Where M_t was the cumulative drug released at time t and M was the initial drug present in the PLGA microparticles-loaded hydrogels. k_1, k_H, and k_{KP} are the first order, Higuchi, and Korsmeyer-Peppas release constant, respectively.

M_t/M_∞ was the fraction of drug released at time t, and n was the diffusional release exponent symbolic of the release mechanism. The rate of oxaliplatin release from the HC12, Guardix-Sol® and HC21-loaded PLGA microparticles were slower and constant compared with the oxaliplatin powder-loaded hydrogels, as indicated by the K_H values of 18.9686, 17.5626, and 20.6559% $h^{1/2}$, respectively. Release constants were determined using the slope of the appropriate plots, and the regression coefficient (R^2) was obtained through linear regression analysis (Table 2). The coefficient of determination (R^2) was used as an indicator of curve fit for each of the considered models [27]. The regression coefficients R^2, from the Korsmeyer-Peppas plots were 0.9342, 0.9554, and 0.9366 for HC12, Guardix-Sol® and HC21, respectively, thus the log of cumulative drug release was proportional to the log of time. The best linear fits were observed for the PLGA microparticles-loaded hydrogels using both the Higuchi and Korsmeyer-Peppas models, suggesting that oxaliplatin release from the PLGA microparticles-loaded hydrogels were diffusive process. Oxaliplatin gradually dissolved into the fluid within the swelled hydrogels, then slowly diffused from polymeric networks of the hydrogels.

Table 2. Release rate constants and regression coefficient R^2 obtained from drug release profile based on kinetic equations.

Equations	Loaded in HC12 Hydrogel		Loaded in Guardix-Sol® Hydrogel		Loaded in HC21 Hydrogel		PLGA Microparticle
	Oxaliplatin Powder	PLGA Microparticle	Oxaliplatin Powder	PLGA Microparticle	Oxaliplatin Powder	PLGA Microparticle	
[a] Higuchi model: k_H (% $h^{1/2}$)	28.5970	18.9686	22.1635	17.5626	24.3401	20.6559	20.0882
R^2	0.6738	0.9611	0.7431	0.9783	0.7746	0.9485	0.8026
[b] First—Order model: k_1 (h^{-1})	0.0302	0.0421	0.0263	0.0469	0.0379	0.0522	0.0219
R^2	0.1639	0.6646	0.2327	0.7224	0.2640	0.6451	0.4145
[c] Korsmeyer—Peppas model: k_{KP}	0.4517	0.5033	0.3750	0.5475	0.5352	0.6308	0.2884
R^2	0.5495	0.9342	0.6099	0.9554	0.6512	0.9366	0.7767

[a] Higuchi model: ($Mt = k_H \times t^{1/2}$); [b] First—Order model: ($\ln M_t = \ln M + k_1 \times t$); [c] Korsmeyer—Peppas model: ($Mt/M\infty = k_{KP} \times t^n$).

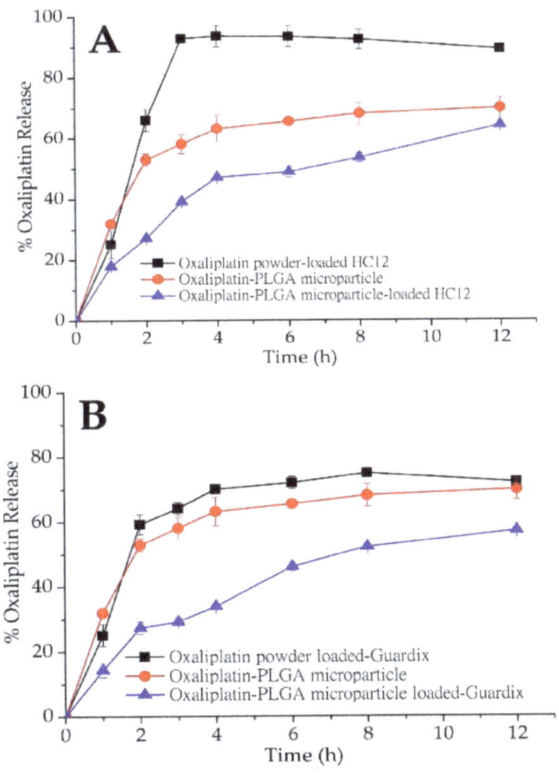

Figure 3. *Cont.*

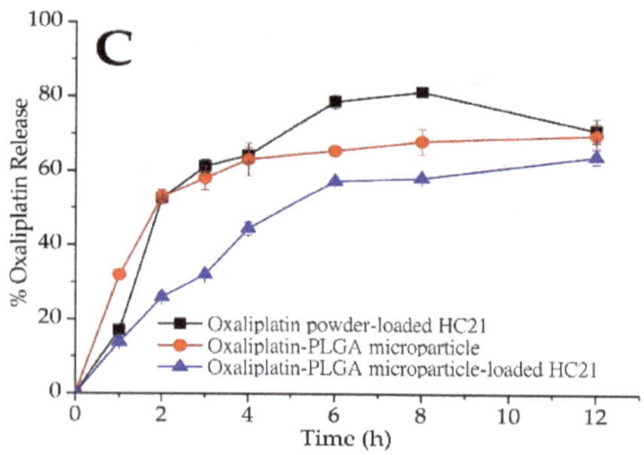

Figure 3. In vitro oxaliplatin release from PLGA microparticles (red, ●). Oxaliplatin release profile from oxaliplatin powder and oxaliplatin-PLGA microparticles-loaded in (**A**) HC12; (**B**) Guardix-Sol®; and (**C**) HC21 hydrogel. Mean ± S.D. (n = 3).

Although hydrogels are swellable materials with high water content, which readily allow the release or leaching of hydrophilic drugs through the channels, high viscosity might hinder this process. Therefore, release may be completed through bioerosion. In this study, three different hydrogel systems—HC12, HC21, and Guardix-Sol®, were loaded with oxaliplatin powder and oxaliplatin-PLGA microparticles. The HC12 hydrogel system (low viscosity) was loaded with oxaliplatin powder and more than 90% oxaliplatin release occurred within 3 h, followed by saturated release behavior up to 12 h. However, oxaliplatin-PLGA microparticles loaded into the HC12 hydrogel showed a slower release pattern than that of the oxaliplatin powder. Approximately 50% oxaliplatin was released after 4 h, followed by 64.2% release up to the end of the experiment ($p < 0.05$). Due to the less hydrophilicity of the PLGA copolymers, they absorb less water, and subsequently degrade more slowly. Therefore, drug release from the PLGA microparticles was delayed. In the case of Guardix-Sol®, with moderate viscosity, a sustained release profile was observed for the oxaliplatin-PLGA microparticles. During the first 2 h of the release study, less than 30% of oxaliplatin was released; however, 59.25% of oxaliplatin was released after the same amount of time when loaded with oxaliplatin powder ($p < 0.05$).

In addition, the HC21 hydrogel system (high viscosity) showed a similar sustained release profile when loaded with oxaliplatin-PLGA microparticles. In all three systems, more rapid oxaliplatin release was observed when oxaliplatin was loaded as a powder compared to that when loaded as microparticles. The release rate was faster than those of both oxaliplatin-PLGA microparticles and oxaliplatin-PLGA microparticles-loaded hydrogels. Additionally, both Guardix-Sol® and HC21 showed similar sustained release patterns up to 12 h. Although PLGA microparticles were generated using the well-known double emulsion method, further studies are necessary to establish process parameters and extensive characterization of the particles.

3.4. Pharmacokinetics in Rats

The bioavailability of oxaliplatin-PLGA microparticles loaded into the HC21 hydrogel was evaluated in rats. Figure 4 shows the mean concentration–time profiles of oxaliplatin in rats after a single dose (5 mg/kg) of oxaliplatin solution, oxaliplatin-PLGA microparticles, and oxaliplatin powder loaded into the HC21 hydrogel. The samples were introduced through a midline incision to open the peritoneum immediately after introducing intra-abdominal adhesions by multiple scraping to mimic postoperative surgical conditions. Intraperitoneal absorption of oxaliplatin solution was obviously higher than that of the hydrogel loaded samples (oxaliplatin-PLGA microparticles and oxaliplatin powder). For oxaliplatin solution $AUC_{0–48h}$, C_{max}, and T_{max} were 8181.51 ± 176.89 ng·h/mL, 2265.28 ± 192.51 ng/mL, and 1.0 h, respectively. In the case of oxaliplatin powder loaded into the HC21 hydrogel, $AUC_{0–48h}$, C_{max}, and T_{max} were 16,571.37 ± 139.13 ng·h/mL, 690.63 ± 140.54 ng/mL, and 1.5 h, respectively. Intraperitoneal bioavailability of oxaliplatin was significantly increased by up to 2-fold in the HC21 hydrogel (Table 3). In particular, 1.9-fold higher bioavailability was observed in the case of oxaliplatin-PLGA microparticles loaded into the HC21 hydrogel compared to that of the oxaliplatin solution. AUC_{0-48h}, C_{max}, and T_{max} were 16,012.12 ± 188.75 ng·h/mL, 528.75 ± 144.50 ng/mL, and 1.5 h, respectively. Moreover, mean residence time (MRT) was increased by 2.7-fold for oxaliplatin-PLGA microparticles when loaded into the HC21 hydrogels ($p < 0.05$). When the oxaliplatin-PLGA microparticles were loaded into the HC21 hydrogel, oxaliplatin release rate decreased due to the multi-layered encapsulation, which was observed from the in vitro release study. Therefore, in the high, moderate, and low viscous hydrogels (HC21, Guardix-Sol®, and HC12, respectively), oxaliplatin release from the PLGA microparticles, followed by release from the hydrogels, was observed in a sustained manner (Figure 3). Furthermore, using sustained-release hydrogels allows a longer residence time of the component at the application site (intraperitoneal after cytoreductive surgery), which offers additional benefits through the prevention of intra-abdominal adhesion and improvement in the delivery of intraperitoneal oxaliplatin from the PLGA microparticles.

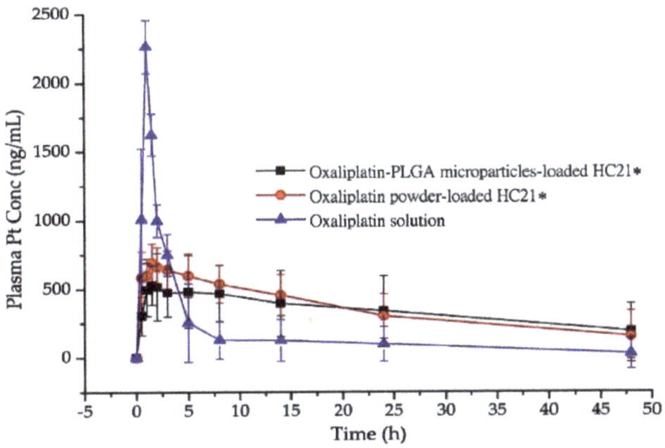

Figure 4. Plasma concentration-time profile of Pt in rats after intra-peritoneal administration of oxaliplatin powder and oxaliplatin-PLGA microparticles-loaded in HC21 hydrogel, and oxaliplatin solution. Data are expressed as the Mean ± standard deviation (n = 5). *, $p < 0.05$ represents a significant difference, two-sided RM ANOVA and Bonferroni test.

Table 3. In vivo pharmacokinetic parameters after intra-peritoneal administration to rats (n = 5).

Formulations	Pharmacokinetic Parameters			
	C_{max} (ng/mL)	T_{max} (h)	AUC_{0-48h} (ng·h/mL)	MRT (h)
Oxaliplatin solution	2265.28 ± 192.51	1	8181.51 ± 176.89	4.36 ± 0.65
Oxaliplatin powder loaded HC21	690.63 ± 140.54	1.5	16571.37 ± 139.13	10.29 ± 0.33
Oxaliplatin-PLGA microparticle loaded HC21	528.75 ± 144.50	1.5	16012.12 ± 188.75	12.02 ± 0.41

3.5. Intraperitoneal Anti-Adhesion Effect

An extensive investigation of the intraperitoneal anti-adhesion efficacy of HC hydrogels was conducted in our previous study, after introducing peritoneal injury to generate peritoneal adhesion [18]. HC hydrogel groups (treated) showed the highest anti-adhesion barrier compared to the control group (non-treated). In the present study, the pharmacokinetic parameters of the PLGA microparticles loaded into the HC21 hydrogel were evaluated and compared with those of oxaliplatin powder loaded into hydrogels. Artificial injury on the left abdominal sidewall was introduced to mimic surgical conditions and observe the anti-adhesion barrier effect of hydrogel samples followed by the intraperitoneal delivery of oxaliplatin. The method was adopted from experienced surgeons certainly feasible in human administration after cytoreductive surgery in colorectal cancer treatment. Intraperitoneal anti-adhesion effect was observed and recorded photographically. Figure 5 shows a photographical representation of adhesion characteristics of the study groups.

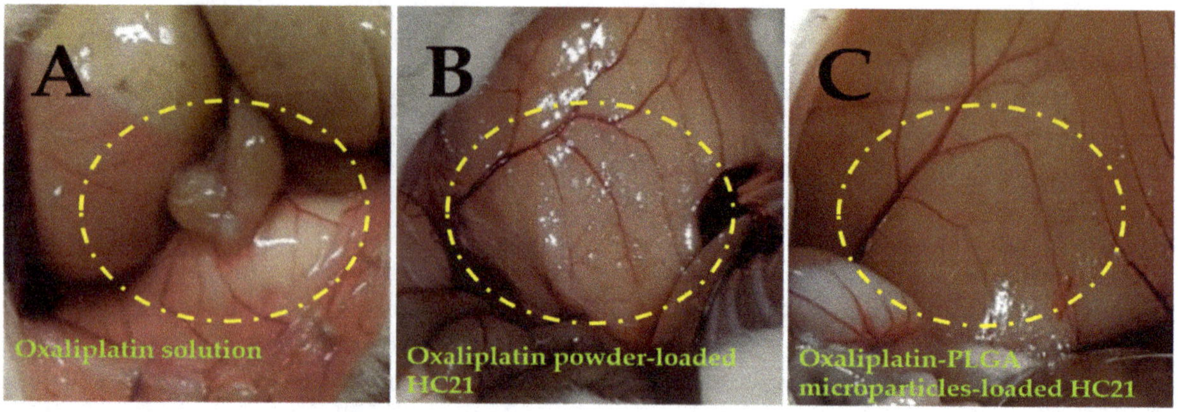

Figure 5. Photographical expression of in vivo anti-adhesion efficacy observed in rats after introducing intra-peritoneal injury. (**A**) oxaliplatin solution; (**B**) oxaliplatin powder-loaded HC21 hydrogel; and (**C**) oxaliplatin-PLGA microparticles-loaded HC21 hydrogel.

HC21 hydrogel samples exhibited an efficient anti-adhesion barrier effect towards the injury. Although hydrogels were not intended to cure the injury, long resident time hydrogels significantly prevented adhesion along with rapid recovery of the injury, possibly due to mechanical separation from the injury site [28]. As reported previously, the washing away or displacement of the oxaliplatin solution from the application site allows less barrier or protection to the injury site [29]. Therefore, dense adhesion on the abdominal wall was observed, and, although current study was not intended to be carried out extensively, adhesion scoring and extent (as disclosed in a previous report) and photographic representation demonstrated the superiority of the hydrogels in terms of the anti-adhesion barrier. In the hydrogel-loaded samples, no or minor adhesion was observed in the treated rat abdomen (Figure 5B,C). Although two different samples were evaluated after loaded in HC21 hydrogel both oxaliplatin powder and oxaliplatin-PLGA microparticles loaded hydrogels showed significant improvement as anti-adhesion barrier. Subsequently, both hydrogel systems showed rapid wound recovery effect may be due to mechanical separation- could be seen from the blood spot in Figure 5C. Instead, oxaliplatin solution presents no barrier to the injure site and dense abdominal adhesion was observed. The HC21 hydrogel-loaded sample showed enhanced anti-adhesion protection to the injury site, suggesting its potential therapeutic application in CRC patients who have undergone cytoreductive surgery. Although the current study evaluated the pharmacokinetic profile of PLGA microparticle-loaded HC hydrogels, a further pharmacodynamics study on a CRC model is required to evaluate the composition of the hydrogels.

4. Conclusions

Oxaliplatin-PLGA microparticles were loaded into hydrogels to improve intraperitoneal chemotherapy with an anti-adhesion barrier effect. In an in vitro release study, we observed sustained oxaliplatin release from PLGA microparticles loaded into hydrogels in comparison with the unloaded sample. Moreover, in the in vivo pharmacokinetics study on rats, PLGA microparticle-loaded hydrogels showed higher bioavailability compared to oxaliplatin solution. Furthermore, visual observations revealed that the HC hydrogels were effective as an intra-abdominal anti-adhesion barrier. Therefore, intraperitoneal delivery of PLGA microparticle-loaded hydrogels, which have an effective intra-abdominal anti-adhesion barrier, is expected to provide an optimized alternative therapy for CRC. Earlier reports of cytotoxicity study for PLGA (RG502H) microparticles exhibited non-cytotoxic at increasing concentration [30]. Additionally, both HA and CMCNa are considered as inert and non-cytotoxic. However, cytotoxicity profile for the novel oxaliplatin-PLGA microparticles-loaded HC hydrogels were yet to revealed. As the investigation undertaken in current study was preliminary, pharmacokinetic and anti-adhesion efficacy of this multi-complex drug delivery system, further studies are required to address cytotoxicity, cell viability, toxicity in liver function, and efficacy in CRC model in vivo.

Author Contributions: Conceptualization, S.M.A., J.-H.A.; Analytical Support, S.M.A., K.S.P.; Methodology, J.-H.A., E.J.P.; Writing—Original Draft Preparation, S.M.A.; Writing—Review and Editing, J.-H.A., E.J.P., S.-J.H., S.H.B.; Supervision, S.H.B., S.-J.H.; Project Administrator, S.-J.H.

Acknowledgments: The authors would like to acknowledge Yonsei Center for Research Facilities (YCRF, Seoul, Korea), Yonsei University for writing assistance.

References

1. Verwaal, V.J.; van Ruth, S.; Witkamp, A.; Boot, H.; van Slooten, G.; Zoetmulder, F.A.N. Long-term survival of peritoneal carcinomatosis of colorectal origin. *Ann. Surg. Oncol.* **2005**, *12*, 65–71. [CrossRef] [PubMed]
2. Koppe, M.J.; Boerman, O.C.; Oyen, W.J.G.; Bleichrodt, R.P. Peritoneal carcinomatosis of colorectal origin—Incidence and current treatment strategies. *Ann. Surg.* **2006**, *243*, 212–222. [CrossRef] [PubMed]
3. Verwaal, V.J.; van Ruth, S.; de Bree, E.; van Slooten, G.W.; van Tinteren, H.; Boot, H.; Zoetmulder, F.A.N. Randomized trial of cytoreduction and hyperthermic intraperitoneal chemotherapy versus systemic chemotherapy and palliative surgery in patients with peritoneal carcinomatosis of colorectal cancer. *J. Clin. Oncol.* **2003**, *21*, 3737–3743. [CrossRef] [PubMed]
4. Diamond, M.P.; Freeman, M.L. Clinical implications of postsurgical adhesions. *Hum. Reprod. Update* **2001**, *7*, 567–576. [CrossRef] [PubMed]
5. Dizerega, G.S. Contemporary Adhesion Prevention. *Fertil. Steril.* **1994**, *61*, 219–235. [CrossRef]
6. Oh, A. Trends of anti-adhesion adjuvant—Review. *Biomater. Res.* **2013**, *17*, 138–145.
7. Lim, W.Q.; Phua, S.Z.F.; Chen, H.Z.; Zhao, Y.L. An oxaliplatin(iv) prodrug-based supramolecular self-delivery nanocarrier for targeted colorectal cancer treatment. *Chem. Commun.* **2018**, *54*, 12762–12765. [CrossRef]
8. Serrano, D.R.; Hernandez, L.; Fleire, L.; Gonzalez-Alvarez, I.; Montoya, A.; Ballesteros, M.P.; Dea-Ayuela, M.A.; Miro, G.; Bolas-Fernandez, F.; Torrado, J.J. Hemolytic and pharmacokinetic studies of liposomal and particulate amphotericin B formulations. *Int. J. Pharm.* **2013**, *447*, 38–46. [CrossRef]
9. Song, N.; Pogue-Geile, K.L.; Gavin, P.G.; Yothers, G.; Kim, S.R.; Johnson, N.L.; Lipchik, C.; Allegra, C.J.; Petrelli, N.J.; O'Connell, M.J.; et al. Clinical Outcome From Oxaliplatin Treatment in Stage II/III Colon Cancer According to Intrinsic Subtypes Secondary Analysis of NSABP C-O7/NRG Oncology Randomized Clinical Trial. *JAMA Oncol.* **2016**, *2*, 1162–1169. [CrossRef]
10. Piche, N.; Leblond, F.A.; Sideris, L.; Pichette, V.; Drolet, P.; Fortier, L.P.; Mitchell, A.; Dube, P. Rationale for Heating Oxaliplatin for the Intraperitoneal Treatment of Peritoneal Carcinomatosis A Study of the Effect of Heat on Intraperitoneal Oxaliplatin Using a Murine Model. *Ann. Surg.* **2011**, *254*, 138–144. [CrossRef]
11. Elias, D.; Raynard, B.; Farkhondeh, F.; Goere, D.; Rouquie, D.; Ciuchendea, R.; Pocard, M.; Ducreux, M. Peritoneal carcinomatosis of colorectal origin—Long-term results of intraperitoneal chemohyperthermia with oxaliplatin following complete cytoreductive surgery. *Gastroen. Clin. Biol.* **2006**, *30*, 1200–1204. [CrossRef]
12. Makkouk, A.; Joshi, V.B.; Wongrakpanich, A.; Lemke, C.D.; Gross, B.P.; Salem, A.K.; Weiner, G.J. Biodegradable Microparticles Loaded with Doxorubicin and CpG ODN for In Situ Immunization Against Cancer. *AAPS J.* **2015**, *17*, 184–193. [CrossRef]
13. Ramasamy, T.; Ruttala, H.B.; Gupta, B.; Poudel, B.K.; Choi, H.G.; Yong, C.S.; Kim, J.O. Smart chemistry-based nanosized drug delivery systems for systemic applications: A comprehensive review. *J. Control. Release* **2017**, *258*, 226–253. [CrossRef]
14. Blasi, P. Poly(lactic acid)/poly(lactic-co-glycolic acid)-based microparticles: An overview. *J. Pharm. Investig.* **2019**, *49*, 337–346. [CrossRef]
15. Taghizadehghalehjoughi, A.; Hacimuftuoglu, A.; Cetin, M.; Ugur, A.B.; Galateanu, B.; Mezhuev, Y.; Okkay, U.; Taspinar, N.; Taspinar, M.; Uyanik, A.; et al. Effect of metformin/irinotecan-loaded poly-lactic-co-glycolic acid nanoparticles on glioblastoma: In vitro and in vivo studies. *Nanomedicine* **2018**, *13*, 1595–1606. [CrossRef]
16. Palileo, A.; Munoz-Sagastibelza, M.; Martello-Rooney, L. Treatment with paclitaxel causes upregulation in resistance protein tubulin beta III in a type 2 human endometrial cancer cell line. *Gynecol. Oncol.* **2019**, *154*, e15. [CrossRef]

17. Dwivedi, P.; Han, S.Y.; Mangrio, F.; Fan, R.; Dwivedi, M.; Zhu, Z.A.; Huang, F.S.; Wu, Q.; Khatik, R.; Cohn, D.E.; et al. Engineered multifunctional biodegradable hybrid microparticles for paclitaxel delivery in cancer therapy. *Mater. Sci. Eng. C-Mater.* **2019**, *102*, 113–123. [CrossRef]
18. Lee, J.E.; Abuzar, S.M.; Seo, Y.; Han, H.; Jeon, Y.; Park, E.J.; Baik, S.H.; Hwang, S.-J. Oxaliplatin-loaded chemically cross-linked hydrogels for prevention of postoperative abdominal adhesion and colorectal cancer therapy. *Int. J. Pharm.* **2019**, *565*, 50–58. [CrossRef]
19. Naghizadeh, Z.; Karkhaneh, A.; Khojasteh, A. Simultaneous release of melatonin and methylprednisolone from an injectable in situ self-crosslinked hydrogel/microparticle system for cartilage tissue engineering. *J. Biomed. Mater. Res. A* **2018**, *106*, 1932–1940. [CrossRef]
20. Khaing, Z.Z.; Agrawal, N.K.; Park, J.H.; Xin, S.J.; Plumton, G.C.; Lee, K.H.; Huang, Y.J.; Niemerski, A.L.; Schmidt, C.E.; Grau, J.W. Localized and sustained release of brain-derived neurotrophic factor from injectable hydrogel/microparticle composites fosters spinal learning after spinal cord injury. *J. Mater. Chem. B* **2016**, *4*, 7560–7571. [CrossRef]
21. Jain, R.A. The manufacturing techniques of various drug loaded biodegradable poly(lactide-co-glycolide) (PLGA) devices. *Biomaterials* **2000**, *21*, 2475–2490. [CrossRef]
22. Liu, L.; Liu, D.R.; Wang, M.; Du, G.C.; Chen, J. Preparation and characterization of sponge-like composites by cross-linking hyaluronic acid and carboxymethylcellulose sodium with adipic dihydrazide. *Eur. Polym. J.* **2007**, *43*, 2672–2681. [CrossRef]
23. Marshall, C.D.; Hu, M.S.; Leavitt, T.; Barnes, L.A.; Cheung, A.T.; Malhotra, S.; Lorenz, H.P.; Longaker, M.T. Creation of Abdominal Adhesions in Mice. *J. Vis. Exp.* **2016**, *144*. [CrossRef]
24. Graham, M.A.; Lockwood, G.F.; Greenslade, D.; Brienza, S.; Bayssas, M.; Gamelin, E. Clinical pharmacokinetics of oxaliplatin: A critical review. *Clin. Cancer Res.* **2000**, *6*, 1205–1218.
25. Milas, M.; Rinaudo, M.; Roure, I.; Al-Assaf, S.; Phillips, G.O.; Williams, P.A. Comparative rheological behavior of hyaluronan from bacterial and animal sources with cross-linked hyaluronan (hylan) in aqueous solution. *Biopolymers* **2001**, *59*, 191–204. [CrossRef]
26. Bittner, B.; Witt, C.; Mader, K.; Kissel, T. Degradation and protein release properties of microspheres prepared from biodegradable poly(lactide-co-glycolide) and ABA triblock copolymers: Influence of buffer media on polymer erosion and bovine serum albumin release. *J. Control. Release* **1999**, *60*, 297–309. [CrossRef]
27. Rehman, F.; Volpe, P.L.O.; Airoldi, C. The applicability of ordered mesoporous SBA-15 and its hydrophobic glutaraldehyde-bridge derivative to improve ibuprofen-loading in releasing system. *Colloid Surf. B* **2014**, *119*, 82–89. [CrossRef]
28. Peppas, N.A.; Bures, P.; Leobandung, W.; Ichikawa, H. Hydrogels in pharmaceutical formulations. *Eur. J. Pharm. Biopharm.* **2000**, *50*, 27–46. [CrossRef]
29. Chen, C.H.; Chen, S.H.; Mao, S.H.; Tsai, M.J.; Chou, P.Y.; Liao, C.H.; Chen, J.P. Injectable thermosensitive hydrogel containing hyaluronic acid and chitosan as a barrier for prevention of postoperative peritoneal adhesion. *Carbohydr. Polym.* **2017**, *173*, 721–731. [CrossRef]
30. Kasturi, S.P.; Qin, H.; Thomson, K.S.; El-Bereir, S.; Cha, S.C.; Neelapu, S.; Kwak, L.W.; Roy, K. Prophylactic anti-tumor effects in a B cell lymphoma model with DNA vaccines delivered on polyethylenimine (PEI) functionalized PLGA microparticles. *J. Control. Release* **2006**, *113*, 261–270. [CrossRef]

12

Design and In Vivo Pharmacokinetic Evaluation of Triamcinolone Acetonide Microcrystals-Loaded PLGA Microsphere for Increased Drug Retention in Knees after Intra-Articular Injection

Myoung Jin Ho [1], Hoe Taek Jeong [1], Sung Hyun Im [1], Hyung Tae Kim [1], Jeong Eun Lee [1], Jun Soo Park [1], Ha Ra Cho [1], Dong Yoon Kim [1], Young Wook Choi [2], Joon Woo Lee [3], Yong Seok Choi [1,*] and Myung Joo Kang [1,*]

1 College of Pharmacy, Dankook University, 119, Dandae-ro, Dongnam-gu, Cheonan-si, Chungcheongnam-do 31116, Korea
2 College of Pharmacy, Chung-Ang University, 84, Heukseok-ro, Dongjak-gu, Seoul 06974, Korea
3 Department of Radiology, Seoul National University Bundang Hospital, 82, Gumi-ro 173beon-gil, Bundang-gu, Seongnam-si, Gyeonggi-do 13620, Korea
* Correspondence: analysc@dankook.ac.kr (Y.S.C.); kangmj@dankook.ac.kr (M.J.K.)

Abstract: A novel polymeric microsphere (MS) containing micronized triamcinolone acetonide (TA) in a crystalline state was structured to provide extended drug retention in joints after intra-articular (IA) injection. Microcrystals with a median diameter of 1.7 μm were prepared by ultra-sonication method, and incorporated into poly(lactic-*co*-glycolic acid)/poly(lactic acid) (PLGA/PLA) MSs using spray-drying technique. Cross-sectional observation and X-ray diffraction analysis showed that drug microcrystals were evenly embedded in the MSs, with a distinctive crystalline nature of TA. In vitro drug release from the novel MSs was markedly decelerated compared to those from the marketed crystalline suspension (Triam inj.®), or even 7.2 μm-sized TA crystals-loaded MSs. The novel system offered prolonged drug retention in rat joints, providing quantifiable TA remains over 28 days. Whereas, over 95% of IA TA was removed from joints within seven days, after injection of the marketed product. Systemic exposure of the steroidal compound was drastically decreased with the MSs, with <50% systemic exposure compared to that with the marketed product. The novel MS was physicochemically stable, with no changes in drug crystallinity and release profile over 12 months. Therefore, the TA microcrystals-loaded MS is expected to be beneficial in patients especially with osteoarthritis, with reduced IA dosing frequency.

Keywords: triamcinolone acetonide; microcrystal; PLGA microsphere; local delivery; spray-drying technique; intra-articular injection; joint retention; systemic exposure

1. Introduction

Intra-articular (IA) injection of corticosteroids, such as triamcinolone acetonide (TA) crystalline suspension, is commonly recommended to alleviate pain and inflammation in knee joints [1,2]. Marketed injectable TA suspensions are intended to be slowly dissolved in the synovial fluid, and the glucocorticoid molecules steadily bind to and activate the glucocorticoid receptors, obstructing the production of inflammation mediators, including prostaglandins, leukotrienes, and pro-inflammatory cytokines [3]. Nevertheless, the analgesic and/or anti-inflammatory effect of the TA crystalline suspension are reported to be weakened within two weeks following IA injection because of a rapid efflux of the drug from the arthritic joint [4–6]. As the synovial lining is ultra-structured with permeable intercellular gaps measuring 0.1–5.5 μm, therapeutic agents injected via the IA route tend to easily escape from the joint [7,8]. Moreover, the steroidal compound is quite soluble in aqueous media (21 μg/mL in phosphate buffered saline at 25 °C) [9], and TA crystals that have decreased to a few microns in size might be readily translocated into systemic circulation. In vitro release experiments showed that the marketed TA crystalline suspension was completely dissolved within 2 h [10].

Several pharmaceutical approaches, including hydrogels, liposomes, nanoparticles, and microparticles (MPs), have been explored to prolong the retention time of steroidal compounds in the synovial tissues, minimizing systemic exposure following IA injection [2,10–15]. When considering the leaky structure of the synovium, one of the sound strategies for localized delivery to the synovial tissues is administering the therapeutic agents to IA after entrapping in a micro-sized carrier system. Biocompatible and biodegradable polymeric MPs generally larger than 10 μm have been reported to be effective for remaining in the synovial cavity and providing a sustained-release profile in the joint [2,9,16]. Actually, a single IA injection of the PLGA MPs was clinically demonstrated to be effective in providing an extended retention time of the corticosteroid in joints while reducing the drug distribution in the bloodstream [17].

We previously formulated a PLGA MS system containing TA as in a stable crystalline form, to achieve the sustained-release profile in joints after IA injection [18]. Compared to the polymeric MS containing TA in an amorphous state, the TA crystals-loaded MSs prepared by layering the suspended drug crystals with PLGA polymer exhibited excellent physicochemical stability under storage condition (25 °C/60% R.H.) in terms of drug crystallinity and drug content in MSs. However, the MS system containing TA crystals with a median diameter of 7 μm could not effectively retard drug release, as the coating layer on the irregular TA crystals was unfair, with insufficient coating thickness; the extent of drug released from the MSs reached 75% for 12 h under sink condition. Thus, we assumed that the additional micronization process of the TA crystals might be beneficial, prior to encapsulation process, to obtain satisfactory coating thickness on the TA crystals, providing sustained-release profile in joints.

Herein, the goals of this study were to construct uniform TA microcrystals and embed the microcrystals in the polymeric MS, providing a prolonged retention profile in the joint following IA injection. The uniform drug microcrystals were prepared by an ultra-sonication method and then encapsulated into the polymeric MS by a spray-drying technique. The physicochemical characteristics of the microcrystals-loaded MSs were evaluated in terms of outer and inner structures, particle size, the drug loading amount, and loading efficiency. In vitro drug release patterns from the MSs were regulated by adjusting the ratio of PLGA to PLA polymers and the ratio of drug to the polymer. The in vivo concentration profile of TA in the plasma and joint tissue following IA injection of the microcrystals-loaded MSs were comparatively evaluated with those of the marketed TA crystalline suspension in rats.

2. Materials and Methods

2.1. Materials

TA powder and Triam inj.® were kindly provided by Shinpoong Pharmaceutical Co. (Seoul, Korea). PLGA polymer with a lactide/glycolide ratio of 50:50 (5050DLG 4A, molecular weight 38,000–54,000 kDa) and PLA polymer (R203H, 18,000–24,000 kDa) were purchased from Lakeshore Biomaterials (Birmingham, AL, USA). Polysorbate 20, polysorbate 80, Sorbian monolaurate (Span 20), poly(ethyleneglycol) 4000 (PEG 4000), polyethylene-polypropylene glycol 188 (Poloxamer 188), cholesterol, benzalkonium chloride (BKC), sodium lauryl sulfate (SLS), and phosphate buffered saline tablets were purchased from Sigma Chemical Co. (St. Louis, MO, USA). Lecithin (L-α-phosphatidylcholine) was obtained from Avanti Polar Lipids, Inc. (Alabaster, AL, USA). Gelatin and glycerol were provided from TCI Chemicals, Co. (Tokyo, Japan). Acetonitrile (ACN), ethyl alcohol, and methanol of HPLC grade were obtained from J.T. Baker (Phillipsburg, NJ, USA). All other reagents were analytical grade.

2.2. *Preparation of TA Microcrystals Using an Ultra-Sonication Method*

Drug microcrystal suspension was fabricated using an ultra-sonication method previously reported with slight modifications [19]. Different kinds of stabilizers (polysorbate 20, polysorbate 80, span 20, PEG 4000, poloxamer 188, cholesterol, and BKC) were dissolved in ACN in the concentration ranges from 0.05 to 0.5 *w/v* % as shown is Table 1. TA powder (100 mg) was then added to the solution and vigorously vortexed for 5 min to disperse the drug powder homogeneously. The ultra-sonicator (Model Vibracell VC-505, Sonics and Materials Inc., Newtown, NC, USA) equipped with a 1/2-inch (13 mm) probe was placed into the TA suspension and it was sonicated for 3 min at 40% amplitude with 3 s pulses (on/off alteration). To prevent temperature elevation, the samples were located inside an ice bath during the sonication procedure. Prepared TA microcrystal suspensions were then stored at room temperature for further experiments.

2.3. *Preparation of TA Microcrystals-Loaded MSs Using a Spray-Drying Technique*

TA microcrystals-loaded MSs were fabricated by a spray-drying technique with a Buchi mini-spray dryer (Model B-290, Buchi Labortechnik AG, Flawil, Switzerland). The feeding solution was prepared by subsequently dissolving PLGA/PLA polymers and lecithin into the BKC-stabilized TA microcrystal suspension. The composition of each microcrystals-embedded MSs is represented in Table 2. The feeding solution was then pumped into the spray dryer nozzle at a feeding rate of 3 mL/min and a stirring rate of 250 rpm. The inlet and outlet temperatures were set to 70 °C and 45 °C, respectively, to evaporate the organic solvent. The atomizing air flow was 246 L/h and the aspirator capacity was 100%. Prepared microcrystals-loaded MS powders were collected and stored in a desiccator (Model OH-3S, As-one, Seoul, Korea) at 25 °C for 24 h to remove the residual organic solvent.

2.4. *Morphological Features of TA Microcrystals and Microcrystals-Loaded MSs*

2.4.1. Appearance f TA Microcrystals and Microcrystals-Loaded MSs

Morphological features of raw material, TA microcrystals, and polymeric MSs were observed by SEM (Model Sigma 500, Carl Zeiss, Oberkochen, Germany). Drug powder and MSs samples were placed on a carbon tape and fixed onto an aluminum stub. The TA microcrystal suspension was dropwise loaded on the carbon tape and then dried for 6 h at room temperature to remove the aqueous vehicle. The platinum coating procedure was then conducted using an automatic sputter coater (Model 108Auto, Cressington, UK) at 15 mA. Appearance of samples was scrutinized by an electron microscope at an accelerated voltage of 15 kV.

2.4.2. Cross-Sectional Image of TA Microcrystals-Loaded MSs

The internal structure of the microcrystals-loaded MSs was scrutinized by SEM after fixing the MSs in the gelatin blocks. At first, the gelatin medium was prepared by dissolving gelatin (20 *w/v* %) and glycerin (5 *w/v* %) in distilled water [20]. Approximately 40 mg of the MSs powder was dispersed in the 3 mL of gelatin medium inside the polystyrene disposable base mold (Tissue-Tek®, 15 × 15 × 5 mm) at 37 °C. The mold was then placed in a deep freezer maintained at −70 °C for 12 h. The frozen gelatin block was mounted to the cryostat stub (Model CM3050S, Leica Microsystems, Wetzlar, Germany) using an optimum cutting temperature compound (Sakura Finetechnical Co., Ltd., Tokyo, Japan). The MS-loaded block was then sectioned at a thickness of 20 μm at −20 °C and was immediately placed on the double-sided carbon tape. Samples were defrosted for 1 h at room temperature and coating and observation procedures were conducted using the same method as described above.

2.4.3. Hyperspectral Mapping Images of TA Microcrystals-Loaded MSs

A hyperspectral microscopy imaging system (Model CytoViva®, Cytoviva Inc., Auburn, AL, USA) was employed to visualize TA microcrystals inside the MSs. The Cytoviva® system included a BX-41 microscope (Olympus Corporation, Tokyo, Japan), a visible-near infrared hyperspectral imaging system, dual fluorescence module, and high-resolution adaptor. Approximately 10 μL of TA microcrystal suspension, blank MSs, and TA microcrystals-loaded MSs suspended in 1 mL of 0.5 *w/v* % polysorbate 80 solution was dropped onto a cover glass and the hyperspectral spectra were analyzed. The mapping process was performed on the TA microcrystals-loaded MS image, with acquired spectra of TA microcrystals and blank MSs (HyperVisual Software ENVI 4.8, ITT Visual Information Solutions, Boulder, CO, USA). The spectra corresponding to TA microcrystals and the blank MSs were expressed as red and yellow, respectively, in the hyperspectral image of TA microcrystals-loaded MSs.

2.5. *Physicochemical Characterization TA Microcrystals and Microcrystals-Loaded MSs*

2.5.1. Crystallinity Analysis

The crystalline state of TA powder, TA microcrystals, blank MSs, and microcrystals-loaded MSs was analyzed using an X-ray diffractometer (XRD, Model Ultima IV, Rigaku, Tokyo, Japan) at 25 °C. For the TA microcrystal suspension, the aqueous vehicle was removed by centrifuging the suspension at 3500 g for 10 min, and subsequently, oven drying at 40 °C for 12 h. Each sample was put on the glass sample plate and the diffraction pattern over a 2θ range of 5–35° was determined using a step size of 0.02°. Voltage, current, and scan speed were set to 40 kV, 30 mA, and 1 s/step, respectively.

2.5.2. Particle Size Analysis

Size distributions of TA microcrystals and MSs were determined by Mastersizer MS 2000 (Malvern Instruments Ltd., Worcestershire, UK) equipped with a Hydro 2000 S automatic dispersion unit. Prior to analysis, MSs powder was suspended in the aqueous medium consisting of 1 *w/v* % PEG 4000 and 0.5 *w/v* % polysorbate 20. The suspended samples were then dropwise added to an automatic dispersion unit to obtain a 10–15% range of obscuration. Sample and background measurement times were set to 5 s and 10 s, respectively, and 5 runs were conducted for each measurement. Mie theory was applied to calculate the size distribution by volume with the refractive index value of 1.52. The resultant particle sizes of the three batches were averaged and presented as mean ± standard deviation (SD) (n = 3). The $d_{0.5}$, $d_{0.9}$, and $d_{0.1}$ indicated the median value defined as the diameter where 50%, 90%, and 10% of the population were below this value, respectively. SPAN value was an indicator representing the homogeneity of the particle size and was calculated by dividing the difference of $d_{0.9}$ and $d_{0.1}$ by $d_{0.5}$ [21].

2.5.3. Determination of Loading Amount and Efficiency of TA Microcrystals in MSs

To dissolve TA microcrystals-loaded MSs, 10 mg of MSs were added to 1 mL of dimethyl sulfoxide and then sonicated with a bath-type sonicator (Model 5510E-DTH, Bransonic, USA) for 10 min. The opaque solution was diluted with ACN and distilled water mixture (3:2 *v/v*) and was subsequently centrifuged at 16,000 *g* for 10 min to remove the precipitates. The concentration of TA in the supernatant was determined by a Waters HPLC system (Waters Corporation, Milford MA, USA) comprised of a pump (Model 515), auto sampler (Model 717 plus), UV detector (Model 486), and equipped with a Capcell Pak C18 column (150 mm × 2.0 mm, 3 μm, Shiseido, Tokyo, Japan). The mobile phase consisted of ACN and distilled water at a volume ratio of 3:2 and was eluted with a flow rate of 1.0 mL/min. The detection wavelength was set to 254 nm. The calibration curve of TA was linear in the concentration range of 1–100 μg/mL, with r^2 values of 0.999. The drug loading amount and loading efficiency were calculated as follows [22]:

$$\text{Drug loading amount} = WL/WT, \quad (1)$$

$$\text{Drug loading efficiency (\%)} = (\text{WL/WF}) \times 100, \tag{2}$$

where W_L, W_T and W_F represent the weight of TA in microcrystals-loaded MSs (mg), total weight of microcrystals-loaded MSs (mg) and feeding weight of TA (mg).

2.6. *In Vitro Drug Release Profiles and Morphological Changes of Microcrystals-Loaded MSs*

In vitro release profiles of TA from the novel MSs were comparatively evaluated with that of a marketed product under accelerated test conditions (45 ± 0.5 °C). To guarantee sink condition during the experiment, 0.5 *w/v* % of SLS and 0.05 *w/v* % of poloxamer 188, were added to 10 mM phosphate buffered saline (pH 7.4). MSs or the marketed product (Triam inj.®, TA 40 mg/mL) containing 20 mg of TA were immersed into 200 mL dissolution medium maintained at 45 ± 0.5 °C and then shaken with an agitation speed of 100 rpm. At predetermined intervals, 1 mL of the release medium was withdrawn and centrifuged at 16,000 *g* for 10 min. The supernatant was diluted two-fold with the mobile phase and TA concentration in the aliquot was determined by HPLC as described above. The equivalent volume of fresh pre-warmed dissolution medium was replenished to maintain a constant medium volume.

The morphological changes of the novel MSs during the in vitro release test were scrutinized by SEM. At predetermined intervals, MSs prepared with the PLGA:PLA ratio of 4:0 (F1), 1:3 (F4), and 0:4 (F5) were withdrawn and centrifuged at 900 *g*. The pelletized MSs were stored at −70 °C for 24 h and lyophilized for 24 h. The appearance of the lyophilized MS samples was observed by SEM with the same procedure described earlier.

2.7. *In Vivo Systemic Exposure and Joint Retention of TA after IA Injection in Rats*

2.7.1. Animals and Experimental Protocols

In Vivo pharmacokinetic studies were performed after approval from the Institutional Animal Care and Use Committee (IACUC) of Seoul National University Bundang Hospital (approval number: BA1608-206/050-01, date of approval: August 9, 2016). Six-week-old male Sprague-Dawley rats (250 ± 20 g) were acquired from Samtako (Kyungki-do, Korea). Four or five rats were housed in each cage and kept in a temperature- and relative humidity-controlled room (23 ± 1 °C and 50 ± 5%, respectively) with a 12-h light-dark cycle. During the acclimatization period, rats were allowed free access to tap water and standardized chow.

After at least three days of the acclimatization period, rats were divided into three groups (n = 9 per group) by a stratified randomization scheme for similar body weights groups. The hair on both hind knee joints was removed using hair removal cream. Prior to IA injection, spray-dried MS (F4 and F8) were re-dispersed in the sterile diluent composed of 0.66 *w/v* % sodium chloride, 0.63 *w/v* % carboxymethylcellulose sodium, and 0.04 *w/v* % polysorbate 80 at the same drug concentration (2.5 mg/mL as TA). Each group received 50 μL of the marketed product, F4, and F8, respectively, using an insulin syringe (31 G) in both knee joints, to administer 125 μg of TA per knee. At the predetermined time, blood samples (approximately 0.2 mL) were collected from the submandibular vein using a 26 G heparinized syringe. Blood samples were centrifuged at 16,000 *g* for 10 min. The obtained plasma samples were then stored at −70 °C until being analyzed by LC-MS/MS assay.

Apart from the systemic exposure evaluation, knee samples were collected to estimate the level of TA in joint tissues. After 3, 7, 21, 28, and 42 days of the IA injection in both knees, two animals from each group were sacrificed, and both knees were removed using bone cutters. After removing any residual substances and adhered tissues, knees were accurately weighed and stored at −70 °C until LC-MS/MS analysis.

2.7.2. LC-MS/MS Analysis of TA Concentration in Plasma and Knee Tissues

The TA concentrations in rat plasma or joint tissue were determined using the LC–MS/MS assay previously reported [23]. In brief, thawed plasma (100 μL) was mixed with 900 μL of methanol and vigorously vortexed for 10 min, to precipitate protein. After centrifuging at 16,000 g, a supernatant

(10 μL) was analyzed through an LC-MS/MS system (Model LC-20 Prominence HPLC, Shimadzu and Model API 2000, AB/SCIEX, Foster City, CA, USA). In the case of articular samples, the frozen knee tissues were thawed and immersed in 2 mL of ACN and shaken overnight to extract TA from the tissue. The extracted solution was centrifuged at 16,000 *g* for 5 min and the supernatant was injected into the LC-MS/MS system. The transitions of 435.1/415.0/15 precursor ion (*m/z*)/product ion (*m/z*)/collision energy (V) were then monitored for TA. Data acquisition/analyses were conducted using Analyst® version 1.5.2 software (ABSciex, Concord, ON, Canada). The assay was validated thoroughly and showed acceptable precision and accuracy, with a lower limit of quantification of 0.2 ng/mL in both rat plasma and knee tissue extract.

2.7.3. Pharmacokinetic Parameters from TA Concentration Profile in Plasma

Pharmacokinetic parameters such as area under the plasma concentration versus time curve ($AUC_{0\text{–}7days}$), maximum plasma concentration (C_{max}), time needed to reach the maximum plasma concentration (T_{max}), and terminal half-life ($T_{1/2}$) in plasma were calculated using the linear trapezoidal rule in the BA Calc 2007 pharmacokinetic analysis program (Korea Food & Drug Administration, Seoul, Korea).

2.8. Physicochemical Stability of TA Microcrystals-Loaded MSs

The long-term storage stability of the novel MSs was evaluated in terms of drug crystallinity, drug content, and in vitro release profile. TA microcrystals-loaded MS (F4) power was placed into the scintillation vial and was stored in the chamber maintained at 25 °C and 60% R.H. After 12 months of storage, the drug crystallinity, drug content, and in vitro release profile were evaluated with the same method as previously described.

2.9. Statistical Analysis

Each experiment was performed at least thrice and the data are presented as the mean ± SD. Statistical significance was determined using a one-way analysis of variance (ANOVA) test and was considered to be significant at $p < 0.05$ unless otherwise indicated.

3. Results and Discussion

3.1. Formulation and Physical Characteristics of TA Microcrystals

Various stabilizers were screened to micronize TA powder in the organic solvent using a probe type ultra-sonicator (Table 1). ACN was employed as the vehicle as it exhibited low solubility for the steroidal compound (<1 mg/mL), and high solvation capacity for PLGA and PLA polymers [18]. When the surface stabilizer was not included in the vehicle, TA powder was not uniformly dispersed in the medium after the homogenization process, rather forming large precipitates. The addition of steric stabilizers, such as polysorbate 20, polysorbate 80, PEG 4000, poloxamer 188, and cholesterol could not provide a uniform dispersion of the split TA microcrystals, forming drug aggregates within 24 h. On the other hand, when BKC was included in the organic vehicle at a concentration of 0.1 to 0.5 *w/v* %, TA microcrystals with a median size below 2.1 μm were shaped with re-dispersibility in the organic solvent (Table 1 and Figure 1A). When the concentration of the cationic surfactant was less than 0.05 *w/v* %, it could not afford the re-dispersibility of TA microcrystals. Thus, BKC at the concentration of 0.1 *w/v* % was employed for further preparation of TA microcrystal suspension in ACN.

The morphological feature of the TA microcrystals stabilized by 0.1 *w/v* % BKC was observed by FE-SEM. TA raw material showed characteristic crystal forms, such as hexahedron, octahedron, and dodecahedrons, with different sizes in the range from 2 to 20 μm (Figure 1C). Whereas, the crystal size was markedly decreased to 1–3 μm by the ultra-sonication process (Figure 1D), coinciding with the crystal size as determined by Mastersizer ($d_{0.5}$, 1.7 μm). In spite of crystal size reduction, no noticeable change to the shape was observed in the TA microcrystals. The crystalline state of TA microcrystals was further evaluated by comparing the X-ray diffraction spectrum of TA microcrystals with that of the raw material (Figure 1B). The spectrum of TA microcrystals was identical to that of drug powder, exhibiting distinctive diffraction peaks at 2θ equal to 9.9°, 14.5°, 17.6°, and 24.7°. On the other hand, the cationic surfactant showed no distinctive diffraction peaks over the 2θ range of 5–35°. Taken together, we concluded that TA powder was effectively micronized to 1–3 μm, with no crystalline changes during the ultra-sonication process.

Table 1. Effects of kinds of stabilizers on size, homogeneity, and dispersibility of TA microcrystals in ACN.

Stabilizer (*w/v* %) [1]	Crystal Size ($d_{0.5}$, μm) [2,3]	Homogeneity (SPAN) [2,4]	Dispersibility [5]
- [6]	7.21 ± 1.02	2.14 ± 0.13	Aggregated
Polysorbate 20 0.5%	6.63 ± 0.82	2.11 ± 0.07	Aggregated
Polysorbate 80 0.5%	7.35 ± 0.91	1.99 ± 0.04	Aggregated
Span 20 0.5%	17.7 ± 6.27	1.81 ± 0.11	Aggregated
PEG 4000 0.5%	7.15 ± 3.07	2.10 ± 0.88	Aggregated
Poloxamer 188 0.5%	5.44 ± 1.84	2.00 ± 0.52	Aggregated
Cholesterol 0.5%	8.72 ± 3.49	1.81 ± 0.60	Aggregated
BKC 0.5%	2.11 ± 0.05	1.32 ± 0.03	Re-dispersible
BKC 0.2%	1.94 ± 0.06	1.20 ± 0.03	Re-dispersible
BKC 0.1%	1.73 ± 0.02	1.21 ± 0.01	Re-dispersible
BKC 0.05%	4.75 ± 0.23	1.99 ± 0.02	Aggregated

[1] Weight per volume concentration in ACN. [2] Expressed as mean ± SD (n = 3). [3] Indicates the volume weighted diameter below which 50% of the total particle. [4] Calculated by dividing the difference between $d_{0.9}$ and $d_{0.1}$ by $d_{0.5}$. $d_{0.9}$ and $d_{0.1}$ indicate the volume weighted diameters below which 90% and 10% of the total particle, respectively. [5] Visually evaluated after 24 h storage at room temperature. [6] Indicates without stabilizer.

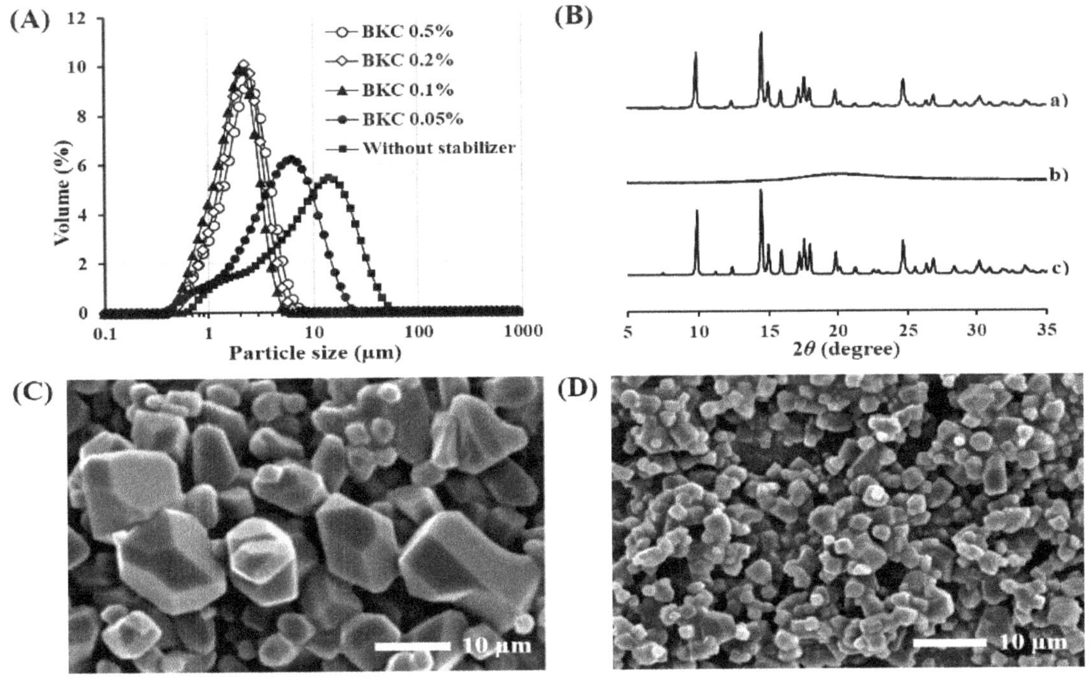

Figure 1. Morphological and physical characteristics of TA microcrystals. (**A**) Size distribution of the drug microcrystals stabilized by BKC, (**B**) XRD patterns of (a) TA raw material, (b) BKC powder, and (c) TA microcrystals, SEM images of (**C**) TA raw material, and (**D**) TA microcrystals stabilized by BKC at the concentration of 0.1 *w/v* %.

3.2. Formulation and Physical Characteristics of TA Microcrystals-Loaded MSs

Various TA microcrystals (1.7 μm median size) or intact TA powder (7.2 μm)-embedded MSs were fabricated using the spray-drying technique, and these particle size, homogeneity, drug loading amount, and loading efficiency are represented in Table 2. The median particle size of MSs prepared ranged from 15.8 to 18.8 μm, with a narrow size distribution possessing a SPAN value below 2.1. The formulation variables, such as TA crystal size, the ratio of PLGA and PLA polymers, and the ratio of drug to polymer, did not cause marked differences in size and homogeneity of TA-loaded MSs (Table 2). The particle size of the novel MS was considered to be suitable for IA prolonged delivery, preventing the trans-synovial efflux of injected TA microcrystals [17,24,25]. There was also no remarkable difference in the drug loading efficiency in the polymeric MSs between the formulas, exhibiting more than 90% drug loading efficiency in all formulations. The absence of the external phase during the spray-drying process might prevent distribution and/or diffusion of TA microcrystals during the external phase, and thus promote TA crystals to be located in the polymeric matrix after solvent evaporation, irrespective of composition variables. On the other hand, the loading amount of TA in MS was adjusted from 0.09 to 0.31 *w/w*, by controlling the drug to polymer weight ratio from 1:2 to 1:10.

Table 2. Compositions and physicochemical characteristics of TA microcrystals-loaded MSs.

	Compositions			Characteristics			
	TA crystal Size (μm) [1,5]	PLGA:PLA Ratio (w:w)	Drug:polymer Ratio (w:w)	Particle Size (μm) [1,5]	SPAN [2,5]	Loading Amount [3,5]	Loading Efficiency (%) [4,5]
F0	7.21 ± 1.02	1:3	1:5	15.9 ± 0.95	2.03 ± 0.04	0.16 ± 0.02	97.2 ± 2.35
F1	1.73 ± 0.02	4:0	1:5	16.2 ± 1.35	1.89 ± 0.05	0.15 ± 0.01	93.5 ± 0.87
F2	1.73 ± 0.02	3:1	1:5	17.2 ± 0.43	1.89 ± 0.02	0.15 ± 0.04	92.7 ± 5.76
F3	1.73 ± 0.02	2:2	1:5	16.1 ± 0.56	2.06 ± 0.02	0.14 ± 0.01	90.9 ± 1.01
F4	1.73 ± 0.02	1:3	1:5	16.9 ± 0.35	1.80 ± 0.01	0.16 ± 0.01	98.1 ± 1.84
F5	1.73 ± 0.02	0:4	1:5	15.9 ± 0.06	2.11 ± 0.01	0.15 ± 0.02	96.3 ± 2.48
F6	1.73 ± 0.02	1:3	1:2	18.9 ± 0.25	1.70 ± 0.01	0.31 ± 0.00	96.0 ± 0.18
F7	1.73 ± 0.02	1:3	1:3	15.8 ± 1.11	2.04 ± 0.07	0.22 ± 0.01	93.7 ± 1.33
F8	1.73 ± 0.02	1:3	1:10	16.9 ± 0.42	1.20 ± 0.01	0.09 ± 0.02	99.5 ± 2.55

[1] Presented as $d_{0.5}$ value; the volume weighted diameter below 50% of the total particle. [2] Calculated by dividing the difference between $d_{0.9}$ and $d_{0.1}$ by $d_{0.5}$: $d_{0.9}$ and $d_{0.1}$ by $d_{0.5}$: $d_{0.9}$ and $d_{0.1}$ are the volume weighted diameters below 90% and 10% of the total particle, respectively. [3] Calculated by dividing the weight of TA in microcrystals-loaded MSs by total weight of microcrystals-loaded MSs (mg). [4] Expressed as the percentage (%) after dividing the weight of TA loaded in MSs by total fed weight of TA (mg). [5] Expressed as mean ± SD (n = 3); Note: Lecithin was included in all formulations at the weight ratio of 5 *w/w* % to the total amount of polymers.

The novel TAs-loaded MSs were further characterized in terms of outer and internal structures and drug crystallinity in MS (Figure 2). The MSs (F4) prepared by the spray-drying technique was highly spherical, with a smooth and homogeneous surface (Figure 2A). In the cross-sectional image, the microcrystals showed different textures from the polymeric matrix and were found to be uniformly embedded in the polymeric matrix (Figure 2B). The number of microcrystals loaded per MS was elucidated by translating the loading amount into the number of MS and TA microcrystals. In the process of converting the weight to a number, the volume of single MS and TA microcrystal was calculated with the assumption that the shape of the MS and microcrystal were spherical and cubic, respectively, with both having a density of 1.0. In the MS formulations prepared with the drug to polymer ratio of 1:2 (F6), 1:3 (F7), 1:5 (F4), and 1:10 (F8), the number of microcrystals embedded in each MS was calculated as 215, 94, 82, and 50, respectively. In the hyperspectral image (Figure 2C), TA microcrystals (red color) were observed to be principally located inside the PLGA/PLA MS (yellow color). However, individual microcrystals were not separately spotted in the image, probably because of the low resolution of Cytoviva®. The characteristic peak of TA microcrystals was identically detected in the microcrystals-load MS (Figure 2D), denoting that TA microcrystals stabilized by BKC were successfully incorporated in the MSs, with no crystalline changes during the fabrication process.

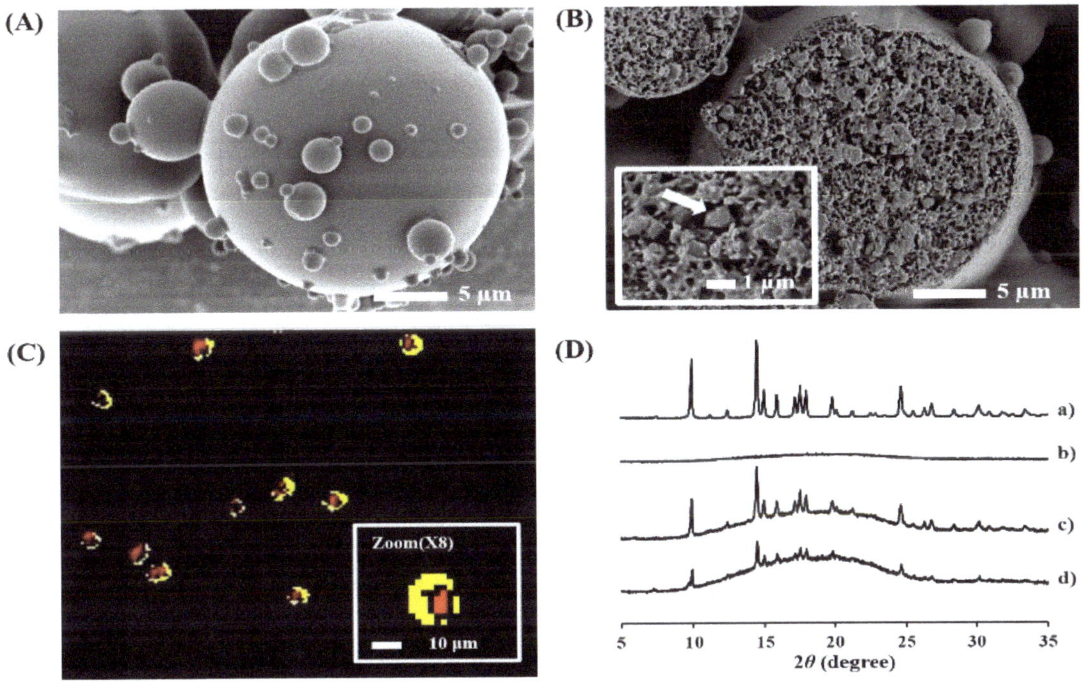

Figure 2. Morphological and physical characteristics of the microcrystals-loaded MSs. Representative micrograph of (**A**) intact and (**B**) cross-sectioned microcrystals-loaded MS (F4), (**C**) hyperspectral image of microcrystals-loaded MSs, and (**D**) XRD patterns of (a) TA microcrystals, (b) blank MS, (c) F4 MS (drug:polymer = 1:5), and (d) F8 MS (1:10); Notes: Inset in (**B**) is ×5000 magnified images and the arrow points to the TA crystal surrounded by the polymeric matrices. In the hyperspectral image (**C**), PLGA/PLA polymers and TA microcrystals are colored as yellow and red, respectively.

3.3. In Vitro Drug Release and Degradation Profiles of TA Microcrystals-Loaded MSs

In Vitro drug release profiles from the marketed product, the drug powder- or micronized TA crystals-loaded MSs were evaluated under accelerated dissolution conditions. Although the synovial fluid does not assure the sink condition for the drug dissolution, the in vitro release test under sink conditions was favored for quicker comparison between the formulations. Moreover, as the drug release profiles from PLGA/PLA MSs could be retarded from days to months at body temperature (37 °C), the liberation pattern of the steroidal compound from the MSs was further facilitated by elevating the temperature of the dissolution media (45 °C), promoting the degradation and/or hydrolysis of the biodegradable polymers [26–28]. Actually, the accelerated test at high temperature was reported to be beneficial for faster comparison of release behavior between MS formulas, with high correlation with that obtained at 37 °C [27]. Shen and Burgess (2012) revealed that the time required to reach 100% drug release from the MSs prepared with PLGA polymer with the glass transition temperature (T_g) of 44–48 °C was determined to be 10, 5, 3, and 1.3 days, respectively, at temperatures of 45, 50, 53, and 60 °C. Herein, the temperature of the dissolution medium was set to 45 °C, which did not exceed the T_g values of both polymers (46–52 °C). When the polymeric MSs were exposed to the medium at temperatures above the T_g of the polymer, the drug diffusion coefficient was drastically increased [29], diminishing the difference between the release profiles between the polymeric particulates.

Under the accelerated condition, the marketed product containing 13 µm-sized TA crystals stabilized by polysorbate 20 and sodium carboxymethyl cellulose was rapidly liquefied in the aqueous medium, showing complete drug release within 90 min (Figure 3A). It coincided with a previous report that showed that the TA crystal suspension was readily dissolved in phosphate buffered saline within 2 h [10]. The drug release from the MS with 7.2-µm-sized TA crystals (F0) was not markedly retarded compared to the intact drug crystal, releasing over 95% of TA within 3 h. The incomplete and/or erratic coating thickness of the polymeric layer on the TA crystals probably could not effectively restrain the dissolution and diffusion procedures of the TA crystals into the aqueous media. On the other hand, drug release from the MSs containing smaller TA crystals (median size of 1.7 μm) was markedly impeded compared to the marketed product or 7.2-μm-sized TA crystal-loaded MS, especially as the ratio of PLA increased in the MS (Figure 3A).

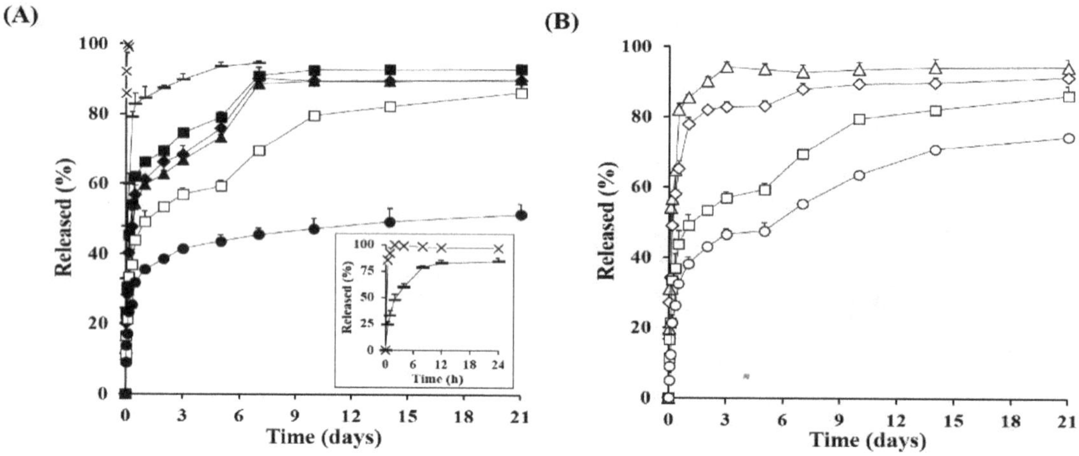

Figure 3. In Vitro release profile of TA from the novel MSs under accelerated conditions (45 °C). (**A**) Drug release profile from the marketed product (×), 7.2 μm-sized TA crystals-loaded MS (F0, –), and 1.7 μm-sized TA crystals-loaded MS prepared with different PLGA:PLA ratios; 4:0 (F1, ■), 3:1 (F2, ♦), 2:2 (F3, ▲), 1:3 (F4, □), and 0:4 (F5, ●) and (**B**) drug release profile from MSs prepared with different drug:polymer ratios; 1:2 (F6, △), 1:3 (F7, ◇), 1:5 (F4, □), and 1:10 (F8, ○); Notes: The inset graph (**A**) is the magnified release profile from the marketed product and 7.2 μm-sized TA crystals-loaded MS. Data are expressed as the mean value (n = 3) and error bars are SDs.

As the glycolic acid has faster hydration/swelling behavior compared to lactic acid [30], MSs prepared with over 50% of PLGA polymers (F1, F2, and F3) showed higher burst release, with over 60% of drug released within 2 days. After the initial burst release, the extent of TA liberated from the F1, F2, and F3 polymers continuously rose, exhibiting over 90% release after 7 days under sink condition. On the other hand, the F4 formula with a PLGA:PLA ratio of 1:3, exhibited a more protracted release profile compared to that of F1, F2, and F3, exhibiting a linear release pattern for 21 days after a 53% initial release in the first 2 days. F5 (PLGA:PLA ratio of 0:4) showed the slowest release profile, displaying only 52% of the accumulated drug release after 21 days. Although there was marked difference in release profile depending on the ratio of PLGA and PLA polymer, the drug release pattern from novel drug microcrystals-loaded MSs were characterized by initial burst release and subsequent slow release profile, which is consistent with the typical release pattern of PLGA/PLA based MPs previous reported [31,32]. In the early phase, TA microcrystals located on or inner compartment near the surface of the MS might be rapidly dissolved by surrounding and/or penetrated aqueous media, and released from polymeric matrix mainly by diffusion mechanism. After initial burst release, the drug release rate tended to be retarded, due to the increased diffusion distance. Afterward, and the remaining steroidal compound in the MSs might be liberated by polymeric degradation and erosion and/or collapse of polymeric MSs.

Different drug release patterns depended on the PLGA:PLA ratio were highly consistent by the morphological changes of TA microcrystals-loaded MSs. As shown in Figure 4, because of the rapid swelling and hydrolysis nature of PLGA polymer, the PLGA MSs (F1) began to collapse and was excavated within three days. Thus, the drug microcrystals embedded in the PLGA MS might be readily exposed to aqueous media, and immediately dissolved under sink condition. On the contrary, because of the greater hydrophobicity of the PLA polymer compared to the PLGA polymer, the hydrolytic degradation of PLA MS (F5, PLGA:PLA = 0:4) progressed slowly. When the MSs were scrutinized at 3 and 7 days, fine pores were formed on the roughed surface and the pore size was gradually enlarged as time elapsed. Nevertheless, the overall globular shape and dimension of MS were retained even at 21 days, supporting the slow and incomplete release profile of TA from the MS (F7). The degradation pattern of F4 prepared with the PLGA:PLA ratio of 1:3 was intermediate between those of MSs prepared with PLGA or PLA polymer F1 and F5, respectively. After surface erosion and pore formation at three days, the MS was then gradually collapsed over 21 days. The drug release rate from F4 was markedly delayed compared to that from F1 but was much faster and higher than that from F5, releasing over 80% of the drug loaded for 21 days. The ratio of PLGA to PLA polymers was fixed to 1:3, expecting the prolonged release pattern for further investigation.

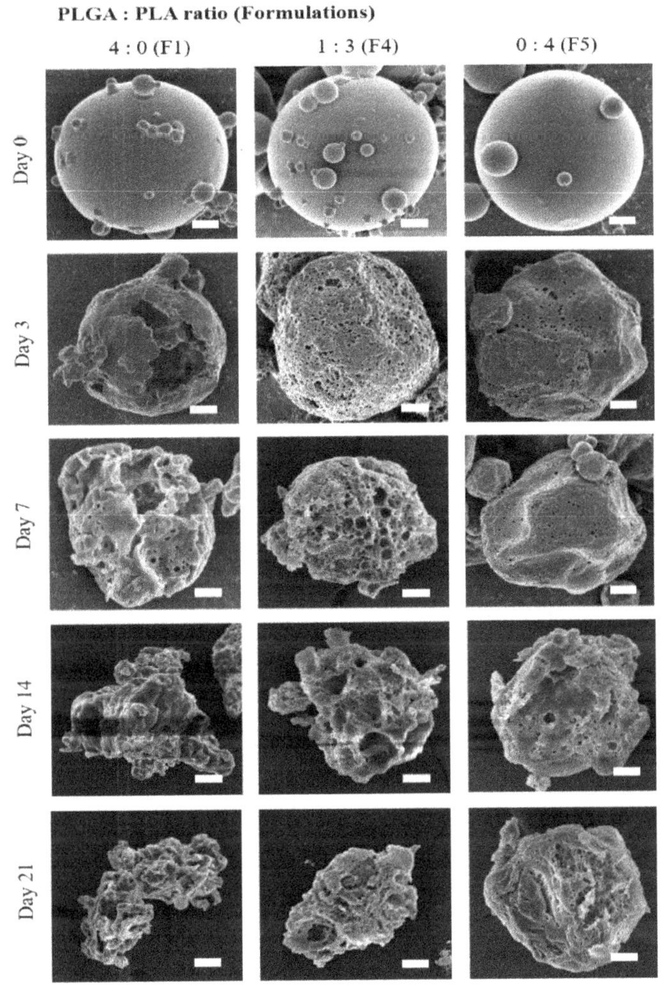

Figure 4. Morphological changes of TA microcrystals-loaded MSs prepared with different PLGA:PLA ratios, 0:4 (F1), 1:3 (F4), 0:4 (F5) under the accelerated release conditions (45 °C); Note: Scale bars in each image indicate 2.0 μm.

The in vitro release profile of TA from the PLGA/PLA MSs prepared with different drug to polymer ratios was further evaluated. As shown in Figure 3B, the initial drug release from the novel MSs were gradually decreased, as the drug to polymer ratio was increased. When the ratio of drug to polymer was 1:2 (F6) or 1:3 (F7), the percentage of drug released for 24 h had reached approximately 86% and 78%, respectively. On the other hand, in the formulations of the drugs:polymer ratio of 1:5 (F4) and 1:10 (F8), the release of the steroidal compound from the MSs were markedly retarded, exhibiting less than 60% of drug release over 5 days. Drug release from the F4 or F8 was steeped after 7 days, probably because of erosion and/or collapse of the MSs, but prolonged for 21 days. Formulas F4 and F8 were further exploited for in vivo pharmacokinetic study in rats, expecting an extended release profile over one month in the knee joint.

3.4. *In Vivo Systemic Exposure and Ioint Retention of TA after IA Injection in Rats*

The systemic exposure and local bioavailability of TA following a single IA injection of the marketed product or the novel MSs (F4 and F8) were evaluated in normal rats. The IA dose of TA treated in all groups was same to 0.25 mg per knee, which was well tolerated in rats [10]. The plasma levels of TA as a function of time following IA injection of the marketed product, F4, and F8 are represented in Figure 5 and the relevant PK parameters are summarized in Table 3. It is recommended that the exposure of the steroidal compound in blood be minimized, as the exogenous corticosteroid can cause Cushing syndrome, incurred impaired wound healing, infection, and muscle weakness [10,33,34]. However, unfortunately, the plasma level of TA was drastically elevated after administration of the marketed product, reaching C_{max} value of 218.7 ng/mL after 3.7 h. This rapid redistribution of TA into the bloodstream is in agreement with earlier reports that intra-articularly injected TA crystals were rapidly absorbed, with a T_{max} value of 4 h in patients with osteoarthritis [6,35,36]. This rapid drug efflux from the knee joint is also correlated with in vitro release profiles, denoting that TA crystalline suspension injected in the joint might be rapidly dissolved and passed out the gap in the synovial membrane. After reaching a C_{max} of 3.7 h, the plasma level of TA sharply decreased below 30 ng/mL after 12 h post-administration of the marketed product.

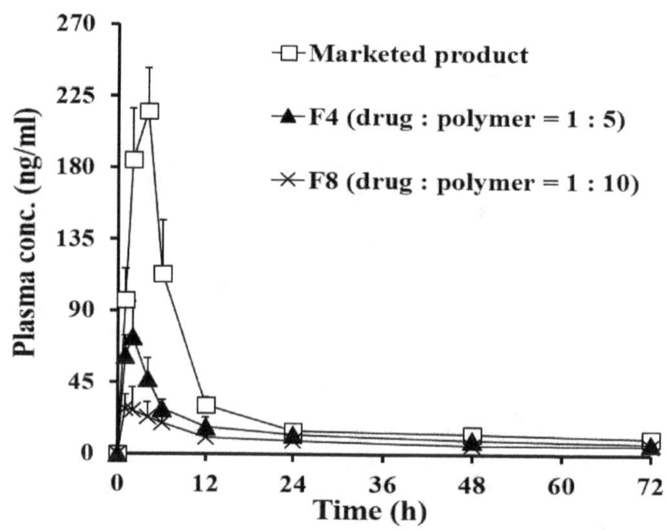

Figure 5. Plasma concentration–time profiles of TA following IA administration of the marketed product, F4 (drug:polymer = 1:5) and F8 (drug:polymer = 1:10) in rats at a dose of 0.5 mg/kg; Note: Each point represents mean ± SD (n = 5).

Table 3. Pharmacokinetic parameters of TA in plasma following IA administration of the marketed product, F4, and F8 in rats.

Parameters	Marketed Product	F4	F8
$AUC_{0\text{–}7day}$ (ng·h/mL)	2787.4 ± 187.4	1500.4 ± 218.9 *	1022.2 ± 161.9 *,**
C_{max} (ng/mL)	218.7 ± 26.6	75.6 ± 17.2 *	32.2 ± 12.0 *,**
T_{max} (h)	3.7 ± 0.8	1.8 ± 0.4 *	1.4 ± 0.5 *
$T_{1/2}$ (h) [1]	5.3 ± 0.1	9.0 ± 0.5 *	13.3 ± 2.7 *,**

[1] Calculated from the plasma concentration–time curve from T_{max} to 24 h after IA injection; Notes: Data are expressed as mean ± SD (n = 5). Statistical analysis was performed using the one-way ANOVA test; * significantly different from the marketed product ($p < 0.05$), ** significantly different from F4 ($p < 0.05$); Abbreviations: $AUC_{0\text{–}7days}$, area under the plasma concentration–time curve until day 7; C_{max}, maximum plasma concentration; T_{max}, time to reach maximum plasma concentration; $T_{1/2}$, elimination half-life of the drug.

In contrast, the systemic exposure of the exogenous corticosteroid was markedly decreased following IA injection of the TA microcrystals-loaded MSs (F4 and F8). The C_{max} values of TA following IA injection of F4 and F8 were determined to 75.6 ng/mL and 32.2 ng/mL, respectively, which were only

34% ($p < 0.05$) and 15% ($p < 0.05$) that of the marketed product. Correspondingly, $AUC_{0-7days}$ values in the F4- and F8-treated groups were drastically decreased to less than 54% ($p < 0.05$) and 37% ($p < 0.05$) of that obtained from the marketed product, respectively. These pharmacokinetic data indicated that the novel MSs remarkably lessened the redistribution of dissolved and/or micronized compound into the bloodstream, prolonging the retention time of TA in the knee. Between the two groups treated with MSs prepared with loading amount of 0.16 (F4) and 0.09 (F8), respectively, the drug exposure to blood was much lowered in the F8-treated group, showing 68% and 42% decreased $AUC_{0-7days}$ and C_{max} values compared to those obtained from the F4-treated group. This pharmacokinetic tendency is explainable with the in vitro release test results, which revealed that the extent of drug released from the polymeric matrix declined as the drug to polymer ratio increased.

The drug remaining in the joint tissue following IA single injection of each formula was further assessed in normal rats (Figure 6). After the IA injection of the marketed product, the drug concentration in the joint at three days post-dosing was only 5.6 μg/g because TA crystals were quickly effluxed from the joint tissue. The percentages of the drug remaining in the joint tissue at 3 and 7 days were calculated to be only 4.5% and 2.4%, respectively. After 21 days, the drug concentration in the joint tissue was below the limit of detection. This result is in line with a previous report that only two of eight patients with osteoarthritis had quantifiable synovial TA concentration at week 6, following IA injection of the marketed product [37]. On the other hand, the novel MS formulations exhibited a markedly profound and prolonged concentration profile in joint tissue compared to the marketed product, exhibiting quantifiable TA concentration over 28 days. Three days after the single administration of F4 or F8, the drug concentration in joints was determined to be 45 μg/g and 67 μg/g, respectively, which is one-third and one-half of the initial dose. In both MSs-treated groups, the TA concentration in the tissue gradually decreased as time elapsed, but approximately 5% of the initial dose was still detected at 28 days. These findings suggested that the retention time of TA in the joint tissue was extended with the sustained-release pattern of the novel MSs.

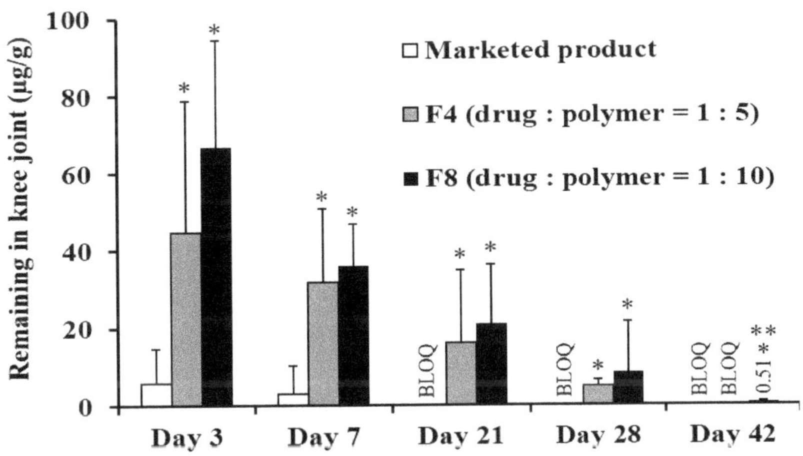

Figure 6. TA remains in rat joint tissue following IA administration of the marketed product, F4, and F8 at a dose of 125 μg of TA per knee; Notes: Vertical bars represent mean ± SD ($n = 6$). Statistical analysis was performed using the one-way ANOVA test; * significantly different from the marketed product ($p < 0.05$), ** significantly different from F4 ($p < 0.05$). BLOQ value of LC-MS/MS analysis was determined to 0.2 ng/mL.

3.5. *Long-Term Stability of TA Microcrystals-Loaded MS*

The physicochemical stability of the novel MS was evaluated after 12 weeks of storage under ambient conditions (25 °C, 60% RH). The storage condition of the MSs was set to ambient condition, as there was morphological change above 40 °C, due to softening of the polymer over T_g. At first, the drug crystallinity in the MS was assessed using XRD because a change in drug crystalline nature may occur during storage, affecting the drug chemical stability and release pattern from the MS. Under ambient conditions, the crystallinity of TA microcrystals embedded in the MS was stably maintained over 12 months, with no changes in diffraction pattern (Figure A1). There was also no change in drug content in F8 MS, displaying over 97% drug content after 12 months of storage. The in vitro dissolution pattern was also comparable with that of MSs immediately prepared, exhibiting a sustained-release profile of over 21 days (Figure A1). From these findings, we concluded that the novel MS system was physicochemically stable at least for one year under ambient conditions.

4. Conclusions

A novel parenteral sustained-release system of TA was successfully prepared by micronizing TA powder into 1.7 μm-sized microcrystals, and subsequently embedding into PLGA/PGA polymeric MSs using a spray-drying technique. TA microcrystals were efficiently entrapped into the polymeric MSs, preserving their distinctive crystalline nature. In vitro drug release from the novel MSs was markedly retarded compared to the marketed product and even 7.2 μm-sized TA crystal-loaded MSs, exhibiting a prolonged release profile over 21 days under accelerated conditions (45 °C). In an in vivo pharmacokinetic study in normal rats, the duration that the TA remained in the joint tissue was markedly extended, providing profound drug remains at 28 days following IA single injection. Moreover, TA microcrystals-loaded MSs drastically decreased the systemic exposure of the steroidal compound compared to the marketed product. Thus, the novel IA long-acting system could be a valuable tool, providing both increased drug retention in the knee and diminished systemic exposure of TA following a single administration.

Author Contributions: Conceptualization, M.J.H. and M.J.K.; Data curation, M.J.H., H.T.J. and J.S.P.; Formal analysis, H.R.C., D.Y.K. and Y.S.C.; Funding acquisition, M.J.K.; Investigation, S.H.I., H.T.K. and J.S.P.; Methodology, M.J.H., H.T.J. and J.W.L.; Project administration, Y.W.C., Y.S.C. and M.J.K.; Resources, H.T.J., S.H.I., H.T.K., J.E.L. and J.S.P.; Supervision, Y.W.C., Y.S.C. and M.J.K.; Validation, H.R.C., D.Y.K. and Y.S.C.; Visualization, M.J.H.; Writing—original draft, M.J.H.; Writing—review & editing, Y.W.C., J.W.L., Y.S.C. and M.J.K.

Appendix A

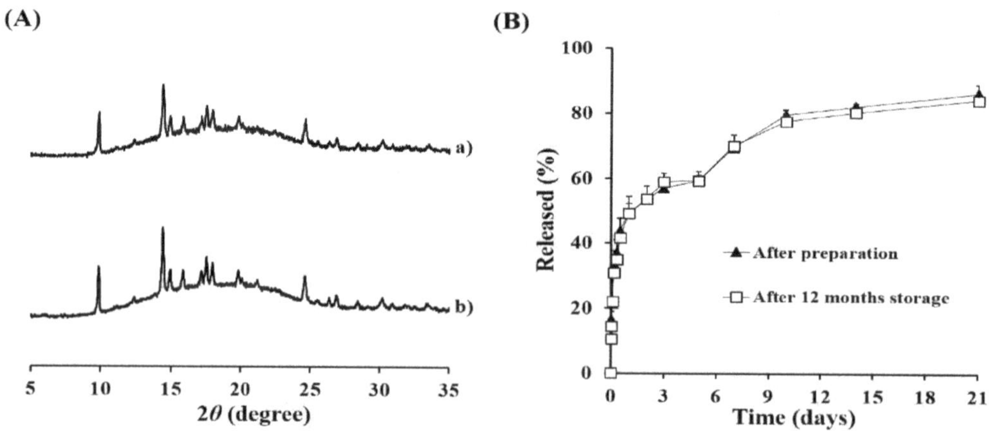

Figure A1. Physicochemical stability of TA microcrystals-loaded MS (F4) after 12 months of storage under ambient conditions. (**A**) XRD patterns of F4 MS (a) after preparation and (b) after 12 months of storage, (**B**) in vitro release profile of F4 after preparation and after 12 months storage under accelerated conditions; Notes: XRD pattern and release profile of F4 MS after preparation are identical to those depicted in Figures 2D and 3B, respectively. Each point in (**B**) in vitro release profile represents mean ± SD ($n = 3$).

References

1. Gerwin, N.; Hops, C.; Lucke, A. Intraarticular drug delivery in osteoarthritis. *Adv. Drug Deliv. Rev.* **2006**, *58*, 226–242. [CrossRef] [PubMed]
2. Luzardo-Álvarez, A.; Lamela-Gómez, I.; Otero-Espinar, F.; Blanco-Méndez, J. Development, characterization, and in vitro evaluation of resveratrol-loaded poly-(ε-caprolactone) microcapsules prepared by ultrasonic atomization for intra-articular administration. *Pharmaceutics* **2019**, *11*, 249. [CrossRef] [PubMed]
3. Creamer, P. Intra-articular corticosteroid injections in osteoarthritis: Do they work and if so, how? *Ann. Rheum. Dis.* **1997**, *56*, 634–636. [CrossRef] [PubMed]
4. Godwin, M.; Dawes, M. Intra-articular steroid injections for painful knees. Systematic review with meta-analysis. *Can. Fam. Physician* **2004**, *50*, 241–248. [PubMed]
5. Bjordal, J.M.; Johnson, M.I.; Lopes-Martins, R.A.; Bogen, B.; Chow, R.; Ljunggren, A.E. Short-term efficacy of physical interventions in osteoarthritic knee pain. a systematic review and meta-analysis of randomised placebo-controlled trials. *BMC Musculoskelet. Disord.* **2007**, *8*, 51. [CrossRef] [PubMed]
6. Ayhan, E.; Kesmezacar, H.; Akgun, I. Intraarticular injections (corticosteroid, hyaluronic acid, platelet rich plasma) for the knee osteoarthritis. *World J. Orthop.* **2014**, *5*, 351. [CrossRef]
7. Knight, A.D.; Levick, J.R. Morphometry of the ultrastructure of the blood-joint barrier in the rabbit knee. *Q. J. Exp. Physiol.* **1984**, *69*, 271–288. [CrossRef]
8. Ayral, X. Injections in the treatment of osteoarthritis. *Best Pract. Res. Clin. Rheumatol.* **2001**, *15*, 609–626. [CrossRef]
9. Kambhampati, S.P.; Mishra, M.K.; Mastorakos, P.; Oh, Y.; Lutty, G.A.; Kannan, R.M. Intracellular delivery of dendrimer triamcinolone acetonide conjugates into microglial and human retinal pigment epithelial cells. *Eur. J. Pharm. Biopharm.* **2015**, *95*, 239–249. [CrossRef]
10. Rudnik-Jansen, I.; Colen, S.; Berard, J.; Plomp, S.; Que, I.; van Rijen, M.; Woike, N.; Egas, A.; van Osch, G.; van Maarseveen, E.; et al. Prolonged inhibition of inflammation in osteoarthritis by triamcinolone acetonide released from a polyester amide microsphere platform. *J. Control. Release* **2017**, *253*, 64–72. [CrossRef]
11. Elron-Gross, I.; Glucksam, Y.; Margalit, R. Liposomal dexamethasone–diclofenac combinations for local osteoarthritis treatment. *Int. J. Pharm.* **2009**, *376*, 84–91. [CrossRef]
12. Rudnik-Jansen, I.; Woike, N.; de Jong, S.; Versteeg, S.; Kik, M.; Emans, P.; Mihov, G.; Thies, J.; Eijkelkamp, N.; Tryfonidou, M.; et al. Applicability of a modified rat model of acute arthritis for long-term testing of drug delivery systems. *Pharmaceutics* **2019**, *11*, 70. [CrossRef]
13. He, Z.; Wang, B.; Hu, C.; Zhao, J. An overview of hydrogel-based intra-articular drug delivery for the treatment of osteoarthritis. *Colloids Surf. B Biointerfaces* **2017**, *154*, 33–39. [CrossRef]
14. Zhang, Z.; Wei, X.; Gao, J.; Zhao, Y.; Zhao, Y.; Guo, L.; Chen, C.; Duan, Z.; Li, P.; Wei, L.; et al. Intra-articular injection of cross-linked hyaluronic acid-dexamethasone hydrogel attenuates osteoarthritis: An experimental study in a rat model of osteoarthritis. *Int. J. Mol. Sci.* **2016**, *17*, 411. [CrossRef]
15. Ho, M.J.; Kim, S.R.; Choi, Y.W.; Kang, M.J. Recent advances in intra-articular drug delivery systems to extend drug retention in joint. *J. Pharm. Investig.* **2019**, *49*, 9–15. [CrossRef]
16. Evans, C.H.; Kraus, V.B.; Setton, L.A. Progress in intra-articular therapy. *Nat. Rev. Rheumatol.* **2014**, *10*, 11–22. [CrossRef]
17. Bodick, N.; Lufkin, J.; Willwerth, C.; Kumar, A.; Bolognese, J.; Schoonmaker, C.; Ballal, R.; Hunter, D.; Clayman, M. An intra-articular, extended-release formulation of triamcinolone acetonide prolongs and amplifies analgesic effect in patients with osteoarthritis of the knee: a randomized clinical trial. *J. Bone Jt. Surg. Am.* **2015**, *97*, 877–888. [CrossRef]
18. Ho, M.J.; Kim, S.R.; Choi, Y.W.; Kang, M.J. a novel stable crystalline triamcinolone acetonide-loaded PLGA microsphere for prolonged release after intra-articular injection. *Bull. Korean Chem. Soc.* **2016**, *37*, 1496–1500. [CrossRef]
19. Ige, P.P.; Baria, R.K.; Gattani, S.G. Fabrication of fenofibrate nanocrystals by probe sonication method for enhancement of dissolution rate and oral bioavailability. *Colloids Surf. B Biointerfaces* **2013**, *108*, 366–373. [CrossRef]
20. Xiao, C.-D.; Shen, X.-C.; Tao, L. Modified emulsion solvent evaporation method for fabricating core–shell microspheres. *Int. J. Pharm.* **2013**, *452*, 227–232. [CrossRef]

21. Ouyang, H.; Zheng, A.; Heng, P.; Chan, L. Effect of lipid additives and drug on the rheological properties of molten paraffin wax, degree of surface drug coating, and drug release in spray-congealed microparticles. *Pharmaceutics* **2018**, *10*, 75. [CrossRef]
22. Naik, J.B.; Waghulde, M.R. Development of vildagliptin loaded Eudragit® microspheres by screening design: In Vitro evaluation. *J. Pharm. Investig.* **2018**, *48*, 627–637. [CrossRef]
23. César, I.C.; Byrro, R.M.D.; de Santana e Silva Cardoso, F.F.; Mundim, I.M.; de Souza Teixeira, L.; de Sousa, W.C.; Gomes, S.A.; Bellorio, K.B.; Brêtas, J.M.; Pianetti, G.A. Determination of triamcinolone in human plasma by a sensitive HPLC-ESI-MS/MS method: Application for a pharmacokinetic study using nasal spray formulation. *J. Mass Spectrom.* **2011**, *46*, 320–326. [CrossRef]
24. Zulian, F.; Martini, G.; Gobber, D.; Plebani, M.; Zacchello, F.; Manners, P. Triamcinolone acetonide and hexacetonide intra-articular treatment of symmetrical joints in juvenile idiopathic arthritis: A double-blind trial. *Rheumatology* **2004**, *43*, 1288–1291. [CrossRef]
25. Zhang, Z.; Bi, X.; Li, H.; Huang, G. Enhanced targeting efficiency of PLGA microspheres loaded with Lornoxicam for intra-articular administration. *Drug Deliv.* **2011**, *18*, 536–544. [CrossRef]
26. Zolnik, B.S.; Leary, P.E.; Burgess, D.J. Elevated temperature accelerated release testing of PLGA microspheres. *J. Control. Release* **2006**, *112*, 293–300. [CrossRef]
27. Shen, J.; Burgess, D.J. Accelerated in vitro release testing of implantable PLGA microsphere/PVA hydrogel composite coatings. *Int. J. Pharm.* **2012**, *422*, 341–348. [CrossRef]
28. Tomic, I.; Vidis-Millward, A.; Mueller-Zsigmondy, M.; Cardot, J.-M. Setting accelerated dissolution test for PLGA microspheres containing peptide, investigation of critical parameters affecting drug release rate and mechanism. *Int. J. Pharm.* **2016**, *505*, 42–51. [CrossRef]
29. Frank, A.; Rath, S.K.; Venkatraman, S.S. Controlled release from bioerodible polymers: Effect of drug type and polymer composition. *J. Control. Release* **2005**, *102*, 333–344. [CrossRef]
30. Stewart, S.; Domínguez-Robles, J.; Donnelly, R.; Larrañeta, E.; Stewart, S.A.; Domínguez-Robles, J.; Donnelly, R.F.; Larrañeta, E. Implantable polymeric drug delivery devices: Classification, manufacture, materials, and clinical applications. *Polymers* **2018**, *10*, 1379. [CrossRef]
31. Witt, C.; Kissel, T. Morphological characterization of microspheres, films and implants prepared from poly(lactide-*co*-glycolide) and ABA triblock copolymers: Is the erosion controlled by degradation, swelling or diffusion? *Eur. J. Pharm. Biopharm.* **2001**, *51*, 171–181. [CrossRef]
32. Makadia, H.K.; Siegel, S.J.; Makadia, H.K.; Siegel, S.J. Poly lactic-*co*-glycolic acid (PLGA) as biodegradable controlled drug delivery carrier. *Polymers* **2011**, *3*, 1377–1397. [CrossRef]
33. Hopkins, R.L.; Leinung, M.C. Exogenous Cushing's syndrome and glucocorticoid withdrawal. *Endocrinol. Metab. Clin. N. Am.* **2005**, *34*, 371–384. [CrossRef]
34. Wernecke, C.; Braun, H.J.; Dragoo, J.L. The Effect of Intra-articular corticosteroids on articular cartilage. *Orthop. J. Sport. Med.* **2015**, *3*, 232596711558116. [CrossRef]
35. Jüni, P.; Hari, R.; Rutjes, A.W.; Fischer, R.; Silletta, M.G.; Reichenbach, S.; da Costa, B.R. Intra-articular corticosteroid for knee osteoarthritis. *Cochrane Database Syst. Rev.* **2015**, *10*, CD005328. [CrossRef]
36. Hepper, C.T.; Halvorson, J.J.; Duncan, S.T.; Gregory, A.J.M.; Dunn, W.R.; Spindler, K.P. The efficacy and duration of intra-articular corticosteroid injection for knee osteoarthritis: a systematic review of level I studies. *J. Am. Acad. Orthop. Surg.* **2009**, *17*, 638–646. [CrossRef]
37. Kraus, V.B.; Conaghan, P.G.; Aazami, H.A.; Mehra, P.; Kivitz, A.J.; Lufkin, J.; Hauben, J.; Johnson, J.R.; Bodick, N. Synovial and systemic pharmacokinetics (PK) of triamcinolone acetonide (TA) following intra-articular (IA) injection of an extended-release microsphere-based formulation (FX006) or standard crystalline suspension in patients with knee osteoarthritis (OA). *Osteoarthr. Cartil.* **2018**, *26*, 34–42. [CrossRef]

13

Photodynamic Therapy of Ovarian Carcinoma Cells with Curcumin-Loaded Biodegradable Polymeric Nanoparticles

Lili Duse [1,†], Michael Rene Agel [1,†], Shashank Reddy Pinnapireddy [1], Jens Schäfer [1], Mohammed A. Selo [2,3], Carsten Ehrhardt [2] and Udo Bakowsky [1,*]

1 Department of Pharmaceutics and Biopharmaceutics, University of Marburg, Robert-Koch-Str. 4, 35037 Marburg, Germany; lili.duse@pharmazie.uni-marburg.de (L.D.); michael.agel@pharmazie.uni-marburg.de (M.R.A.); shashank.pinnapireddy@pharmazie.uni-marburg.de (S.R.P.); j.schaefer@staff.uni-marburg.de (J.S.)

2 School of Pharmacy and Pharmaceutical Sciences and Biomedical Sciences Institute, Trinity College Dublin, Dublin 2, Ireland; mohammeda.mohsin@uokufa.edu.iq (M.A.S.); ehrhardc@tcd.ie (C.E.)

3 Faculty of Pharmacy, University of Kufa, 31001 Kufa, Iraq

* Correspondence: ubakowsky@aol.com

† Both authors contributed equally to this work.

Abstract: Accumulation of photosensitisers in photodynamic therapy in healthy tissues is often the cause of unwanted side effects. Using nanoparticles, improved bioavailability and site-specific drug uptake can be achieved. In this study, curcumin, a natural product with anticancer properties, albeit with poor aqueous solubility, was encapsulated in biodegradable polymeric poly(lactic-*co*-glycolic acid) (PLGA) nanoparticles (CUR-NP). Dynamic light scattering, laser Doppler anemometry and atomic force microscopy were used to characterise the formulations. Using haemolysis, serum stability and activated partial thromboplastin time tests, the biocompatibility of CUR-NP was assessed. Particle uptake and accumulation were determined by confocal laser scanning microscopy. Therapeutic efficacy of the formulation was tested in SK-OV-3 human ovarian adenocarcinoma cells post low level LED irradiation by determining the generation of reactive oxygen species and cytotoxicity. Pharmacologic inhibitors of cellular uptake pathways were used to identify the particle uptake mechanism. CUR-NP exhibited better physicochemical properties such as stability in the presence of light and improved serum stability compared to free curcumin. In addition, the novel nanoformulation facilitated the use of higher amounts of curcumin and showed strong apoptotic effects on tumour cells.

Keywords: PLGA; nanoscaled drug delivery; LED; cancer; serum stability; reactive oxygen species; cellular uptake

1. Introduction

Light has long been used in the treatment of diseases as different as psoriasis, rickets or cancer [1]. With an alarming mortality rate, cancer is one of the most prevalent causes of death worldwide [2]. Hence, tremendous efforts have been made to develop novel safe, selective and effective cancer therapies. One such treatment, photodynamic therapy, exemplifies a novel minimally invasive tumour targeting therapy, in which tumour tissues can be selectively destroyed by three main mechanisms [3,4]. In the first case there is a combination of three individually inert entities viz. a photoactive drug molecule (photosensitiser; PS), oxygen and a light source of a specific wavelength, which upon combining, activate the photosensitiser and exhibit toxicity towards cancer cells and tissues [5,6]. This process of photosensitisation hugely relies upon the presence of molecular oxygen and forms the basis for a successful photodynamic therapy (PDT) [7]. After absorbing energy from the light source, the PS interacts with molecular oxygen via energy transfer process or electron transfer process and generates reactive oxygen species (ROS), which oxidise cellular and subcellular organelles to induce either apoptosis or necrosis leading to cell death [8,9]. Since cytotoxic ROS occurs only after irradiation of the PS, tumour tissues can be targeted with high precision. Due to its high reactivity and short half-life, ROS generation only targets cells lying in close proximity of the site of irradiation [1]. The half-life of singlet oxygen in biological systems is ~0.01–0.04 μs, with a restricted site of action of a radius spanning 0.01–0.02 μm [5,10]. PDT can also damage the tumour-associated vasculature, leading to tumour infarction. Finally, PDT can activate the immune response against tumour cells. All three mentioned mechanisms can also influence each other and act synergistically. PDT has an added advantage of almost no or minimal effect towards healthy tissues, making this therapy site specific [11]. It could also be combined with other therapies or immune-stimulatory agents like microbial adjuvants or cytokine for T-cell therapy and adoptive cellular therapy, respectively [1]. Another advantage of PDT is its effectiveness against otherwise chemoresistant cell types [12]. Furthermore, the photosensitiser can be administered by various means, such as systemically, locally or topically [1].

For the success of any PDT, it is important to choose an optimal PS. Despite many studies performed using different PS, only a few have reached the stage of advanced human clinical trials or even U.S. Food and Drug Administration (FDA) approval for clinical use [13]. A very promising photosensitiser for photodynamic treatment of tumours is curcumin. Curcumin (diferuloylmethane), is a naturally occurring yellowish polyphenol extract from the rhizomes of turmeric (*Curcuma longa*), which is cultivated widely in south and southeast tropical Asia [14]. Curcumin is the most active component of turmeric, making up approx. 0.5–3.14% of the dry weight of turmeric powder. Curcumin is used for a variety of therapeutic activities against many different diseases and conditions such as skin diseases, pulmonary and gastrointestinal systems, aches, pains, wounds, sprains, and liver disorders [15].

Offering a variety of potential applications, curcumin has been commonly used as a food-colouring agent (E100) as well as in pharmaceutical research due to its anti-inflammatory, anti-oxidative, anti-carcinogenic and anti-microbial effects [16,17]. It is a proven anticancer agent and therefore a perfect choice for a photosensitiser [18]. However, curcumin exhibits a very low level of bioavailability, since it is a highly lipophilic substance (solubility 11 ng/mL in phosphate buffer saline, PBS; pH 5) [19]. Systemically absorbed curcumin is prone to an extensive first-pass metabolism and undergoes a fast metabolic reduction with biliary excretion [20]. In 1978, Wahlstrom and Blennow observed the uptake of curcumin using Sprague–Dawley rats. After oral administration of 1 g/kg curcumin only negligible amounts of curcumin could be found in blood plasma [21].

These limitations can be overcome by the use of polymeric nanoparticles such as carrier systems, wherein the active substance is protected from degradation in the physiological environment and the bio-membrane permeability and cellular uptake of highly hydrophobic molecules are facilitated [17]. Several studies have revealed a remarkable enhancement of curcumin's phototoxicity through nanoparticle encapsulation [22–26]. One such polymer is PLGA, which is an FDA and European Medicines Agency (EMA) approved biocompatible and biodegradable polymer [27,28]. In the body, PLGA undergoes hydrolysis wherein the endogenous metabolite monomers lactic acid and glycolic acid are and easily metabolised by the body (to water and carbon dioxide) via Krebs cycle [27,29,30]. The degradation time of PLGA and the release of drug from the nanoparticles mainly depends on the nature of copolymer composition [31]. In this study, PLGA 50:50 was chosen due to its ability to hydrolyse much faster than other types of PLGA with a half-life (50% loss of molecular weight) of 15 days for microspheres [32,33].

Another important aspect in PDT is the choice of the irradiation device. There is an array of radiation devices available for PDT such as lasers or lamps [13]. In the current study, with an aim to make PDT more cost effective, efficient and safe, we have utilised a custom manufactured prototype low level light emitting diode (LED) array for the irradiation of PS [34]. LEDs are energy efficient, generate less thermal energy in the form of heat and are versatile in terms of structural form. They have the ability to emit light over a wide area with a relatively homogenous output, which enables treatment of larger lesions in fewer therapy sessions. Using a combination of curcumin loaded PLGA nanoparticles and LED-based PDT, superficial tumours (melanomas and lymphomas) and accessible adenocarcinomas (such as ovarian and cervical) could be treated effectively. The PLGA nanoparticles can be administered intratumourally or could be surface modified to enable systemic application.

In the present study, we have exploited the combination of biodegradable PLGA nanoparticles and LED-based PDT using curcumin as a photosensitiser. The nanoparticles have been characterised for their size and surface charge using Dynamic light scattering (DLS) and laser Doppler anemometry (LDA), respectively. Structural morphology was analysed using atomic force microscopy (AFM) and transmission electron microscopy (TEM). The photo-destructive effects have been evaluated in vitro by cytotoxicity assays and confocal laser scanning microscopy (CLSM). The cellular uptake in SK-OV-3 cells was also analysed using three different uptake inhibitors. Irradiation experiments were carried out in SK-OV-3 tumour cells and the oxidative stress induced during the irradiation was analysed by determining the inhibition of ROS. Furthermore, haemolysis assays using fresh blood, serum stability using serum and activated partial thromboplastin time tests (aPTT) using plasma were used to demonstrate the biocompatibility of the curcumin-loaded polymeric nanoparticles.

2. Materials and Methods

2.1. Materials

Curcumin (95% purity) was obtained from Alfa Aesar (Ward Hill, MA, USA); PLGA (Resomer RG 503 H) was supplied by Evonik (Essen, Germany); poly(vinyl alcohol) (PVA, Mowiol 4-88) was purchased from Kuraray (Hattersheim, Germany); polysorbate 80 (Tween 80), 3-(4,5-dimethylthiazol-2-yl)-2,5-diphenyltetrazolium bromide (MTT), 2′,7′-dichlorofluorescin diacetate (DCFDA) and tert-butyl hydroperoxide (TBHP) were obtained from Sigma-Aldrich Chemie (Taufkirchen, Germany). Inhibitors of cellular uptake, viz. Filipin III, chlorpromazine and dynasore were also obtained from Sigma Aldrich. Ultrapure water, generated by a PURELAB flex 4 device (ELGA LabWater, High Wycombe, UK) was used for all experiments. For cell culture studies, ultrapure water was additionally autoclaved and filter-sterilised using 0.2 µm polyethersulphone membrane filters (Sarstedt, Nümbrecht, Germany) prior to use. HPLC-grade ethyl acetate (VWR, Darmstadt, Germany) was used to prepare the organic phases. All other chemicals used were of analytical grade. All buffers used in this study were prepared in the laboratory, unless stated otherwise.

2.2. Light Source

The LED device used in this study was custom made by Lumundus (Eisenach, Germany) to be usable with microtiter plates. The device is equipped with an array of two different LEDs, capable of emitting light at wavelengths of 457 nm and 620 nm, respectively. Irradiation time, current (i.e., 20, 40, 60, 80, and 100 mA) and wavelength settings are adjustable as per the energy requirement. Radiation intensity was calculated based on the current and irradiation time.

2.3. Cell culture

The human ovarian adenocarcinoma cell line SK-OV-3 was procured from American Type Culture Collection (ATCC, Manassas, VA, USA). SK-OV-3 cells were cultivated in Iscove's modified Dulbecco's medium (Capricorn Scientific, Ebsdorfergrund, Germany) supplemented with 10% foetal bovine serum (Sigma-Aldrich, Taufkirchen, Germany) at 37 °C and 7% CO_2 in humidified atmosphere. The medium was replaced every other day and the cells were sub-cultured upon reaching 80% confluency.

2.4. Formulation of Nanoparticles

Curcumin-loaded nanoparticles (CUR-NP) and unloaded PLGA nanoparticles (NP) were prepared from PLGA by the emulsion–diffusion–evaporation technique as previously described by Kumar et al. [35]. In a pilot study, the method was optimised by varying formulation parameters (e.g., concentration of PLGA, PVA and curcumin; homogenisation speed and time). Briefly, 200 mg of PLGA were dissolved in 5 mL ethyl acetate at room temperature. Curcumin stock solution was prepared by dissolving curcumin in ethyl acetate (2 mg/mL). Equal volumes of PLGA and curcumin stock solutions were mixed and filtered through a 0.45 μm nylon syringe filter (Pall Corporation, New York, NY, USA). The organic solution was added dropwise to an aqueous solution of 2% PVA (*w*/*w*) and the resulting emulsion was stirred in a sealed tube for about 3 h, before homogenising for 10 min at 13,400 rpm using an Ultra-Turrax T25 homogeniser (IKA-Werke, Staufen, Germany). Nanoprecipitation was induced by adding water at a constant rate of 120 mL/h using a syringe pump (Perfusor, B. Braun, Melsungen, Germany). Finally, the organic solvent was evaporated by stirring overnight at room temperature in a dark environment. The nanosuspension was adjusted to a final volume of 50 mL and a concentration of 0.1 mg/mL curcumin. Unloaded nanoparticles were prepared by the same protocol, except that pure ethyl acetate was used instead of the curcumin stock solution. To remove agglomerates, the nanoformulations were centrifuged at 2000× *g* for 45 s using an Eppendorf Centrifuge 5418 (Eppendorf, Hamburg, Germany). The resulting pellet was discarded, and the supernatant was washed three times with water to separate the nanospheres from non-encapsulated curcumin. Between each washing step, centrifugation at 16,000× *g* for 45 min was performed. For prolonged storage, the CUR-NP were freeze-dried using an Alpha 1-4LSC lyophiliser (Martin Christ Gefriertrocknungsanlagen, Osterode am Harz, Germany) using 0.5% PVA as a cryoprotectant. Afterwards the nanoformulations were stored at 4 °C protected from light.

2.5. *Dynamic Light Scattering and Laser Doppler Anemometry*

To determine particle size distribution and zeta (ζ)-potential of the particles, DLS and LDA were used, respectively (Zetasizer Nano ZS, Malvern Instruments, Malvern, UK). A viscosity of 0.88 mPa × s and a refractive index of 1.33 of water at 25 °C were assumed for data interpretation. Measurement position and laser attenuation were automatically adjusted by the instrument. The instrument performs 15 size runs per measurement with each lasting 10 s. For ζ-potential measurements, the instrument automatically performs 15–100 runs per measurement, depending upon the sample. All samples were diluted with filtered PBS buffer (1:100) [36]. Data from at least three independent experiments were measured for both DLS and LDA analysis.

2.6. *Morphological Characterisation*

To investigate the morphology of CUR-NP and to confirm size data obtained by DLS measurements, AFM was performed using a Nanowizard 3®(JPK Instruments, Berlin, Germany) and a Digital Nanoscope IV Bioscope (Veeco Instruments, Santa Barbara, CA, USA), respectively. Formulations were diluted 1:100 with water and 20 μL of the diluted sample were placed onto a silica wafer or an untreated microscopic glass slide. The samples were left to settle onto the surface for a few minutes and the remaining fluid was absorbed by a lint-free wipe (Kimtech Precision Wipes, Kimberly-Clark, Fullerton, CA, USA). Measurements were performed in tapping mode, in which the cantilever oscillated with determined amplitude close to its resonance frequency, with scan rates from 0.5 to 1 Hz. A HQ:NSC16/AL_BS (Anfatec Instruments, Oelsnitz, Germany) cantilever was used [37]. Data were processed using JPKSPM data processing software (v. 5.1.8, JPK instruments).

For the TEM analysis, the nanoparticle suspension was applied onto 300-mesh copper grids. Samples were then negative stained thrice with 2% uranyl acetate (pH 4.2), which was alternated by washing steps with water. The samples were then allowed to dry overnight before being examined under the TEM (LEO 912 AB, Carl Zeiss, Jena, Germany) [22].

2.7. *Yield, Encapsulation Efficiency and Loading Capacity*

The freeze-dried nanoparticles were weighted, and the percentage yield was calculated using the following equation

$$\%\text{Yield} = \frac{\text{Dry weight of nanoparticles}}{\text{Weight of drug and polymer used for NP preparation}} \times 100 \quad (1)$$

The encapsulation efficiency (%EE) was determined by extracting curcumin from nanospheres that were previously washed and separated from free curcumin, as previously described in Section 2.4. The nanosuspension was mixed with an equal volume of acetonitrile (a solvent for PLGA and curcumin) and sonicated for 20 min. The absorbance of this solution was measured spectrophotometrically at 425 nm using a Multiskan GO micro plate reader (Thermo Fischer Scientific, Waltham, MA, USA), and the amount of drug quantified using a calibration curve recorded with known curcumin concentrations. For determination of the total drug content, nanoparticles without any washing procedure were measured in the same way. The %EE (*w*/*w*) was calculated as follows:

$$\%\text{EE} = \frac{\text{Drug}_{\text{encapsulated}}}{\text{Drug}_{\text{total}}} \times 100 \quad (2)$$

In addition, the loading capacity (LC) was calculated using the equation:

$$\%\text{LC} = \frac{\text{Drug}_{\text{encapsulated}}}{\text{Dry weight of nanoparticles}} \times 100 \quad (3)$$

2.8. *In Vitro Drug Release*

For determination of drug release, 10 mg lyophilised nanoparticles were redispersed in 30 mL PBS buffer (pH 5.5 and pH 7.4) containing 1% polysorbate 80 (*v*/*v*) to assure sink conditions. This dispersion was stored under absence of light in a shaking incubator (TH 15/KS 15, Edmund Bühler, Bodelshausen, Germany) at 37 °C under slight agitation (50 rpm). For the following seven days, 500 µL samples were drawn and replaced with fresh medium. The samples were centrifuged for 10 min at 16,000× *g* (Centrifuge 5418, Eppendorf AG) and the amount of curcumin present in the supernatant was determined spectrophotometrically at 425 nm, using Multiskan GO micro plate reader (Thermo Fischer Scientific).

2.9. *Serum Stability*

To study the stability of the formulations in physiologically relevant conditions, 2 mL serum was diluted with 20 mM HEPES (pH 7.4) to make a 60% serum solution. Curcumin-loaded PLGA nanoparticles were added in a ratio of 1:5 (*v*/*v*). The mixture was incubated at 37 °C in a shaking incubator at 100 rpm for 24 h. Samples were further diluted to a ratio of 1:20 (*v*/*v*) with 20 mM HEPES (pH 7.4) prior to DLS and LDA analyses at different time points. All measurements were carried out in triplicates [38].

2.10. *In Vitro Irradiation Experiments*

Cells were seeded onto in 96-well plates (10,000 cells/0.35 cm^2 (per well); Nunclon Delta, Thermo Fisher Scientific, Waltham, MA, USA) and were allowed to adhere overnight. Various concentrations of CUR-NP and free curcumin (dissolved in DMSO) were added to the wells and incubated for 4 h. Irradiation was performed at a wavelength of 457 nm with a radiation fluence of 8.6 J/cm^2 and the plates were incubated overnight. Dark (un-irradiated) plates were used as control [39]. Subsequently, the medium was replaced with fresh medium containing MTT dye and cells were incubated for 4 h. Absorbance of the resulting formazan crystals dissolved in DMSO was measured using a plate reader

(FLUOstar Optima; BMG Labtech, Offenburg, Germany) at 570 nm. Viability of untreated cells was considered as 100%.

2.11. *Cellular Uptake Studies*

To determine the cellular uptake mechanism, SK-OV-3 cells were seeded at a density of 10,000 cells/0.35 cm^2 (per well) in 96-well plates (Nunclon Delta, Nunc/Thermo Fischer Scientific, Waltham, MA, USA) and incubated overnight. The next day, cells were washed with PBS containing Ca^{2+} and Mg^{2+} (pH 7.4) and were incubated for 30 min with pharmacological inhibitors of different endocytic mechanisms viz. dynasore (80 μM), chlorpromazine (14 μM) and Filipin III (8 mM) [40]. After incubation with the uptake inhibitors, cells were washed again with PBS and exposed to 50 μM CUR-NP or free curcumin (dissolved in DMSO) for 4 h. After irradiation at 457 nm with a radiation fluence of 8.6 J/cm^2, cells were incubated with MTT and the absorbance from resulting formazan crystals (dissolved in DMSO) was determined at 570 nm as described above.

2.12. *Reactive Oxygen Species*

ROS were determined using 2′,7′-dichlorofluorescin diacetate (DCFDA, Abcam, Cambridge, UK) according to the supplier's protocol with slight modifications [34]. Briefly, SK-OV-3 cells were seeded in 96-well plates as mentioned above. The next day, cells were incubated with CUR-NP for 4 h. Tert-butyl hydroperoxide (TBHP, 50 μM) was used as positive control. Cells were subsequently washed using PBS containing Ca^{2+} and Mg^{2+} (pH 7.4) and supplemented with fresh medium. Irradiation was carried out at 457 nm with a radiation fluence of 8.6 J/cm^2. The cells were washed again with PBS and incubated with culture medium (IMDM without phenol red) containing 25 μM DCFDA for 1 h. Cell culture lysis reagent (Promega, Mannheim, Germany) was used to lyse the cell and fluorescence was recorded using a FLUOstar Optima plate reader (λ_{ex} 480 nm/λ_{em} 520 nm).

2.13. *Intracellular Visualisation of PDT*

Cells were seeded onto 12-well plates (90,000 cells/3.5 cm^2 (per well); Nunclon Delta) containing cover slips (15 mm in diameter). The plates were incubated for 24 h, before being used for the experiments. CUR-NP suspension was added dropwise to each well. After 4 h, the supernatant was removed and cells were washed twice with PBS containing Ca^{2+} and Mg^{2+} (pH 7.4). Cell were treated with a 4% formaldehyde solution for 20 min to fix them. The nucleus was counterstained with 0.1 μg/mL 4′,6-diamidino-2-phenylindole (DAPI) for 20 min. Finally, the cells were washed again with PBS (pH 7.4) and the cover slips were mounted onto slides. Samples were examined under a LSM700 confocal laser-scanning microscope (Carl Zeiss Microscopy, Jena, Germany).

2.14. *Activated Partial Thromboplastin Time Test*

An aPTT test was performed as previously described, using a Coatron M1 coagulation analyser (Teco, Neufahrn, Germany) to determine the effect of the formulations on blood coagulation [41]. Briefly, 25 μL of plasma was mixed with 25 μL each of sample and of aPTT reagent followed by addition of an equal volume of pre-warmed 0.025 M calcium chloride solution to activate coagulation. Coagulation was determined spectrophotometrically.

2.15. *Haemolysis Assay*

To determine the effect of the formulations on blood, human erythrocytes were isolated from fresh blood as described previously [42]. Briefly, following prior consent from the donor, whole blood was collected into EDTA tubes as centrifuged to separate the red blood cell (RBC) pellet. The RBC pellet was washed thrice with PBS buffer (pH 7.4) and diluted to a ratio of 1:50 with PBS. The erythrocytes were incubated together with the formulations in V-bottom microtiter plates placed in an orbital shaker KS4000 IC (IKA Werke) for 1 h at 37 °C. Supernatants were collected from the plates following centrifugation and the absorbance was determined at 540 nm using a plate reader (FLUOstar Optima). PBS (pH 7.4) and 1% Triton X-100 were used as controls.

2.16. Statistical Analysis

All experiments were performed in triplicates and data are presented as mean ± standard deviation, unless otherwise stated. Two-tailed Student's *t*-test was performed to identify statistical significance differences.

3. Results

3.1. Physicochemical Characterisation

Preliminary experiments were performed to determine an ideal stabiliser concentration, homogenisation speed and curcumin content. In emulsion–diffusion–evaporation technique, PVA acts as a stabiliser of the nanodroplets and is one of the widely used emulsifier for polymeric nanoparticle preparations. Both, particle size and size distribution are affected by the concentration of PVA in the aqueous phase during particle preparation [35]. After testing different PVA concentrations, we narrowed down to 2% PVA considering the physicochemical properties of the resultant nanoformulations. The Z-average data from DLS as well as LDA results are summarised in Table 1. CUR-NP and NP showed a narrow size distribution indicating a high reproducibility. No extensive change in particle size was noticeable after curcumin loading. This was also the case for lyophilised samples, thereby showing that lyophilisation has no deleterious effects on the physicochemical characteristics. Furthermore, LDA revealed a slightly negative ζ-potential at pH 7.4, regardless of curcumin loading for both formulations.

Table 1. Hydrodynamic diameter, polydispersity index (PDI) and ζ-potential of curcumin-loaded poly(lactic-*co*-glycolic acid) (PLGA) nanoparticles (CUR-NP) and unloaded PLGA nanoparticles (NP). Lyophilised samples represent samples resuspended after lyophilisation. Hydrodynamic diameters are expressed as a measure of particle size distribution by intensity. All samples were measured in triplicates ($n = 9$, independent formulations) and results are expressed as means ± SD.

Sample	Diameter [nm]	PDI	ζ-potential [mV]
NP	194.7 ± 8.7	0.09 ± 0.05	−5.33 ± 0.88
CUR-NP	203.6 ± 7.8	0.08 ± 0.04	−5.24 ± 0.86
Lyophilised NP	195.0 ± 6.9	0.09 ± 0.05	−5.09 ± 0.73
Lyophilised CUR-NP	201.8 ± 6.0	0.09 ± 0.03	−5.43 ± 0.67

PLGA in an aqueous environment undergoes hydrolysis spanning over several weeks, depending on the ratio of lactic acid to glycolic acid. The PLGA 50:50 used in this study therefore exhibits the fastest degradation [43]. To increase the storage stability the nanoparticles were lyophilised, using PVA as cryoprotectant. Freeze-dried and resuspended nanoparticles showed no extensive change in particle size (CUR-NP +0.3 nm, NP −1.8 nm) or polydispersity index (data not shown).

For the determination of encapsulation efficiency, a direct method of dissolving the purified particles and measuring the actual amount of curcumin available in the nanoparticle formulation was used. Since curcumin is near to insoluble in water, un-encapsulated free curcumin should exist in crystalline form. In this case the crystals would sediment during ultracentrifugation and be present in the pellet. Hence discarding the supernatant would not lead to sufficient separation of nanoparticles from crystalline curcumin. Therefore (in contrast to NP), a first separation step of centrifugation with a relatively low force of 2000× *g* is necessary to sediment the larger crystals. The optimised formulation of CUR-NP showed a relatively high encapsulation efficiency (EE) with an actual loading capacity of 2% (Table 2). The good EE results can be explained by the fact that PLGA and curcumin are both soluble in ethyl acetate, which was employed for the nanoparticle preparation process. Moreover, PLGA's ability to effectively encapsulate curcumin has been demonstrated in previous studies [44–46].

Table 2. Theoretical load, percentage of yield, encapsulation efficiency and loading capacity of curcumin-loaded poly(lactic-*co*-glycolic acid) (PLGA) nanoparticles (CUR-NP) and unloaded PLGA nanoparticles (NP). All samples were measured in triplicates ($n = 9$, independent formulations) and results are expressed as means ± SD.

Sample	Theoretical Load [%] [a]	%Yield	%EE	%LC
NP	-	80.5 ± 2.3	-	-
CUR-NP	2.5	87.5 ± 0.7	80.4 ± 10.6	2.0 ± 0.3

[a] % *w/w* loading of curcumin to polymer; EE, encapsulation efficiency; LC, loading capacity.

3.2. Morphological Characterisation

In all images (Figure 1), round-shaped CUR-NP with a monomodal size distribution are clearly visible. Due to dilution of pure nanoparticle samples, even single CUR-NPs with a smooth surface indicating that the curcumin is completely incorporated could be visualised. The AFM size analysis was in agreement with the DLS measurements. It should however be noted that the differences in size arising from the DLS and AFM measurements is because the hydrodynamic diameter is obtained in aqueous conditions whereas the latter is measured under atmospheric conditions [47]. Furthermore, a PVA corona was noticeable in TEM micrographs (Figure 1C). While free PVA was removed through centrifugation and washing of the redispersed nanoparticles prior to each experiment, it is a known fact, that small quantities of PVA still remain on the surface of PLGA nanoparticles, which cannot be removed even by extensive washing. This strong adsorption of PVA may be caused by hydrophobic bonding of PVA's hydroxyl groups to the acetyl groups of PLGA [48].

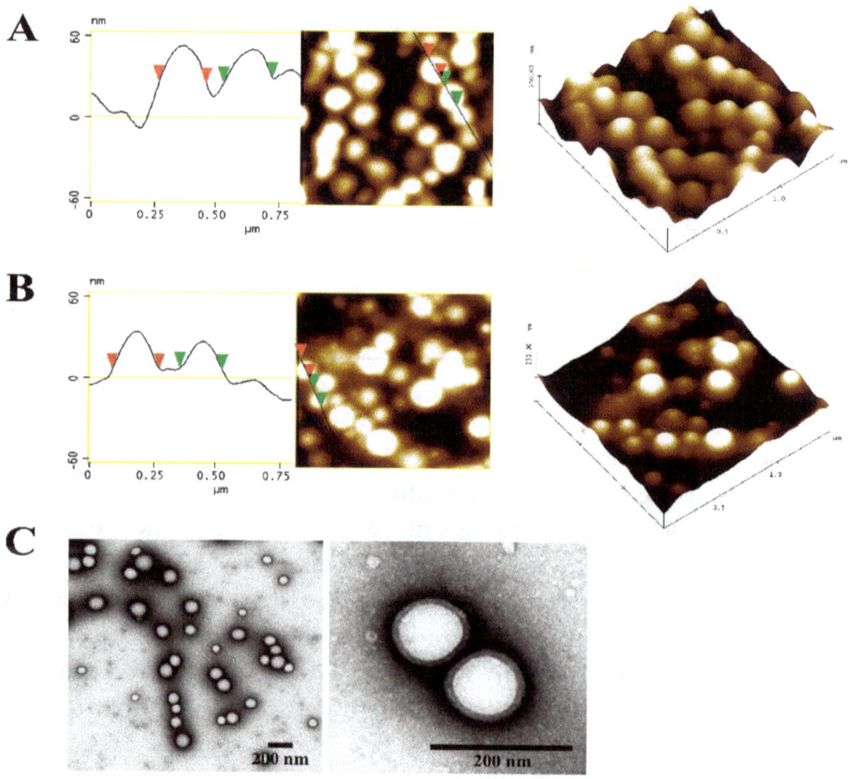

Figure 1. Morphology of representative curcumin-loaded poly(lactic-*co*-glycolic acid) (PLGA) nanoparticles (CUR-NP) shown by atomic force microscopy (AFM) (**A**,**B**) and transmission electron microscopy (TEM) (**C**). (**A**) Freshly prepared nanoparticles, (**B**,**C**) nanoparticles post lyophilisation. All AFM micrographs are presented in height mode. Samples were negatively stained with 2% uranyl acetate prior to TEM measurement. Scale bars in TEM micrographs represent 200 nm.

3.3. In Vitro Drug Release

Different mechanisms were reported for the drug release from PLGA nanoparticles: (i) desorption of drug absorbed on the particles surface, (ii) diffusion through the polymer matrix, (iii) erosion of the polymer matrix, and (iv) a combination of erosion and diffusion processes [29,49].

The cumulative drug release of curcumin from CUR-NP at pH 5.5 and 7.4 is shown in Figure 2. Due to curcumin's low water solubility (~0.01 μg/mL at pH 5 and ~0.4 μg/mL at pH 7.3) and low stability at neutral to basic pH, the addition of a solubility-enhancing component was necessary to assure sink conditions and to achieve UV/VIS detectable concentrations [50]. We chose polysorbate 80 for this purpose, since it is reported, that it is capable of increasing the solubility of hydrophobic drugs and protecting them against degradation through the formation of micelles [51].

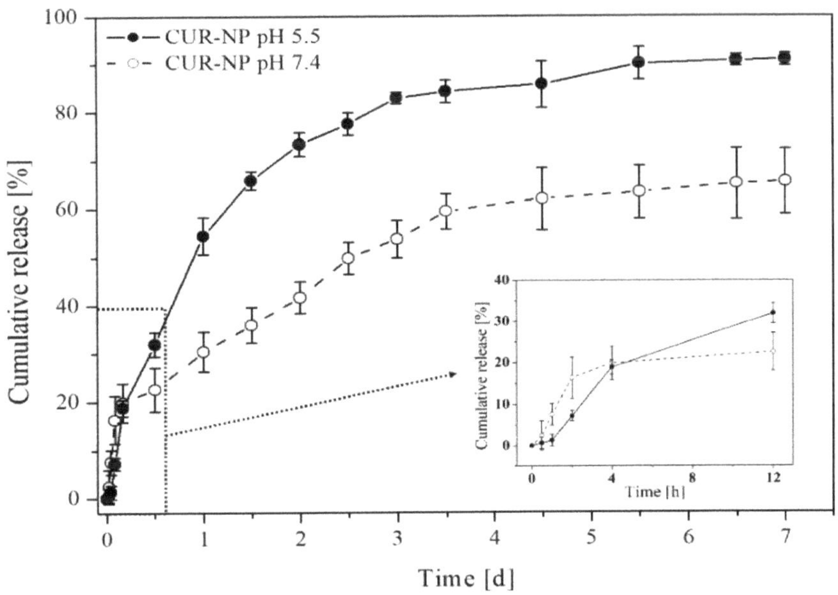

Figure 2. Cumulative in vitro drug release of curcumin from CUR-NP in phosphate buffer (pH 5.5 and 7.4) containing 1% polysorbate 80 to assure sink conditions. The inset represents the first 12 h of the release study in a different scale (hours instead of days).

CUR-NP showed a typical biphasic release pattern of PLGA nanoparticles with a burst release of around 20% loading within the initial 4 h, followed by controlled release of 90% drug loading over the following 7 days. Burst release is most likely attributed to the drug absorbed to the particle's surface, while controlled release might be induced through a combination of erosion and diffusion processes [52,53]. Furthermore, drug release was much faster in acidic medium compared to pH 7.4 which could be caused by a faster degradation rate of PLGA under acidic conditions [33].

Tumour cells often exhibit an extracellular pH of around 6.5, which would lead to a faster release of curcumin in this acidic environment and therefore an increased cytotoxicity compared to healthy tissue [54,55]. Since the pH of endosomes is even lower (pH ~5.5), drug release of internalised nanoparticles would proceed even faster, leading to higher intracellular curcumin concentration and enhanced tumour damage [56]. Both mechanisms could be used for passive tumour-targeting strategy.

3.4. Serum Stability

Serum stability assay was performed to evaluate the susceptibility of the formulations. For this purpose, DLS and LDA analyses were performed after incubating the nanoparticles in serum. The experiments were carried at 37 °C in a shaking incubator to simulate physiological conditions. The results show shrinkage in the nanoparticle size after 24 h incubation time in serum (Table 3). This could be related to a release of curcumin bound to the particle surface, which leads to particle erosion [57]. Furthermore, the decrease in particle size could be caused by osmotic forces, as reported previously [58].

The increase in the PDI of the nanoparticles could be attributed to the decrease in homogeneity in the presence of serum. After an initial increase (as compared to DLS measurements from native particles), the ζ-potential decreased to more negative values. The initial increase could be due to the accumulation of plasma proteins on the surface of the NP and the subsequent decrease could be attributed to the drug release (curcumin) onto the surface of the NP [59].

Table 3. Physicochemical changes of poly(lactic-*co*-glycolic acid) (PLGA) nanoparticles containing 0.1 mg/mL curcumin. Particles were incubated for 24 h in serum at a volume ratio of 5:1. The hydrodynamic diameter is expressed as a measure of particle size distribution by intensity. All samples were measured in triplicates ($n = 9$, independent formulations) and data are expressed as means ± SD.

Time [h]	Diameter [nm]	PDI	ζ-potential [mV]
0	183.50 ± 2.11	0.19 ± 0.01	2.19 ± 0.49
1	180.80 ± 3.70	0.19 ± 0.01	−8.30 ± 0.21
4	180.45 ± 3.32	0.22 ± 0.01	−12.65 ± 0.35
24	173.57 ± 2.21	0.22 ± 0.01	−13.30 ± 0.10

3.5. *Irradiation Experiments*

For the photo destructive effect of PDT, SK-OV-3 ovarian carcinoma cells were incubated with different concentrations of CUR-NP und free curcumin for 4 h and were irradiated with different radiation fluence. The efficacy of the irradiation was determined by MTT assay. As shown in Figure 3A, after treatment of cells, curcumin-loaded biodegradable nanoparticles and free curcumin dissolved in DMSO show a high photocytotoxic effect. There is a remarkable difference between the dark (non-irradiated) and irradiated plates. An incubation time of 4 h was found to be ideal among all the formulations, since burst release of around 20% curcumin loading from CUR-NP was found within 4 h of drug release studies (Figure 2). In the initial studies, a radiation fluence of 1.4, 4.3, 8.6 and 13.2 J/cm^2 were tested using CUR-NP and for the subsequent studies, the fluence was narrowed down to 8.6 J/cm^2 for the LED induced PDT (data not shown). Beyond a curcumin concentration of 50 μM, there was no further difference in the effect of PDT. It can also be seen that free curcumin dissolved in DMSO, induced a higher photocytotoxicity effect, which could be attributed to controlled release properties of PLGA nanoparticles, as this might be a rate limiting step for the drug being available for light activation. Nevertheless, since DMSO-dissolved curcumin is not suitable for therapeutic applications and due to its hydrophobic nature, we have used a biodegradable polymeric PLGA nanoformulation to increase the bioavailability of curcumin and to make it suitable for therapeutic applications [60]. The internalisation and subsequent localisation of the photosensitiser within the tumour determine the outcome of the therapy.

3.6. *Subcellular Localisation of Curcumin*

To visualise the effect of PDT on tumour cells, qualitative fluorescence microscopic analysis was performed after irradiation (457 nm; 8.6 J/cm^2) of the cells with 50 μM CUR-NP and free curcumin dissolved in DMSO. The cells were fixed with 4% formaldehyde solution and the cell nucleus was counterstained with 300 nM DAPI. Substantial intracellular localisation of curcumin near the cell's nucleus could be seen in both dark and irradiated samples, as shown in Figure 3B. Upon irradiation, photo-destruction induced by PDT could be clearly observed in the micrographs, which is evident from the nuclear perforation. This might be due to the chromatin condensation and DNA fragmentation caused by the curcumin induced PDT [8]. Comparing free curcumin dissolved in DMSO with curcumin-loaded nanoparticles reveals that CUR-NPs indeed damage the nucleus while only free curcumin alone is not as damaging although the micrographs show a cellular uptake of curcumin by both the samples. This confirms the hypothesis that curcumin particles are internalised by uptake mechanisms such as endocytosis and free curcumin penetrates the cells by diffusion and loses its effect (Section 3.6). It could also be seen that upon irradiation, the fluorescence of free curcumin increased and was more distributed than the CUR-NP. Furthermore, the irradiated blank/untreated cells show no photo-destruction.

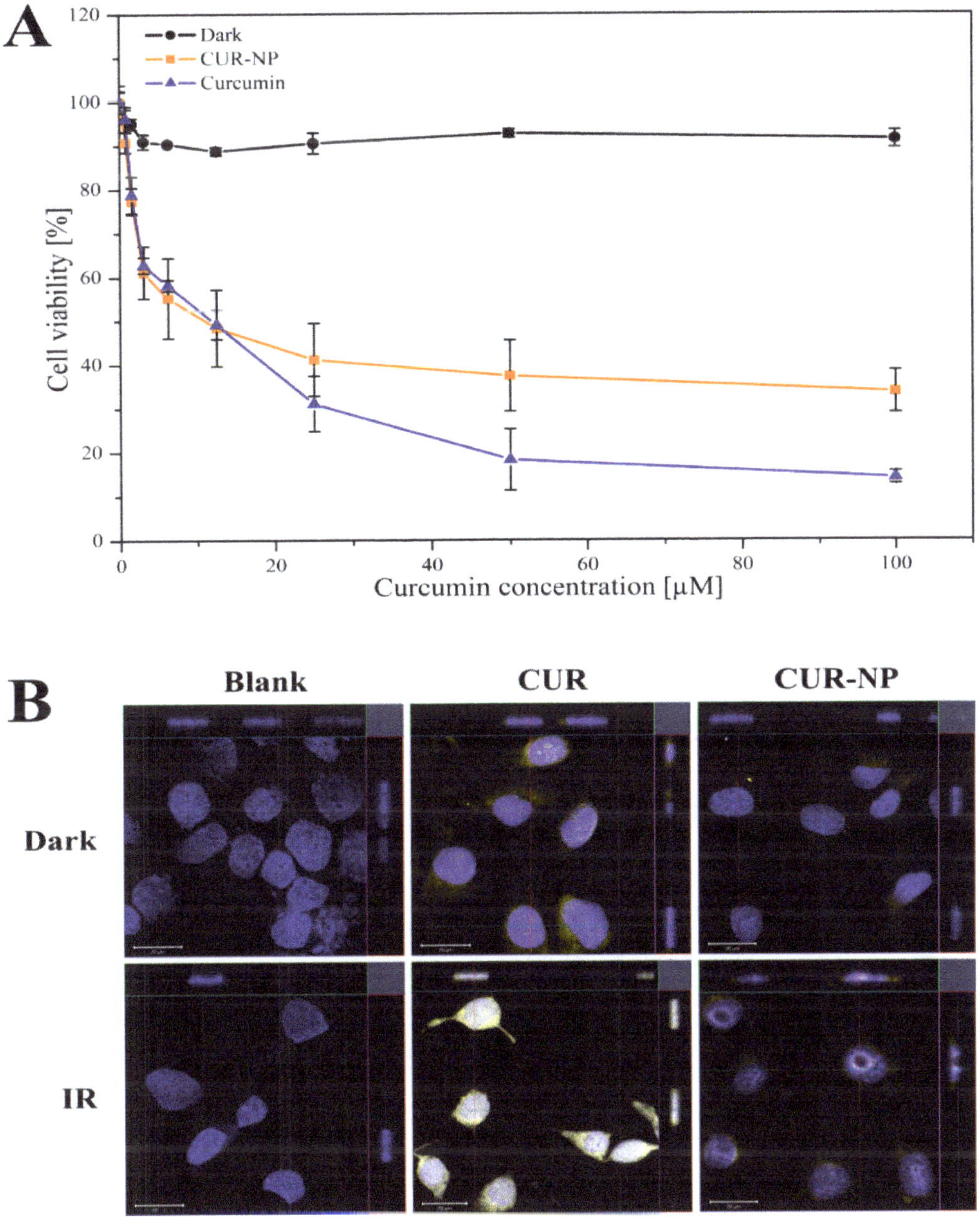

Figure 3. Phototoxic effect of curcumin-loaded poly(lactic-*co*-glycolic acid) PLGA nanoparticles (CUR-NP) and free curcumin dissolved in DMSO (CUR) on SK-OV-3 ovarian carcinoma cells: (**A**) for the MTT-assay, either the nanoformulation or free curcumin was incubated for 4 h at 37 °C and were irradiated at 457 nm with a radiation fluence of 8.6 J/cm^2. Dark was used as negative control and represents cells without irradiation. All samples contain 0.1 mg/mL curcumin and were measured in triplicates (n = 9, independent formulations). Results are expressed as means ± SD. (**B**) CLSM micrographs of SK-OV-3 cells incubated with CUR-NP or free curcumin for 4 h at 37 °C and subsequent irradiation (457 nm, 8.6 J/cm^2). The cell nucleus was counterstained with 0.1 μg/mL DAPI and was fixed with 4% formaldehyde solution. The curcumin concentration in CUR-NP was 50 μM. Nuclear damage is clearly witnessed in the irradiated samples whereas in the dark, the nucleus is intact. Dark was used as negative control and represents cells without irradiation. Scale bars denote 20 μm.

3.7. Cellular Uptake

Different cells use different endocytic pathways for the internalisation of nanoparticles. To study cellular uptake, several different inhibitors of endocytic pathways were utilised. For this purpose, the dynamin-, clathrin- and clathrin-independent endocytosis pathways were considered. Dynasore, a GTPase inhibitor rapidly and reversibly inhibits dynamin activity, which is essential for membrane fission during clathrin-mediated endocytosis (CME). Chlorpromazine also causes a block in CME by inducing the assembly of adaptor proteins and clathrin, leading to the formation of endosomes which then fuse with lysosomes [61]. Chlorpromazine also interferes with the intracellular clathrin processing [62]. Filipin III derived from *Streptomyces filipensis* is a polyene macrolide antibiotic, which inhibits the raft/caveolae endocytosis pathway. It interacts with cholesterol whose presence and state influence endocytic functions [63]. Figure 4 shows a substantial inhibition of CUR-NP by Filipin III and chlorpromazine. The uptake mechanism is dependent on the cell line and hence the data should be regarded cautiously. In our case, chlorpromazine exhibited an 80–90% inhibition of clathrin-dependent endocytosis of CUR-NP and Filipin III a marked 100% inhibition of caveolae-mediated and lipid-raft mediated endocytosis but both could not inhibit free curcumin. Free curcumin dissolved in DMSO does not seem to be internalised by any of these endocytic pathways suggesting a different internalisation mechanism such as diffusion [64]. The inhibition by dynamin dependant endocytosis by Dynasore showed no effect on the CUR-NP.

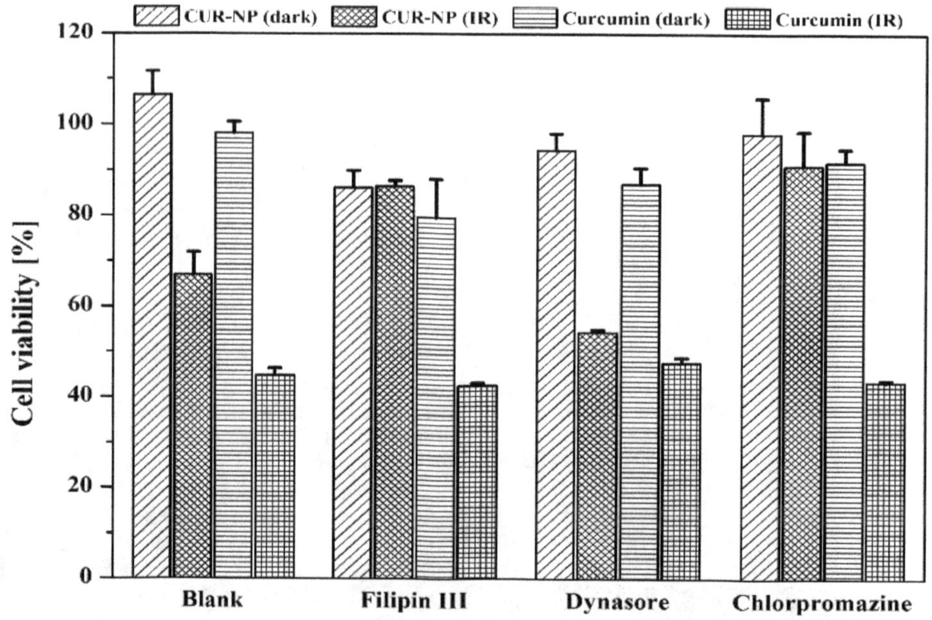

Figure 4. Cellular uptake of curcumin-loaded poly(lactic-*co*-glycolic acid) (PLGA) nanoparticles (CUR-NP) and free curcumin (dissolved in DMSO) in SK-OV-3 cells in presence of three specific inhibitors. After 30 min incubation time with different inhibitors (i.e., 8 μM Filipin III, 80 μM Dynasore and 14 μM chlorpromazine), cells were incubated with 50 μM of either CUR-NP or free curcumin dissolved in DMSO for 4 h at 37 °C and were irradiated at 457 nm with a radiation fluence of 8.6 J/cm^2 (IR). The MTT assay was performed at the end of the experiment to determine the effect of the pathway inhibits on internalisation. Viability of untreated cells was considered as 100%. Dark was used as negative control and represents unirradiated samples. Blank represents cells without any inhibitor. All samples were measured in triplicates (n = 9, independent formulations) and results are expressed as means ± SD.

3.8. Reactive Oxygen Species

ROS generation is the backbone of PDT and is a determining factor in the efficacy of the therapy. As shown in Figure 5, curcumin induced the production of cytotoxic reactive oxygen species after cells were irradiated (50 μM curcumin; 8.6 J/cm^2 radiation fluence). ROS was determined by the measurement of the fluorescence from the lysed cells. Upon incubation with cells, a deacetylated form of DCFDA is oxidised by the resulting ROS to form fluorescent DCF [65]. As expected, curcumin-loaded biodegradable PLGA polymeric nanoparticles exhibited the highest ROS generation followed by free curcumin dissolved in DMSO thereby corresponding to the results of the PDT. The fact that CUR-NP caused the maximum damage to the tumour cells can be explained by the ROS generation, which in this case was intracellular and could be only detected from the cells, which have internalised. Since free curcumin was not internalised by the endocytic pathways, mentioned in Figure 4, the uptake from CUR-NP seems to be higher. As expected, blank (negative control) did not show any ROS generation.

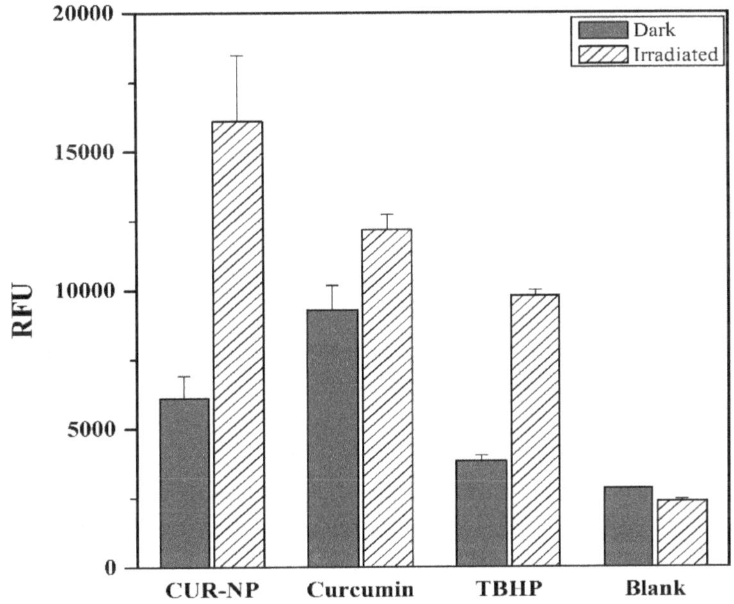

Figure 5. Production of cellular reactive oxygen species (ROS) in response to curcumin-loaded poly(lactic-*co*-glycolic acid) (PLGA) nanoparticles (CUR-NP) or free curcumin (0.1 mg/mL). ROS was measured in SK-OV-3 cells after exposure (for 45 min) to 2′,7′-dichlorofluorescin diacetate (25 μM) and incubation with CUR-NP or free curcumin for 4 h at 37 °C with subsequent irradiation (457 nm, 8.6 J/cm^2). Tert-butyl hydroperoxide (TBHP) was used as positive control and non-irradiated cells served as negative control (Dark), whereas Blank represents untreated cells. Values are represented in relative fluorescence units (RFU). All samples were measured in triplicates (n = 9, independent formulations) and results are expressed as means ± SD.

3.9. Haemocompatibility

To study the effect of the nanoformulation on human erythrocytes, haemolysis assay, which determines the amount of haemoglobin released from the erythrocytes upon exposure to NPs (Figure 6A) was performed. To determine the change in coagulation time upon addition of NPs, aPTT was determined (Figure 6B). Upon its release from erythrocytes, haemoglobin reacts with the atmospheric oxygen to form oxyhaemoglobin [66]. The CUR-NP used in the study showed a minimal haemolytic potential. An increase in the aPTT time was also found to be minimal in the case of CUR-NP. The aPTT analysis revealed that the encapsulated curcumin increased the coagulation time by only 4.01 s, whereas upon addition of free curcumin alone, the coagulation time increased to 120.13 s suggesting an interaction of curcumin with the intrinsic proteins or coagulation factors. The normal coagulation time for the plasma was tested to be 32.2 ± 0.1 s and was found to be in the normal range [67]. Coagulation time between 30 and 40 s is considered within acceptable range and coagulation time above 70 s denotes spontaneous and continuous bleeding leaving the patients with the risk of haemorrhage [67–69].

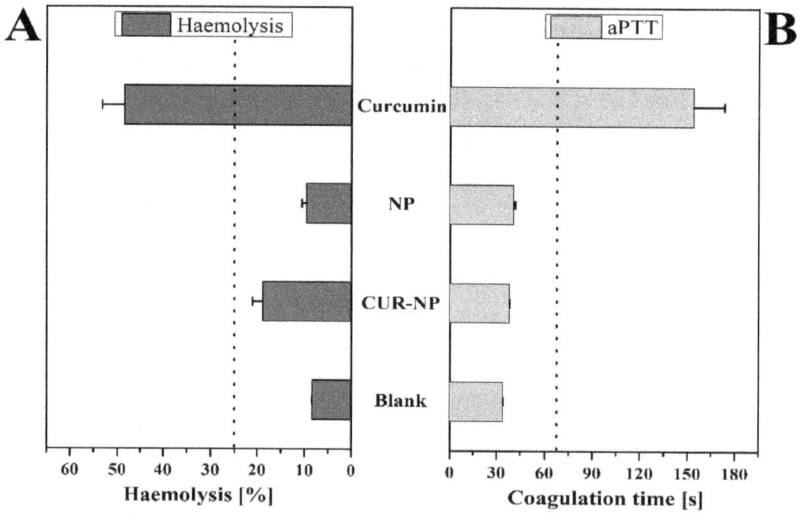

Figure 6. Blood compatibility of curcumin-loaded poly(lactic-*co*-glycolic acid) (PLGA) nanoparticles (CUR-NP), unloaded PLGA nanoparticles (NP) or free curcumin: (**A**) haemolysis assay and (**B**) aPTT test were performed. Where applicable, curcumin was used at a concentration of 0.1 mg/mL. Blank represents erythrocytes in the haemolysis assay and blood plasma in the aPTT test, respectively. Triton X-100 was used as positive control in (**A**) and is considered as 100% haemolysis. All samples were measured in triplicates ($n = 9$, independent formulations) and results are expressed as means ± SD. Dotted lines indicate the tolerance/threshold limits.

4. Conclusions

In this study, curcumin-loaded biodegradable PLGA nanoparticles (CUR-NP) were formulated for photodynamic therapy using a custom manufactured prototype low power LED device. CUR-NP exhibited better physicochemical properties compared to free curcumin, such as improved serum stability. Furthermore, haemocompatibility of curcumin was improved through polymeric encapsulation, minimising the risk of haemorrhages in patients. Successful cellular uptake of CUR-NP was demonstrated with the aid of confocal laser scanning microscopy, which showed photo-destruction and nuclear perforation. Nanoformulation facilitated the use of higher amounts of curcumin, which would otherwise be impossible due to its poor solubility and stability in aqueous media. Curcumin, which elsewise is safe for normal cells, showed cytotoxic effects on tumour cells upon irradiation at a low intensity therefore selectively inhibiting tumour growth. Since production of ROS occurs only upon irradiation of the intracellular photosensitiser, tumour tissues can be targeted with precision. Using LED as an irradiation source offers a number of advantages such as portability, durability and economical compared to lasers. Moreover, LED's have the ability to irradiate a relatively larger area, which could be beneficial for the treatment of large tumours or even skin cancer. The use of visible light of low-energy makes this therapy safer for both the patient and the operator. Finally, the good biocompatibility of this well-documented and highly reproducible formulation process of polymeric nanoparticles are significant advantages of this anti-tumour therapy. Transforming this novel strategy into a safe and effective therapy by combining PDT with other therapies would be our prime research interest in the future.

Author Contributions: Study conceptualization, U.B.; methodology, L.D. and M.R.A.; validation, L.D. and M.R.A.; investigation, L.D. and M.R.A.; data curation, L.D. and M.R.A.; visualisation, S.R.P.; manuscript drafting, L.D. and M.R.A.; manuscript review and editing, U.B., C.E., S.R.P., and M.A.S.; project supervision, J.S.

Acknowledgments: The authors would like to thank Eva Maria Mohr for her help and technical assistance, Thomas Anders for performing the serum stability studies and Elias Baghdan for his support and motivation. The authors are also grateful to Lumundus GmbH for developing the prototype LED device used in this study and would like to express their gratitude towards Martin Hardt and Sabine Agel from imaging unit of Justus-Liebig-University Gießen.

References

1. Dolmans, D.E.J.G.J.; Fukumura, D.; Jain, R.K. Photodynamic therapy for cancer. *Nat. Rev. Cancer* **2003**, *3*, 380–387. [CrossRef] [PubMed]
2. Ferlay, J.; Shin, H.-R.; Bray, F.; Forman, D.; Mathers, C.; Parkin, D.M. Estimates of worldwide burden of cancer in 2008: GLOBOCAN 2008. *Int. J. Cancer* **2010**, *127*, 2893–2917. [CrossRef] [PubMed]
3. Delaney, T.F.; Sindelar, W.F.; Tochner, Z.; Smith, P.D.; Friauf, W.S.; Thomas, G.; Dachowski, L.; Cole, J.W.; Steinberg, S.M.; Glatstein, E.; et al. Phase I study of debulking surgery and photodynamic therapy for disseminated intraperitoneal tumors. *Int. J. Radiat. Oncol. Biol. Phys.* **1993**, *25*, 445–457. [CrossRef]
4. Pass, H.I.; Delaney, T.F.; Tochner, Z.; Smith, P.E.; Temeck, B.K.; Pogrebniak, H.W.; Kranda, K.C.; Russo, A.; Friauf, W.S.; Cole, J.W.; et al. Intrapleural photodynamic therapy: Results of a phase I trial. *Ann. Surg. Oncol.* **1994**, *1*, 28–37. [CrossRef] [PubMed]
5. Dougherty, T.J.; Gomer, C.J.; Henderson, B.W.; Jori, G.; Kessel, D.; Korbelik, M.; Moan, J.; Peng, Q. Photodynamic Therapy. *JNCI J. Natl. Cancer Inst.* **1998**, *90*, 889–905. [CrossRef] [PubMed]
6. Stewart, F.; Baas, P.; Star, W. What does photodynamic therapy have to offer radiation oncologists (or their cancer patients)? *Radiother. Oncol.* **1998**, *48*, 233–248. [CrossRef]
7. Brown, S.B.; Brown, E.A.; Walker, I. The present and future role of photodynamic therapy in cancer treatment. *Lancet Oncol.* **2004**, *5*, 497–508. [CrossRef]
8. Ahn, J.-C.; Kang, J.-W.; Shin, J.-I.; Chung, P.-S. Combination treatment with photodynamic therapy and curcumin induces mitochondria-dependent apoptosis in AMC-HN3 cells. *Int. J. Oncol.* **2012**, *41*, 2184–2190. [CrossRef]
9. Atchison, J.; Kamila, S.; McEwan, C.; Nesbitt, H.; Davis, J.; Fowley, C.; Callan, B.; McHale, A.P.; Callan, J.F. Modulation of ROS production in photodynamic therapy using a pH controlled photoinduced electron transfer (PET) based sensitiser. *Chem. Commun. (Camb. Engl.)* **2015**, *51*, 16832–16835. [CrossRef] [PubMed]
10. Moan, J.; Berg, K. The Photodegradation of Photodegradation of Porphyrins in Cell can be used to Estimate the Liftime of Singlet Oxygen. *Photochem. Photobiol.* **1991**, *53*, 549–553. [CrossRef]
11. Banerjee, S.; Dixit, A.; Karande, A.A.; Chakravarty, A.R. Remarkable Selectivity and Photo-Cytotoxicity of an Oxidovanadium(IV) Complex of Curcumin in Visible Light. *Eur. J. Inorg. Chem.* **2015**, *2015*, 447–457. [CrossRef]
12. Konopka, K.; Goslinski, T. Photodynamic therapy in dentistry. *J. Dent. Res.* **2007**, *86*, 694–707. [CrossRef] [PubMed]
13. Brancaleon, L.; Moseley, H. Laser and non-laser light sources for photodynamic therapy. *Lasers Med. Sci.* **2002**, *17*, 173–186. [CrossRef] [PubMed]
14. Shishodia, S.; Sethi, G.; Aggarwal, B.B. Curcumin: Getting back to the roots. *Ann. N. Y. Acad. Sci.* **2005**, *1056*, 206–217. [CrossRef] [PubMed]
15. Aggarwal, B.B.; Sundaram, C.; Malani, N.; Ichikawa, H. Curcumin: The Indian solid gold. *Adv. Exp. Med. Biol.* **2007**, *595*, 1–75. [CrossRef] [PubMed]
16. Epstein, J.; Sanderson, I.R.; Macdonald, T.T. Curcumin as a therapeutic agent: The evidence from in vitro, animal and human studies. *Br. J. Nutr.* **2010**, *103*, 1545–1557. [CrossRef] [PubMed]
17. Naksuriya, O.; Okonogi, S.; Schiffelers, R.M.; Hennink, W.E. Curcumin nanoformulations: A review of pharmaceutical properties and preclinical studies and clinical data related to cancer treatment. *Biomaterials* **2014**, *35*, 3365–3383. [CrossRef] [PubMed]
18. Wilken, R.; Veena, M.S.; Wang, M.B.; Srivatsan, E.S. Curcumin: A review of anti-cancer properties and therapeutic activity in head and neck squamous cell carcinoma. *Mol. Cancer* **2011**, *10*, 12. [CrossRef]
19. Kaminaga, Y.; Nagatsu, A.; Akiyama, T.; Sugimoto, N.; Yamazaki, T.; Maitani, T.; Mizukami, H. Production of unnatural glucosides of curcumin with drastically enhanced water solubility by cell suspension cultures of Catharanthus roseus. *FEBS Lett.* **2003**, *555*, 311–316. [CrossRef]
20. Shaikh, J.; Bhosale, R.; Singhal, R. Microencapsulation of black pepper oleoresin. *Food Chem.* **2006**, *94*, 105–110. [CrossRef]
21. Anand, P.; Kunnumakkara, A.B.; Newman, R.A.; Aggarwal, B.B. Bioavailability of curcumin: Problems and promises. *Mol. Pharm.* **2007**, *4*, 807–818. [CrossRef] [PubMed]

22. Agel, M.R.; Baghdan, E.; Pinnapireddy, S.R.; Lehmann, J.; Schäfer, J.; Bakowsky, U. Curcumin loaded nanoparticles as efficient photoactive formulations against gram-positive and gram-negative bacteria. *Colloids Surf. B Biointerfaces* **2019**, *178*, 460–468. [CrossRef] [PubMed]
23. Singh, S.P.; Sharma, M.; Gupta, P.K. Enhancement of phototoxicity of curcumin in human oral cancer cells using silica nanoparticles as delivery vehicle. *Lasers Med. Sci.* **2014**, *29*, 645–652. [CrossRef] [PubMed]
24. Duse, L.; Baghdan, E.; Pinnapireddy, S.R.; Engelhardt, K.H.; Jedelská, J.; Schaefer, J.; Quendt, P.; Bakowsky, U. Preparation and Characterization of Curcumin Loaded Chitosan Nanoparticles for Photodynamic Therapy. *Phys. Status Solidi A* **2018**, *215*, 1700709. [CrossRef]
25. Tsai, W.-H.; Yu, K.-H.; Huang, Y.-C.; Lee, C.-I. EGFR-targeted photodynamic therapy by curcumin-encapsulated chitosan/TPP nanoparticles. *Int. J. Nanomed.* **2018**, *13*, 903–916. [CrossRef]
26. Jiang, S.; Zhu, R.; He, X.; Wang, J.; Wang, M.; Qian, Y.; Wang, S. Enhanced photocytotoxicity of curcumin delivered by solid lipid nanoparticles. *Int. J. Nanomed.* **2017**, *12*, 167–178. [CrossRef] [PubMed]
27. Danhier, F.; Ansorena, E.; Silva, J.M.; Coco, R.; Le Breton, A.; Préat, V. PLGA-based nanoparticles: An overview of biomedical applications. *J. Control. Release* **2012**, *161*, 505–522. [CrossRef] [PubMed]
28. Patel, J.; Amrutiya, J.; Bhatt, P.; Javia, A.; Jain, M.; Misra, A. Targeted delivery of monoclonal antibody conjugated docetaxel loaded PLGA nanoparticles into EGFR overexpressed lung tumour cells. *J. Microencapsul.* **2018**, *35*, 204–217. [CrossRef]
29. Kumari, A.; Yadav, S.K.; Yadav, S.C. Biodegradable polymeric nanoparticles based drug delivery systems. *Colloids Surf. B Biointerfaces* **2010**, *75*, 1–18. [CrossRef]
30. Michlovská, L.; Vojtová, L.; Mravcová, L.; Hermanová, S.; Kučerík, J.; Jančář, J. Functionalization Conditions of PLGA-PEG-PLGA Copolymer with Itaconic Anhydride. *Macromol. Symp.* **2010**, *295*, 119–124. [CrossRef]
31. Hariharan, S.; Bhardwaj, V.; Bala, I.; Sitterberg, J.; Bakowsky, U.; Ravi Kumar, M.N.V. Design of estradiol loaded PLGA nanoparticulate formulations: A potential oral delivery system for hormone therapy. *Pharm. Res.* **2006**, *23*, 184–195. [CrossRef] [PubMed]
32. Anderson, J.M.; Shive, M.S. Biodegradation and biocompatibility of PLA and PLGA microspheres. *Adv. Drug Deliv. Rev.* **1997**, *28*, 5–24. [CrossRef]
33. Jain, R.A. The manufacturing techniques of various drug loaded biodegradable poly (lactide-co-glycolide) (PLGA) devices. *Biomaterials* **2000**, *21*, 2475–2490. [CrossRef]
34. Duse, L.; Pinnapireddy, S.R.; Strehlow, B.; Jedelská, J.; Bakowsky, U. Low level LED photodynamic therapy using curcumin loaded tetraether liposomes. *Eur. J. Pharm. Biopharm.* **2018**, *126*, 233–241. [CrossRef]
35. Ravi Kumar, M.N.V.; Bakowsky, U.; Lehr, C.M. Preparation and characterization of cationic PLGA nanospheres as DNA carriers. *Biomaterials* **2004**, *25*, 1771–1777. [CrossRef]
36. Bhatt, P.; Lalani, R.; Vhora, I.; Patil, S.; Amrutiya, J.; Misra, A.; Mashru, R. Liposomes encapsulating native and cyclodextrin enclosed paclitaxel: Enhanced loading efficiency and its pharmacokinetic evaluation. *Int. J. Pharm.* **2018**, *536*, 95–107. [CrossRef]
37. Schaefer, J.; Schulze, C.; Marxer, E.E.J.; Schaefer, U.F.; Wohlleben, W.; Bakowsky, U.; Lehr, C.-M. Atomic force microscopy and analytical ultracentrifugation for probing nanomaterial protein interactions. *ACS Nano* **2012**, *6*, 4603–4614. [CrossRef]
38. Senior, J.; Gregoriadis, G. Stability of small unilamellar liposomes in serum and clearance from the circulation: The effect of the phospholipid and cholesterol components. *Life Sci.* **1982**, *30*, 2123–2136. [CrossRef]
39. Plenagl, N.; Duse, L.; Seitz, B.S.; Goergen, N.; Pinnapireddy, S.R.; Jedelska, J.; Brüßler, J.; Bakowsky, U. Photodynamic therapy–Hypericin tetraether liposome conjugates and their antitumor and antiangiogenic activity. *Drug Deliv.* **2019**, *26*, 23–33. [CrossRef]
40. Tariq, I.; Pinnapireddy, S.R.; Duse, L.; Ali, M.Y.; Ali, S.; Amin, M.U.; Goergen, N.; Jedelská, J.; Schäfer, J.; Bakowsky, U.; et al. Lipodendriplexes: A promising nanocarrier for enhanced gene delivery with minimal cytotoxicity. *Eur. J. Pharm. Biopharm.* **2019**, *135*, 72–82. [CrossRef]
41. Pinnapireddy, S.R.; Duse, L.; Strehlow, B.; Schäfer, J.; Bakowsky, U. Composite liposome-PEI/nucleic acid lipopolyplexes for safe and efficient gene delivery and gene knockdown. *Colloids Surf. B Biointerfaces* **2017**, *158*, 93–101. [CrossRef] [PubMed]
42. Evans, B.C.; Nelson, C.E.; Yu, S.S.; Beavers, K.R.; Kim, A.J.; Li, H.; Nelson, H.M.; Giorgio, T.D.; Duvall, C.L. Ex vivo red blood cell hemolysis assay for the evaluation of pH-responsive endosomolytic agents for cytosolic delivery of biomacromolecular drugs. *J. Vis. Exp.* **2013**, e50166. [CrossRef] [PubMed]

43. Makadia, H.K.; Siegel, S.J. Poly Lactic-co-Glycolic Acid (PLGA) as Biodegradable Controlled Drug Delivery Carrier. *Polymers (Basel)* **2011**, *3*, 1377–1397. [CrossRef] [PubMed]
44. Yallapu, M.M.; Gupta, B.K.; Jaggi, M.; Chauhan, S.C. Fabrication of curcumin encapsulated PLGA nanoparticles for improved therapeutic effects in metastatic cancer cells. *J. Colloid Interface Sci.* **2010**, *351*, 19–29. [CrossRef]
45. Shaikh, J.; Ankola, D.D.; Beniwal, V.; Singh, D.; Kumar, M.N.V.R. Nanoparticle encapsulation improves oral bioavailability of curcumin by at least 9-fold when compared to curcumin administered with piperine as absorption enhancer. *Eur. J. Pharm. Sci.* **2009**, *37*, 223–230. [CrossRef] [PubMed]
46. Raschpichler, M.; Agel, M.R.; Pinnapireddy, S.R.; Duse, L.; Baghdan, E.; Schäfer, J.; Bakowsky, U. In situ intravenous photodynamic therapy for the systemic eradication of blood stream infections. *Photochem. Photobiol. Sci.* **2019**, *18*, 304–308. [CrossRef] [PubMed]
47. Sitterberg, J.; Ozcetin, A.; Ehrhardt, C.; Bakowsky, U. Utilising atomic force microscopy for the characterisation of nanoscale drug delivery systems. *Eur. J. Pharm. Biopharm.* **2010**, *74*, 2–13. [CrossRef] [PubMed]
48. Murakami, H.; Kobayashi, M.; Takeuchi, H.; Kawashima, Y. Preparation of poly(dl-lactide-co-glycolide) nanoparticles by modified spontaneous emulsification solvent diffusion method. *Int. J. Pharm.* **1999**, *187*, 143–152. [CrossRef]
49. Singh, R.; Lillard, J.W. Nanoparticle-based targeted drug delivery. *Exp. Mol. Pathol.* **2009**, *86*, 215–223. [CrossRef] [PubMed]
50. Tonnesen, H. Studies on curcumin and curcuminoids. XIV. Effect of curcumin on hyaluronic acid degradation in vitro. *Int. J. Pharm.* **1989**, *50*, 91–95. [CrossRef]
51. Shahani, K.; Panyam, J. Highly loaded, sustained-release microparticles of curcumin for chemoprevention. *J. Pharm. Sci.* **2011**, *100*, 2599–2609. [CrossRef] [PubMed]
52. Magenheim, B.; Levy, M.Y.; Benita, S. A new in vitro technique for the evaluation of drug release profile from colloidal carriers—Ultrafiltration technique at low pressure. *Int. J. Pharm.* **1993**, *94*, 115–123. [CrossRef]
53. Baghdan, E.; Raschpichler, M.; Lutfi, W.; Pinnapireddy, S.R.; Pourasghar, M.; Schäfer, J.; Schneider, M.; Bakowsky, U. Nano spray dried antibacterial coatings for dental implants. *Eur. J. Pharm. Biopharm.* **2019**, *139*, 59–67. [CrossRef] [PubMed]
54. Webb, B.A.; Chimenti, M.; Jacobson, M.P.; Barber, D.L. Dysregulated pH: A perfect storm for cancer progression. *Nat. Rev. Cancer* **2011**, *11*, 671–677. [CrossRef] [PubMed]
55. Yang, R.; Shim, W.-S.; Cui, F.-D.; Cheng, G.; Han, X.; Jin, Q.-R.; Kim, D.-D.; Chung, S.-J.; Shim, C.-K. Enhanced electrostatic interaction between chitosan-modified PLGA nanoparticle and tumor. *Int. J. Pharm.* **2009**, *371*, 142–147. [CrossRef] [PubMed]
56. Li, B.; Xu, H.; Li, Z.; Yao, M.; Xie, M.; Shen, H.; Shen, S.; Wang, X.; Jin, Y. Bypassing multidrug resistance in human breast cancer cells with lipid/polymer particle assemblies. *Int. J. Nanomed.* **2012**, *7*, 187–197. [CrossRef]
57. Li, Y.-P.; Pei, Y.-Y.; Zhang, X.-Y.; Gu, Z.-H.; Zhou, Z.-H.; Yuan, W.-F.; Zhou, J.-J.; Zhu, J.-H.; Gao, X.-J. PEGylated PLGA nanoparticles as protein carriers: Synthesis, preparation and biodistribution in rats. *J. Control. Release* **2001**, *71*, 203–211. [CrossRef]
58. Wolfram, J.; Suri, K.; Yang, Y.; Shen, J.; Celia, C.; Fresta, M.; Zhao, Y.; Shen, H.; Ferrari, M. Shrinkage of pegylated and non-pegylated liposomes in serum. *Colloids Surf. B Biointerfaces* **2014**, *114*, 294–300. [CrossRef]
59. Nafee, N.; Schneider, M.; Schaefer, U.F.; Lehr, C.-M. Relevance of the colloidal stability of chitosan/PLGA nanoparticles on their cytotoxicity profile. *Int. J. Pharm.* **2009**, *381*, 130–139. [CrossRef]
60. Hebling, J.; Bianchi, L.; Basso, F.G.; Scheffel, D.L.; Soares, D.G.; Carrilho, M.R.O.; Pashley, D.H.; Tjäderhane, L.; de Souza Costa, C.A. Cytotoxicity of dimethyl sulfoxide (DMSO) in direct contact with odontoblast-like cells. *Dent. Mater.* **2015**, *31*, 399–405. [CrossRef]
61. Schäfer, J.; Höbel, S.; Bakowsky, U.; Aigner, A. Liposome-polyethylenimine complexes for enhanced DNA and siRNA delivery. *Biomaterials* **2010**, *31*, 6892–6900. [CrossRef] [PubMed]
62. Wang, L.H.; Rothberg, K.G.; Anderson, R.G. Mis-assembly of clathrin lattices on endosomes reveals a regulatory switch for coated pit formation. *J. Cell Biol.* **1993**, *123*, 1107–1117. [CrossRef] [PubMed]
63. Orlandi, P.A.; Fishman, P.H. Filipin-dependent Inhibition of Cholera Toxin: Evidence for Toxin Internalization and Activation through Caveolae-like Domains. *J. Cell Biol.* **1998**, *141*, 905–915. [CrossRef] [PubMed]

64. Kunwar, A.; Barik, A.; Mishra, B.; Rathinasamy, K.; Pandey, R.; Priyadarsini, K.I. Quantitative cellular uptake, localization and cytotoxicity of curcumin in normal and tumor cells. *Biochim. Biophys. Acta* **2008**, *1780*, 673–679. [CrossRef] [PubMed]
65. McLennan, H.R.; Degli Esposti, M. The Contribution of Mitochondrial Respiratory Complexes to the Production of Reactive Oxygen Species. *J. Bioenerg. Biomembr.* **2000**, *32*, 153–162. [CrossRef] [PubMed]
66. Dobrovolskaia, M.A.; McNeil, S.E. *Handbook of Immunological Properties of Engineered Nanomaterials*; World Scientific: Singapore, 2016; Volume 1, p. 692.
67. Lenaham, J.G.; Frye, S.; Phillips, G.E. Use of the activated partial thromboplastin time in the control of heparin administration. *Clin. Chem.* **1966**, *12*, 263–268. [PubMed]
68. Greer, J.P. *Wintrobe's Clinical Hematology*; Lippincott Williams & Wilkins: Philadelphia, PA, USA, 2008; p. 1272.
69. Pinnapireddy, S.R.; Duse, L.; Akbari, D.; Bakowsky, U. Photo-Enhanced Delivery of Genetic Material Using Curcumin Loaded Composite Nanocarriers. *Clin. Oncol.* **2017**, *2*, 1323.

Permissions

All chapters in this book were first published by MDPI; hereby published with permission under the Creative Commons Attribution License or equivalent. Every chapter published in this book has been scrutinized by our experts. Their significance has been extensively debated. The topics covered herein carry significant findings which will fuel the growth of the discipline. They may even be implemented as practical applications or may be referred to as a beginning point for another development.

The contributors of this book come from diverse backgrounds, making this book a truly international effort. This book will bring forth new frontiers with its revolutionizing research information and detailed analysis of the nascent developments around the world.

We would like to thank all the contributing authors for lending their expertise to make the book truly unique. They have played a crucial role in the development of this book. Without their invaluable contributions this book wouldn't have been possible. They have made vital efforts to compile up to date information on the varied aspects of this subject to make this book a valuable addition to the collection of many professionals and students.

This book was conceptualized with the vision of imparting up-to-date information and advanced data in this field. To ensure the same, a matchless editorial board was set up. Every individual on the board went through rigorous rounds of assessment to prove their worth. After which they invested a large part of their time researching and compiling the most relevant data for our readers.

The editorial board has been involved in producing this book since its inception. They have spent rigorous hours researching and exploring the diverse topics which have resulted in the successful publishing of this book. They have passed on their knowledge of decades through this book. To expedite this challenging task, the publisher supported the team at every step. A small team of assistant editors was also appointed to further simplify the editing procedure and attain best results for the readers.

Apart from the editorial board, the designing team has also invested a significant amount of their time in understanding the subject and creating the most relevant covers. They scrutinized every image to scout for the most suitable representation of the subject and create an appropriate cover for the book.

The publishing team has been an ardent support to the editorial, designing and production team. Their endless efforts to recruit the best for this project, has resulted in the accomplishment of this book. They are a veteran in the field of academics and their pool of knowledge is as vast as their experience in printing. Their expertise and guidance has proved useful at every step. Their uncompromising quality standards have made this book an exceptional effort. Their encouragement from time to time has been an inspiration for everyone.

The publisher and the editorial board hope that this book will prove to be a valuable piece of knowledge for researchers, students, practitioners and scholars across the globe.

List of Contributors

Gauri Gangapurwala, Antje Vollrath and Ulrich S. Schubert
Laboratory of Organic and Macromolecular Chemistry (IOMC), Friedrich Schiller University Jena, Fürstengraben 1, 07743 Jena, Germany
Jena Center for Soft Matter (JCSM), Friedrich Schiller University Jena, Philosophenweg 7, 07743 Jena, Germany

Alicia De San Luis
Laboratory of Organic and Macromolecular Chemistry (IOMC), Friedrich Schiller University Jena, Fürstengraben 1, 07743 Jena, Germany
Jena Center for Soft Matter (JCSM), Friedrich Schiller University Jena, Philosophenweg 7, 07743 Jena, Germany
POLYMAT and Kimika Aplikatua Saila, Kimika Fakultatea, University of the Basque Country UPV/EHU, Joxe Mari Korta Zentroa, Tolosa Hiribidea 72, 20018 Donostia-San Sebastián, Spain

Shang Li
Jiangsu Key Laboratory of New Drug Research and Clinical Pharmacy, Xuzhou Medical University, Xuzhou 221004, China

Jinglei Wang, Zhaorong Liu and Zhiru Zheng
Department of Pharmaceutics, School of Pharmacy, Xuzhou Medical University, Xuzhou 221004, China

Xiaonan Li and Yanzhuo Zhang
Jiangsu Key Laboratory of New Drug Research and Clinical Pharmacy, Xuzhou Medical University, Xuzhou 221004, China
Department of Pharmaceutics, School of Pharmacy, Xuzhou Medical University, Xuzhou 221004, China

Ki-Taek Kim
College of Pharmacy and Natural Medicine Research Institute, Mokpo National University, Muan-gun, Jeonnam 58554, Korea

Jae-Young Lee
College of Pharmacy, Chungnam National University, Daejeon 34134, Korea

Dae-Duk Kim
College of Pharmacy and Research Institute of Pharmaceutical Sciences, Seoul National University, Seoul 08826, Korea

In-Soo Yoon
Department of Manufacturing Pharmacy, College of Pharmacy, Pusan National University, Busan 46241, Korea

Hyun-Jong Cho
College of Pharmacy, Kangwon National University, Chuncheon 24341, Korea

Maria João Ramalho, Joana A. Loureiro, Manuel A. N. Coelho and Maria Carmo Pereira
LEPABE—Laboratory for Process Engineering, Environment, Biotechnology and Energy, Faculty of Engineering, University of Porto, Rua Dr. Roberto Frias, 4200-465 Porto, Portugal

Lucia Morelli, Lucia Salvioni, Maria Guizzetti, Barbara Colzani and Miriam Colombo
NanoBioLab, Dipartimento di Biotecnologie e Bioscienze, Università di Milano-Bicocca, Piazza della Scienza 2, 20126 Milano, Italy

Sara Gimondi, Marta Sevieri, Laura Talamini, Lavinia Morosi, Massimo Zucchetti, Martina Bruna Violatto, Luca Russo, Mario Salmona and Paolo Bigini
IRCCS Mario Negri Institute for Pharmacological Research; Via Mario Negri 2, 20157 Milano, Italy

Luca Palugan and Anastasia Foppoli
Dipartimento di Scienze Farmaceutiche, Università di Milano, Via Giuseppe Colombo 71, 20133 Milano, Italy

Davide Prosperi
NanoBioLab, Dipartimento di Biotecnologie e Bioscienze, Università di Milano-Bicocca, Piazza della Scienza 2, 20126 Milano, Italy
Nanomedicine Laboratory, ICS Maugeri S.p.A. SB, Via S. Maugeri 10, 27100 Pavia, Italy

Patricia García-García and Elisabet Segredo-Morales
Department of Chemical Engineering and Pharmaceutical Technology, University of La Laguna, 38206 La Laguna, Spain

Edgar Pérez-Herrero, Araceli Delgado and Carmen Évora
Department of Chemical Engineering and Pharmaceutical Technology, University of La Laguna, 38206 La Laguna, Spain
Institute of Biomedical Technologies (ITB), University of La Laguna, 38206 La Laguna, Spain

Ricardo Reyes
Institute of Biomedical Technologies (ITB), University of La Laguna, 38206 La Laguna, Spain
Department of Biochemistry, Microbiology, Cell Biology and Genetics, University of La Laguna, 38206 La Laguna, Spain

Woo Mi Ryu and Chang Hee Min
Interdisciplinary Program in Bioengineering, College of Engineering, Seoul National University, Seoul 08826, Korea

Se-Na Kim
Institute of Medical & Biological Engineering, Medical Research Center, Seoul National University, Seoul 03080, Korea

Young Bin Choy
Interdisciplinary Program in Bioengineering, College of Engineering, Seoul National University, Seoul 08826, Korea
Institute of Medical & Biological Engineering, Medical Research Center, Seoul National University, Seoul 03080, Korea
Department of Biomedical Engineering, Seoul National University College of Medicine, Seoul 03080, Korea

Norbert Varga and Árpád Turcsányi
Interdisciplinary Excellence Centre, Department of Physical Chemistry and Materials Science, University of Szeged, Rerrich B. square 1, H-6720 Szeged, Hungary

Viktória Hornok
Interdisciplinary Excellence Centre, Department of Physical Chemistry and Materials Science, University of Szeged, Rerrich B. square 1, H-6720 Szeged, Hungary
Department of Physical Chemistry and Materials Science, MTA Premium Post Doctorate Research Program, University of Szeged, Rerrich B. Square 1, H-6720 Szeged, Hungary

Edit Csapó
Interdisciplinary Excellence Centre, Department of Physical Chemistry and Materials Science, University of Szeged, Rerrich B. square 1, H-6720 Szeged, Hungary
MTA-SZTE Biomimetic Systems Research Group, Department of Medical Chemistry, University of Szeged, Dóm square 8, H-6720 Szeged, Hungary

Teresa del Castillo-Santaella
Biocolloid and Fluid Physics Group, Department of Applied Physics, University of Granada, 18071 Granada, Spain

Inmaculada Ortega-Oller, Miguel Padial-Molina and Pablo Galindo-Moreno
Department of Oral Surgery and Implant Dentistry, University of Granada, 18071 Granada, Spain

Francisco O'Valle
Department of Pathology, School of Medicine & IBIMER, University of Granada, 18071 Granada, Spain

Ana Belén Jódar-Reyes
Biocolloid and Fluid Physics Group, Department of Applied Physics, University of Granada, 18071 Granada, Spain
Excellence Research Unit "Modeling Nature" (MNat), University of Granada, 18071 Granada, Spain

José Manuel Peula-García
Biocolloid and Fluid Physics Group, Department of Applied Physics, University of Granada, 18071 Granada, Spain
Department of Applied Physics II, University of Malaga, 29071 Malaga, Spain

Christopher Janich, Ligia E. de Souza and Karsten Mäder
Institute of Pharmacy, Faculty of Biosciences, Martin Luther University Halle-Wittenberg, 06120 Halle (Saale), Germany

Andrea Friedmann and Christian E. H. Schmelzer
Department of Biological and Macromolecular Materials, Fraunhofer Institute for Microstructure of Materials and Systems IMWS, 06120 Halle (Saale), Germany

Juliana Martins de Souza e Silva and Cristine Santos de Oliveira
Institute of Physics, Martin Luther University Halle-Wittenberg, 06120 Halle (Saale), Germany

Dan Rujescu
Department of Psychiatry, Psychotherapy and Psychosomatics, Martin Luther University Halle-Wittenberg, 06120 Halle (Saale), Germany

Christian Hildebrandt and Moritz Beck-Broichsitter
MilliporeSigma a Business of Merck KGaA, 64293 Darmstadt, Germany

Sharif Md Abuzar, Jun-Hyun Ahn and Sung-Joo Hwang
College of Pharmacy, Yonsei University, 85 Songdogwahak-ro, Yeonsu-gu, Incheon 21983, Korea
Yonsei Institute of Pharmaceutical Sciences, Yonsei University, 85 Songdogwahak-ro, Yeonsu-gu, Incheon 21983, Korea

Kyung Su Park
Advanced Analysis Center, Korea Institute of Science and Technology, Hwarang-ro, Seongbuk-gu, Seoul 02792, Korea

Eun Jung Park and Seung Hyuk Baik
Division of Colon and Rectal Surgery, Department of Surgery, Gangnam Severance Hospital, Yonsei University College of Medicine, Seoul 06273, Korea

Myoung Jin Ho, Hoe Taek Jeong, Sung Hyun Im, Hyung Tae Kim, Jeong Eun Lee, Jun Soo Park, Ha Ra Cho, Dong Yoon Kim, Yong Seok Choi and Myung Joo Kang
College of Pharmacy, Dankook University, 119, Dandae-ro, Dongnam-gu, Cheonan-si, Chungcheongnam-do 31116, Korea

Young Wook Choi
College of Pharmacy, Chung-Ang University, 84, Heukseok-ro, Dongjak-gu, Seoul 06974, Korea

Joon Woo Lee
Department of Radiology, Seoul National University Bundang Hospital, 82, Gumi-ro 173beon-gil, Bundang-gu, Seongnam-si, Gyeonggi-do 13620, Korea

Lili Duse, Michael Rene Agel, Shashank Reddy Pinnapireddy, Jens Schäfer and Udo Bakowsky
Department of Pharmaceutics and Biopharmaceutics, University of Marburg, Robert-Koch-Str. 4, 35037 Marburg, Germany

Carsten Ehrhardt
School of Pharmacy and Pharmaceutical Sciences and Biomedical Sciences Institute, Trinity College Dublin, Dublin 2, Ireland

Mohammed A. Selo
School of Pharmacy and Pharmaceutical Sciences and Biomedical Sciences Institute, Trinity College Dublin, Dublin 2, Ireland
Faculty of Pharmacy, University of Kufa, 31001 Kufa, Iraq

Index

Printed in the USA
CPSIA information can be obtained
at www.ICGtesting.com
LVHW080051211023
761596LV00010BA/2009

9 781646 465583